2007
YEAR BOOK OF
OPHTHALMOLOGY®

The 2007 Year Book Series

Year Book of Anesthesiology and Pain Management™: Drs Chestnut, Abram, Black, Gravlee, Lee, Mathru, and Roizen

Year Book of Cardiology®: Drs Gersh, Cheitlin, Elliott, Graham, Sundt, and Waldo

Year Book of Critical Care Medicine®: Drs Dellinger, Parrillo, Balk, Bekes, Dorman, and Dries

Year Book of Dentistry®: Drs McIntyre, Belvedere, Buhite, Davis, Henderson, Johnson, Ohrbach, Olin, Scott, Spencer, and Zakariasen

Year Book of Dermatology and Dermatologic Surgery™: Drs Thiers and Lang

Year Book of Diagnostic Radiology®: Drs Osborn, Abbara, Birdwell, Dalinka, Elster, Gardiner, Levy, Oestreich, and Rosado de Christenson

Year Book of Emergency Medicine®: Drs Hamilton, Bruno, Handly, Quintana, and Werner

Year Book of Endocrinology®: Drs Mazzaferri, Bessesen, Clarke, Howard, Kennedy, Leahy, Meikle, Molitch, Rogol, and Schteingart

Year Book of Family Practice®: Drs Bowman, Apgar, Bouchard, Dexter, Neill, Scherger, and Zink

Year Book of Gastroenterology™: Drs Lichtenstein, Chang, Dempsey, Drebin, Jaffe, Katzka, Kochman, Makar, Morris, Osterman, Rombeau, Shah, and Stein

Year Book of Hand and Upper Limb Surgery®: Drs Chang and Steinmann

Year Book of Medicine®: Drs Barkin, Berney, Frishman, Garrick, Loehrer, Mazzaferri, Phillips, and Snydman

Year Book of Neonatal and Perinatal Medicine®: Drs Fanaroff, Ehrenkranz, and Stevenson

Year Book of Neurology and Neurosurgery®: Drs Kim and Verma

Year Book of Nuclear Medicine®: Drs Coleman, Blaufox, Royal, Strauss, and Zubal

Year Book of Obstetrics, Gynecology, and Women's Health®: Dr Shulman

Year Book of Oncology®: Drs Loehrer, Arceci, Glatstein, Gordon, Hanna, Morrow, and Thigpen

Year Book of Ophthalmology®: Drs Rapuano, Cohen, Eagle, Flanders, Hammersmith, Myers, Nelson, Penne, Sergott, Shields, Tipperman, and Vander

Year Book of Orthopedics®: Drs Morrey, Beauchamp, Huddleston, Peterson, Swiontkowski, and Trigg

Year Book of Otolaryngology-Head and Neck Surgery®: Drs Paparella, Gapany, and Keefe

Year Book of Pathology and Laboratory Medicine®: Drs Raab, Parwani, Bejarano, and Bissell

Year Book of Pediatrics®: Dr Stockman

Year Book of Plastic and Aesthetic Surgery™: Drs Miller, Bartlett, Garner, McKinney, Ruberg, Salisbury, and Smith

Year Book of Psychiatry and Applied Mental Health®: Drs Talbott, Ballenger, Buckley, Frances, Jensen, and Markowitz

Year Book of Pulmonary Disease®: Drs Phillips, Barker, Lewis, Maurer, Tanoue, and Willsie

Year Book of Rheumatology, Arthritis, and Musculoskeletal Disease™: Drs Panush, Furst, Hadler, Hochberg, Lahita, and Paget

Year Book of Sports Medicine®: Drs Shephard, Cantu, Feldman, Jankowski, McCrory, Nieman, Pierrynowski, Rowland, and Shrier

Year Book of Surgery®: Drs Copeland, Bland, Daly, Eberlein, Fahey, Jones, Mozingo, Pruett, and Seeger

Year Book of Urology®: Drs Andriole and Coplen

Year Book of Vascular Surgery®: Dr Moneta

2007

The Year Book of
OPHTHALMOLOGY®

Editor-in-Chief
Christopher J. Rapuano, MD
Professor of Ophthalmology, Jefferson Medical College of Thomas Jefferson University; Co-Director, Cornea Service; Co-Director, Refractive Surgery Department, Wills Eye Institute, Philadelphia, Pennsylvania

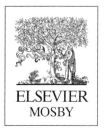

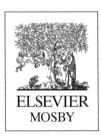

ELSEVIER
MOSBY

Vice President, Continuity: John A. Schrefer
Associate Developmental Editor: Yonah Korngold
Production Supervisor: Donna M. Adamson
Electronic Article Manager: Travis L. Ross
Illustrations and Permissions Coordinator: Linda S. Jones

2007 EDITION
Copyright 2007, Mosby, Inc. All rights reserved.

Printed in the United States of America
Composition by Thomas Technology Solutions, Inc.
Printing/binding by Sheridan Books, Inc.

Editorial Office:
Elsevier
1600 John F. Kennedy Blvd.
Suite 1800
Philadelphia, PA 19103-2899

International Standard Serial Number: 0084-392X
International Standard Book Number: 978-0-323-04655-8

Editorial Board

Table of Contents

Journals Represented

Journals represented in this YEAR BOOK are listed below.

American Journal of Ophthalmology
Anesthesiology
Annals of Neurology
Archives of Ophthalmology
British Journal of Health Psychology
British Journal of Ophthalmology
Clinical Therapeutics
Cornea
Current Opinion in Opthalmology
Freakonomics in The New York Times
Indian Journal of Ophthalmology
Investigative Ophthalmology and Visual Science
Journal of Cataract and Refractive Surgery
Journal of Neuro-Ophthalmology
Journal of Pediatric Ophthalmology and Strabismus
Journal of Refractive Surgery
Journal of the American Association for Pediatric Ophthalmology and
    Strabismus
Journal of the American Medical Association
Medical Care
Nature Genetics
New England Journal of Medicine
Ophthalmic Epidemiology
Ophthalmic Plastic and Reconstructive Surgery
Ophthalmology
Retina
Survey of Ophthalmology

STANDARD ABBREVIATIONS

The following terms are abbreviated in this edition: acquired immunodeficiency syndrome (AIDS), cardiopulmonary resuscitation (CPR), central nervous system (CNS), cerebrospinal fluid (CSF), computed tomography (CT), deoxyribonucleic acid (DNA), diopter (D), electrocardiography (ECG), health maintenance organization (HMO), human immunodeficiency virus (HIV), intensive care unit (ICU), intramuscular (IM), intravenous (IV), magnetic resonance (MR) imaging (MRI), ribonucleic acid (RNA), ultrasound (US), and ultraviolet (UV).

NOTE

The YEAR BOOK OF OPHTHALMOLOGY® is a literature survey service providing abstracts of articles published in the professional literature. Every effort is made to assure the accuracy of the information presented in these pages. Neither the editors nor the publisher of the YEAR BOOK OF OPHTHALMOLOGY® can be responsible for errors in the original materials. The editors' comments are their own opinions. Mention of specific products within this publication does not constitute endorsement.

To facilitate the use of the YEAR BOOK OF OPHTHALMOLOGY® as a reference tool, all illustrations and tables included in this publication are now identified as they appear in the original article. This change is meant to help the reader recognize that any illustration or table appearing in the YEAR BOOK OF OPHTHALMOLOGY® may be only one of many in the original article. For this reason, figure and table numbers will often appear to be out of sequence within the YEAR BOOK OF OPHTHALMOLOGY®.

Foreword

I am again delighted that my Editorial team has done such an excellent job with the 2007 edition of the YEAR BOOK OF OPHTHALMOLOGY! The goal of the YEAR BOOK is to provide a concise summary of the most important peer-reviewed journal articles covering the span of ophthalmic subspecialties from the previous year. The summary is accompanied by a brief discussion of the relevance (or irrelevance) of the paper to practicing ophthalmologists. I believe it does just that!

With the ever-expanding number of peer-reviewed journals, not to mention "throw-away" journals, it is getting harder and harder to not only keep up with the latest developments, but also to sift through the literature to find what is important. The YEAR BOOK OF OPHTHALMOLOGY accomplishes that task AND puts it into perspective. For those of us with hardly enough time to review the important literature in our own sub-specialties, the YEAR BOOK can't be beat for keeping us abreast of the significant issues in other sub-specialties.

I encourage readers to contact me (via e-mail is the best, at cjrapuano @willseye.org) with comments, criticisms, and suggestions. Your input continues to help mold the YEAR BOOK into what is most useful for our readers. I look forward to hearing from you.

Christopher J. Rapuano, MD

1 Cataract Surgery

Year in Review

by Richard Tipperman, MD

This chapter on cataract surgery in the 2007 edition of the YEAR BOOK OF OPHTHALMOLOGY includes a wide variety of articles from numerous journals. As usual, I have tried to include articles that would be relevant to any anterior segment surgeon's clinical practice. In addition to articles dealing with descriptions of techniques, outcomes, and complications the 2007 YEAR BOOK OF OPHTHALMOLOGY also has articles covering psychosocial aspects of cataracts and cataract surgery that do not appear in the "standard" ophthalmic literature. I hope this overview of broad topics will provide a meaningful summary of the literature on cataract surgery which appeared in 2006.

One of the more important topics discussed, both in the ophthalmic literature as well as in numerous meetings, was Toxic Anterior Segment Syndrome (TASS). TASS is used to describe an acute, sterile inflammatory response of the anterior segment, which typically follows uneventful cataract and anterior segment surgery. The symptoms and clinical findings will typically develop within 12 to 24 hours of the surgery, and can include cell and flare with associated fibrin and even hypopyon formationThe previous sentence is unclear.. Patients can develop diffuse corneal edema and pupillary abnormalities, including iris atrophy. Obviously, it is critical to differentiate this sterile postoperative inflammatory process from an infectious endophthalmitis as management of these two distinct entities is very different.

Although there have been numerous hypotheses as to the causative factors of TASS, it is likely that in many situations the causes may be multifactorial. One of the articles reviewed in the current YEAR BOOK is by Dr. Nick Mammalis, who has been a leader in the evaluation and analysis of this clinical syndrome. I would encourage practicing anterior segment surgeons to not only read the review in the YEAR BOOK, but the original source article as well.

Another area of cataract surgery that continues to garner increased interest is the use of multifocal intraocular lens implants (IOLs). Although there are no articles included on specific lens platforms, I have included several articles on surgical techniques which would be beneficial for all cataract surgeons, especially those utilizing multifocal IOLs.

One of the potential problems for all patients who undergo cataract surgery is the development of clinically significant posterior capsule opacification. Vasavada et al (Abstract 1-7) in 2006 described a study using human cadaveric eyes which examined the effect of cortical cleaving hydrodissection alone versus cortical cleaving hydrodissection combined with nucleus rotation. The authors noted that combining the two procedures produced a statistically significant lessening of residual epithelial cells. In clinical practice this should lead to less posterior capsule opacification. Since lesser degrees of posterior capsule opacification can cause greater visual difficulties for patients with multifocal IOLs, this surgical maneuver may confer a clinical advantage.

In 2006 there were two papers that examined the effects of polishing of the anterior capsule. One by Bolz and Menapace et al (Article 1-13) demonstrates that less contraction of the anterior capsule occurs postoperatively when polishing is performed intraoperatively. The second by Mackool and Mackool (Article 1-10) demonstrates that polishing the anterior capsule makes it easier to explant an IOL in the late postoperative period. Both of these findings are important for any cataract surgeon, but they are especially valuable for those utilizing multifocal IOLs since capsular and positional stability of the IOL is essential for success. It is also comforting to know that the IOL can still be explanted if necessary.

Hopefully, those reading this chapter will find it a helpful review and summary of some of the more important topics in cataract surgery in 2006, and will be exposed to some interesting articles in less common journals.

IOL Calculations/Refractive

Simple regression formula for intraocular lens power adjustment in eyes requiring cataract surgery after excimer laser photoablation
Masket S, Masket SE (Univ of California Los Angeles)
J Cataract Refract Surg 32:430-434, 2006   1–1

Purpose.—To develop a simple and accurate method for determining appropriate intraocular lens (IOL) power in cataract patients who had prior excimer laser photoablation for myopia or hyperopia, because laser vision corrective surgery interferes with traditional keratometry and corneal topography, rendering IOL power calculations inaccurate.

Setting.—Private Practice in Century City (Los Angeles), California, and free-standing outpatient surgery centers with institutional review boards.

Methods.—Based on the empiric experience of the senior author, an IOL power correction factor that was proportional to the prior laser photoablation was determined and applied to the IOL power calculated by the IOLMaster (Zeiss). It was necessary to add to the predicted IOL power in eyes with prior myopic laser ablation, whereas eyes having prior hyperopic laser vision correction required a reduction in the IOL power. The correction factor was applied to 30 eyes that required cataract surgery at some time after laser refractive surgery; 23 eyes had prior treatment for myopia, and the remaining 7 eyes had prior hyperopic laser ablation. A regression formula was generated from the IOL power correction factor that was used in the 30 eyes.

Results.—Using the correction factor for 30 eyes, the mean deviation from the desired postcataract refractive outcome was −0.15 diopter (D) ± 0.29 (SD); 28 of 30 eyes were within ±0.5 D of the intended goal; the remaining 2 eyes were both −0.75 D from the desired optical result of cataract surgery. Fourteen of the 30 eyes were emmetropic.

Conclusions.—A simple IOL power corrective adjustment regression formula allowed accurate determination of IOL power after laser refractive photoablation surgery. The weakness of the current method is that knowledge of the amount of prior laser vision correction is necessary.

▶ Although there are numerous formulas and mechanisms for determining the most appropriate IOL power in a patient with previous refractive surgery, none of these is ideal. Some of the formulas require specific topography devices, whereas others require historic data that may not be readily available. This approach by Dr Masket is unique in that it is a simple linear regression formula that can be easily applied to determine the appropriate IOL power in post–refractive surgery patients. Although this formula does require knowledge of the amount of prior laser vision correction, it does not require prerefractive keratometry measurements.

R. Tipperman, MD

Postop/Complications

Severe photic phenomenon
Ernest PH (TCL Eye Care of Michigan, Jackson)
J Cataract Refract Surg 32:685-686, 2006   1–2

Background.—Dysphotopsia after intraocular lens (IOL) implantation has been known for many years, and both positive and negative dysphotopsia have been observed. Dysphotopsia has been reported to occur with several IOL types and designs. In most cases the symptoms will disappear over time. However, some cases may persist, and treatments to reduce the pupil size in these cases have provided mixed results. In this case a new procedure was used to manage a severe case of photic phenomenon

> *Case Report.*—Man, 69, with no significant medical history underwent cataract surgery in the right eye in early September 2003, followed by surgery on the right eye approximately 3 weeks later. Both lenses were well centered in the capsular bag; however, the capsulorrhexis edge was not completely centered on the IOL optic. Visual acuity was 20/15 without correction after surgery. The patient presented postoperatively with positive dysphotopsia. Lens exchange was considered, and the patient had a trial course of brimonidine, followed by pilocarpine. Neither treatment was effective, and the pilocarpine treatment resulted in headaches. A decision was made to insert a piggyback IOL in the patient's left eye. A multipiece

silicone IOL was inserted through the original implantation site. The optic of the new lens was placed on the optic of the original lens, and the haptics were adjusted in the sulcus. Four days after surgery, the patient reported complete satisfaction with his vision in the operated eye. The dysphotopsia continued in the right eye and a piggyback IOL was placed in that eye 1 week later with a similar result. The patient returned several months later with symptoms of dysphotopsia reappearing in the left eye. It was determined that the piggyback lens in the left eye was decentered temporally by 2.0 to 3.0 mm. The lens was repositioned, and the patient's symptoms again vanished.

Conclusions.—Severe positive dysphotopsia was completely eliminated by piggybacking a lens in the sulcus.

▶ Photic phenomena, or dysphotopsias, remain a vexing problem for both the cataract surgeon and patient. Unwanted optical images have been reported with virtually all manufactured IOLs, and the management of them can be problematic. This article is important because it describes a heretofore undescribed approach to managing this problem.

R. Tipperman, MD

The Effectiveness of Nd/YAG Laser Capsulotomy for the Treatment of Posterior Capsule Opacification in Children With Acrylic Intraocular Lenses

Stager DR Jr, Wang X, Weakley DR Jr, et al (Univ of Texas, Dallas; Retina Found of the Southwest, Dallas)
J AAPOS 10:159-163, 2006   1–3

Introduction.—Acrylic intraolcular lenses (IOLs) may result in lower rates of posterior capsular opacification (PCO) than poly(methyl methacrylate) lenses in children. Nonetheless, PCO frequently occurs eventually, especially in younger children. Here, we evaluated the success of neodymium-doped yttrium-aluminum-garnet (Nd:YAG) laser capsulotomy for the management of PCO after acrylic IOL implantation without primary capsulectomy.

Methods.—We reviewed 73 eyes in 57 children (age 23 months to 12 years; median, 6.4 years) who underwent Nd:YAG laser capsulotomy after AcrySof IOL implantation and who had at least 3 months follow-up (range, 3-92 months; median, 25 months). The effectiveness of laser treatment was evaluated in terms of the need for repeat laser procedures or intraocular surgery to clear the visual axis.

Results.—Fifty-one eyes (70%) maintained a clear visual axis after a single Nd:YAG procedure, 10 eyes (84% cumulative) after 2 Nd:YAG procedures, and another 3 eyes (88% cumulative) after 3 Nd:YAG procedures. Six eyes (8%) required pars plana membrane removal to clear the visual axis, whereas 3 eyes (4%) continue to need treatment. Life table analysis showed that the probability of continuing success after 24 months with a single Nd:YAG procedure is 68% (95% confidence interval 53-83%). In younger children (age < 4 years), this rate probability was lower than in older children (35% vs. 74%; P = 0.022). Two eyes developed mild transient elevated intraocular pressure. In 1 eye, the IOL was dislocated and replaced.

Discussion.—Nd:YAG laser capsulotomy is an acceptable option for the management of PCO after AcrySof IOL implantation in children and produces complications infrequently.

▶ Advances in surgical technique and lens design have produced a decrease in the incidence of symptomatic capsular opacification in adults. Pediatric patients, however, have a much higher rate of capsular opacification and, as a result, primary capsulotomy at the time of cataract surgery is often advocated. One approach is to perform a primary posterior capsule capsulorrhexis and capture the IOL through the rhexis to keep the visual axis open. Additionally, the same techniques and technologies that lead to the reduction of capsular opacification in adults should reduce the rate in children as well.

This study demonstrates, however, that when the capsule does opacify, it is possible to perform a YAG capsulotomy to clear the visual axis.

R. Tipperman, MD

Daily Changes in the Morphology of Elschnig Pearls
Neumayer T, Findl O, Buehl W, et al (Med Univ of Vienna)
Am J Ophthalmol 141:517-523, 2006   1–4

Purpose.—To observe and document the daily changes in the morphology of Elschnig pearls.

Design.—A prospective cohort study.

Methods.—Twenty-nine pseudophakic eyes with pronounced, regeneratory posterior capsule opacification (PCO) were included in this prospective study. Retroillumination images were taken at days 0, 1, 2, and 14. A square grid was laid over the images. Increase, decrease, appearance, and disappearance of pearls between the follow-up images were quantified.

Results.—A total of 1371 areas (mean: 53/eye) of 26 eyes were analyzed between days 0 and 1 and 1 and 2, and 896 areas (50/eye) of 18 eyes between days 0 and 14. Between days 0 and 1, days 1 and 2, and days 0 and 14, we observed "no change" in pearl size in 72%, 77%, and 32%, a "minor increase" in 16%, 14%, and 10%, a "major increase" in 4%, 3%, and 42%, a "minor decrease" in 14%, 11%, and 11%, and a "major decrease" in 4%, 3%, and 37%, respectively. Appearance of newly formed pearls was found in 1%, 1%, and 9% and disappearance of pearls in 1%, 1%, and 5%, respectively.

Conclusions.—Significant changes in the morphology of Elschnig pearls were observed within time intervals of only 24 hours. Appearance and disappearance of pearls, as well as progression and regression of pearls within these short intervals illustrate the dynamic behavior of regeneratory PCO.

These findings may contribute to a better understanding of PCO and have implications on pharmaceutical interventions for PCO.

▶ The results of this article were quite striking to me, as I was surprised that significant changes could be seen in the morphology of Elschnig pearls within time intervals of only 24 hours. These findings may likely explain why sometimes patients may give a history of very symptomatic visual problems related to a secondary membrane when they do not have much capsular opacification. When viewed at another date, however, the capsular opacification may be more obvious. These findings may contribute not only to a better understanding of PCO, but also to a better understanding of long-term refractive stability after cataract surgery.

R. Tipperman, MD

Toxic anterior segment syndrome
Mamalis N, Edelhauser HF, Dawson DG, et al (Univ of Utah, Salt Lake City; Emory Univ, Atlanta, Ga)
J Cataract Refract Surg 32:324-333, 2006   1–5

Toxic anterior segment syndrome (TASS) is a sterile postoperative inflammatory reaction caused by a noninfectious substance that enters the anterior segment, resulting in toxic damage to intraocular tissues. The process typically starts 12 to 48 hours after cataract/anterior segment surgery, is limited to the anterior segment of the eye, is always Gram stain and culture negative, and usually improves with steroid treatment. The primary differential diagnosis is infectious endophthalmitis. Review of the literature indicates that possible causes of TASS include intraocular solutions with inappropriate chemical composition, concentration, pH, or osmolality; preservatives; denatured ophthalmic viscosurgical devices; enzymatic detergents; bacterial endotoxin; oxidized metal deposits and residues; and factors related to intraocular lenses such as residues from polishing or sterilizing compounds. An outbreak of TASS is an environmental and toxic control issue that requires complete analysis of all medications and fluids used during surgery, as well as complete review of operating room and sterilization protocols.

▶ I chose this article because TASS is a clinical entity that gained prominence in the past year. It is fascinating that a search of the national medical publication archives for the term yields only 9 articles—8 of which were written in 2006 (the sole remaining article was from 2005).

It is likely that TASS occurred in prior years; however, it is unclear if the "increase" is a true increase or merely one of increased recognition.

Although TASS seems to occur in outbreaks or clusters, attempts to identify a single causative agent have not been successful. Instead, it appears that there may be multifactorial causes, including contaminants, sterilization processes, endotoxins, and even enzymatic detergents.

This is a topic of importance to all ophthalmic surgeons, and I would encourage them to read the original source article.

R. Tipperman, MD

Outbreak of toxic anterior segment syndrome associated with glutaraldehyde after cataract surgery
Ünal M, Yücel i, Akar Y, et al (Akdeniz Univ, Antalya, Turkey)
J Cataract Refract Surg 32:1696-1701, 2006   1–6

Purpose.—To present clinical findings of a cluster of cases of toxic anterior segment syndrome (TASS) after uneventful phacoemulsification cataract surgery.

Setting.—Department of Ophthalmology, Akdeniz University, Antalya, Turkey.

Methods.—Six eyes of 6 patients developed TASS after uneventful phacoemulsification cataract surgery with implantation of a 3-piece acrylic IOL performed by 2 ophthalmologists on the same day. Clinical findings included corneal edema, Descemet's membrane folds, anterior chamber reaction, fibrin formation, and irregular, dilated, and unreactive pupils.

Results.—Glutaraldehyde 2% solution was used inadvertently by the operating room staff who cleaned and sterilized reusable ocular instruments before autoclaving. None of the affected corneas improved. Additional surgical procedures were required and included penetrating keratoplasty, trabeculectomy, and glaucoma tube implantation.

Conclusions.—Glutaraldehyde in concentrations generally used for cold sterilization is highly toxic to the corneal endothelium. The operating room staff involved in sterilizing instruments should be well educated about and careful to follow the protocols to properly clean and sterilize reusable ocular instruments.

▶ I chose this article not just because of the importance of recognizing and including TASS in the differential diagnosis of postoperative inflammation, but also because it demonstrates one of the many different etiologic factors that can induce this clinical condition. In many of the clusters of outbreaks of TASS, one step in the cleaning or sterilizing of the surgical instruments is often identified as the potential cause. It is important that all operating room personnel understand this phenomenon as well as the surgeon.

R. Tipperman, MD

Surgical Techniques

Effect of hydrodissection alone and hydrodissection combined with rotation on lens epithelial cells: Surgical approach for the prevention of posterior capsule opacification

Vasavada AR, Raj SM, Johar K, et al (Iladevi Cataract & IOL Research Centre, Ahmedabad, India)

J Cataract Refract Surg 32:145-150, 2006   1–7

Purpose.—To evaluate the impact of corticocleaving hydrodissection alone and hydrodissection combined with rotation on lens epithelial cells (LECs) and residual cortical fibers (RCFs).

Setting.—Iladevi Cataract and IOL Research Center, Ahmedabad, India.

Methods.—An experimental laboratory study of 20 fresh human cadaver eyes (10 pairs) was conducted. A single eye from each pair was assigned to the control group, in which no hydrodissection and no rotation were performed (control). The other eye was randomized to corticocleaving hydrodissection alone (Group 1) or corticocleaving hydrodissection with rotation (Group 2). Cataract extraction was standardized. Capsule polishing was omitted. Area of LEC loss (%) in the preequatorial zone (PZ) and equatorial zone (EZ) was calculated as: [Area of capsule without cells/Total area of capsule] $\times$ 100. Area of presence of RCFs (%) was calculated as: [Circumference of EZ of capsule with RCF/Total circumference of EZ of the capsule] $\times$ 100. The Mann-Whitney U and the Wilcoxon signed rank tests were applied.

Results.—In the control group, area of cell loss (%) was 3.9 ± 3.2 in the PZ and 2.7 ± 0.8 in the EZ; presence of RCFs (%) was 83.8 ± 1.7. Area of LEC loss (%) in Groups 1 and 2 was 24.8 ± 4.5 and 42.6 ± 5.4 ($P = .008$) in the PZ and 22.4 ± 2.1 and 54 ± 2.5 ($P = .008$) in the EZ, respectively. Area of presence of RCFs (%) in Groups 1 and 2 was 34.2 ± 3.7 and 23.7 ± 3.7 ($P = .008$), respectively.

Conclusion.—Corticocleaving hydrodissection combined with rotation removed significant quantities of LECs and RCFs.

▶ Advances in both surgical technique and IOL design have led to reduced rates of capsular opacification. Conversely, rising patient expectations and advanced-technology IOLs have required long-term capsular clarity and IOL/refractive stability. This article is interesting, in that relatively simple and low-technology maneuvers can be shown to lessen the quantities of lens epithelial cells and residual cortical fibers. Presumably, these approaches will also lessen the incidence of capsular opacification.

R. Tipperman, MD

Effect of a closed foldable equator ring on capsular bag shrinkage in cataract surgery

Kurz S, Krummenauer F, Dumbach C, et al (Johannes Gutenberg-Univ, Mainz, Germany; Technical Univ of Dresden, Germany)
J Cataract Refract Surg 32:1615-1620, 2006   1–8

Purpose.—To evaluate the effect of a closed foldable equator ring (CFER) versus a conventional capsular tension ring (CTR) on capsular bag shrinkage.

Setting.—Department of Ophthalmology, Johannes Gutenberg-University, Mainz, Germany.

Methods.—In this prospective study, 70 eyes of 70 patients were randomized to 2 groups using a 1:1 block scheme. After uneventful cataract surgery, a capsular measuring ring was implanted in all eyes to measure the capsular bag diameter in vivo. In Group 1, a CTR was implanted in the capsular bag. In Group 2, a CFER was inserted. Biometric characteristics such as axial length and the horizontal and vertical corneal radii were measured preoperatively. The capsular bag diameter and capsulorrhexis diameter were measured intraoperatively and 2 or 3 days as well as 1 and 3 months postoperatively.

Results.—There were no statistically significant or clinically relevant between-group differences in covariants such as axial length, vertical and horizontal corneal radii, and capsulorrhexis diameter. Eyes with the CTR had slight but statistically significant capsular bag shrinkage from a median of 10.4 to a median of 10.2 mm after 3 months ($P<.001$). Eyes with the CFER also had slight but statistically significant capsular bag shrinkage from a median of 10.3 to a median of 10.2 mm 3 months postoperatively ($P = .021$). At baseline, the CTR group had a larger capsular bag diameter, but there were no statistically significant differences between the groups at the 3-month follow-up ($P = .669$).

Conclusions.—No clinically relevant capsular bag shrinkage was observed after implantation of a CFER or a CTR. The expected capsular bag shrinkage was the same in both groups.

▶ As cataract surgery becomes increasingly refined and patients expectations become increasingly higher, there has been a concomitant increased interest in long-term capsular bag stability and its potential influence on the refractive outcome of cataract surgery. This is especially true for patients receiving presbyopic or multifocal intraocular lenses.

One way surgeons have advocated increasing the long-term capsular stability (and therefore the postoperative refraction) is to place a capsular tension ring. In this well-designed study, both a closed ring and open-loop ring were compared. Although not immediately intuitive, both rings performed equally well. This should help with further design and use of capsular tension rings to help support long-term capsular stability.

R. Tipperman, MD

Effect of the Morcher capsular tension ring on refractive outcome

Boomer JA, Jackson DW (Univ of Oklahoma, Oklahoma City)
J Cataract Refract Surg 32:1180-1183, 2006   1-9

Purpose.—To evaluate the effect of the Morcher capsular tension ring (CTR) on refractive outcome in patients having cataract extraction by phacoemulsification complicated by zonular instability.

Setting.—Dean A. McGee Eye Institute, Oklahoma City, Oklahoma, USA.

Methods.—A retrospective case-control series of 19 eyes of 19 patients with a CTR were compared with a control population of 24 eyes without zonular instability having routine cataract surgery. A subset of 9 patients with a CTR in 1 eye but milder zonular instability in the contralateral eye not requiring a CTR was analyzed. The main outcome measures were the mean arithmetic and absolute refractive prediction errors (ArRPE, AbRPE) and variances used to gauge accuracy and precision.

Results.—The CTR and control groups were compared using SRK/T and Holladay 2. There was no statistically significant difference in ArRPE or AbRPE, but lower variances in eyes with a CTR were identified. The CTR subset demonstrated a trend toward more accurate outcomes when using Holladay 2 but not SRK/T when compared with contralateral eyes without a CTR. Both formulas showed lower variances in the CTR eyes than in the contralateral eyes.

Conclusions.—In this small population, there was no consistent effect on refractive outcome when a Morcher CTR was placed that would necessitate modification of intraocular lens power calculations. The eyes with a CTR had refractive outcomes as accurate as and more precise than the outcomes in the contralateral eyes with milder zonular instability and the control population of eyes without zonular instability in either eye. The Morcher CTR is not only a tool to assist in complicated cataract surgeries, but a device that can deliver more accurate and precise refractive outcomes.

▶ This article demonstrates many important points, not the least of which is how far cataract surgery has advanced over time. It is no longer just a concern to have surgery in patients with loose or weak zonules completed successfully or with intraocular lens implantation, but we are now studying the ability to achieve predicted and long-term intraocular lens power accuracy in these patients.

Obviously, patients with compromised zonular or capsular support systems would be most likely to have problems with both initial intraocular lens power accuracy as well as long-term stability. If the CTR can help with refractive predictability in this high-risk or compromised population, then it is even more likely to be effective in the routine or noncomplex patient. This may become important as advanced technology and presbyopic lenses become more commonplace for our patients.

R. Tipperman, MD

Removal of lens epithelial cells to delay anterior capsule–intraocular lens adherence

Mackool RJ, Mackool RJ Jr (Mackool Eye Inst, Astoria, NY)
J Cataract Refract Surg 32:1766-1767, 2006   1–10

Background.—The purpose of this study was to test the theory that removal of lens epithelial cells at cataract extraction with intraocular lens (IOL) implantation or refractive lens exchange could decrease the rate at which the anterior capsule becomes adherent to the lens optic postoperatively. Several studies have reported that IOLs, particularly hydrophobic acrylic IOLs, may quickly develop strong adherence to the lens capsule after cataract-IOL surgery. It can be difficult to separate the capsule from the IOL optic with preservation of the capsule for placement in the new IOL, should removal or exchange of the IOL become necessary. It was thought that removal of the lens epithelial cells (LECs) from beneath the anterior capsule at the initial procedure might delay postoperative adhesion of the anterior capsule to the IOL. This technique was performed in approximately 200 eyes considered likely to require postoperative IOL exchange. In 4 eyes that underwent an IOL procedure 6 to 12 weeks after the primary procedure, the anterior capsule was nonadherent or weakly adherent to the lens optic.

> *Case Report.*—Four patients ages 66, 55, 38, and 72 years were treated with refractive lens exchange procedures with insertion of a single-piece acrylic IOL. Intraoperatively, LECs were removed from the undersurface of the anterior capsule immediately after the cortex had been removed. Subepithelial cells were removed from the entire area of visible anterior capsule, except for the quadrant that was directly beneath the incision through which the phacoemulsification procedure was performed. The patients required IOL exchange at 6, 7, 8, and 12 weeks, respectively, because of a postoperative refractive error.

Conclusions.—Adhesion of the lens capsule to IOLs is a well-documented event that desirably fixes the IOL in the capsular bag. However, the adhesion can make surgical procedures difficult if not impossible to accomplish. It is suggested from the findings in 4 patients presented here that removal of the LECs from the anterior capsule during cataract removal or the RLE procedure may reduce the rate at which this adhesion occurs.

▶ This article by an internationally renowned surgeon demonstrates one of the clinical advantages of performing polishing of the anterior capsule. In cases where the surgeons are concerned that there may be a potential need for IOL exchange (eg, multifocal IOL or cataract surgery in the presence of previous lasik surgery), this may be a technique the operating surgeon would want to use.

R. Tipperman, MD

Effect of lens epithelial cell aspiration on postoperative capsulorrhexis contraction with the use of the AcrySof intraocular lens: Randomized clinical trial

Hanson RJ, Rubinstein A, Sarangapani S, et al (Oxford Eye Hosp, England; Stoke Mandeville Hosp, Aylesbury, England)
J Cataract Refract Surg 32:1621-1626, 2006   1–11

Purpose.—To determine whether aspiration of lens epithelial cells (LECs) from under the anterior capsule reduces postoperative contraction of the capsulorrhexis aperture.

Setting.—Stoke Mandeville Hospital, Aylesbury, Buckinghamshire, United Kingdom.

Methods.—This prospective randomized observer-masked study comprised 100 patients who had routine phacoemulsification by the same surgeon at a district general hospital in the United Kingdom. The postoperative changes in capsulorrhexis apertures and anterior capsule opacification (ACO) between Group A (aspiration of LECs) and Group B (control) were compared. Digital retroillumination images of the capsulorrhexis aperture were taken 1 week and 3 months postoperatively. The area of capsulorrhexis aperture was determined with computer software, and capsule opacification was graded subjectively.

Results.—Three months postoperatively, the mean decrease in capsulorrhexis aperture was 1.9% in Group A and 5.6% in Group B ($P = .02$). The ACO at 3 months was grade 2 in 44% of eyes in Group A and in 61% in Group B ($P = .13$).

Conclusion.—Aspiration of LECs from the anterior capsule was a safe procedure that reduced capsulorrhexis aperture contraction 3 months after cataract surgery.

▶ This is yet another article that examines the effect of aspiration of lens epithelial cells from the underside of the anterior capsule. This article studies a different long-term effect of this maneuver and demonstrates that it leads to reduced contraction of the capsulorrhexis aperture. Theoretically, this should help lead to long-term intraocular lens stability. This consequence of the technique of anterior capsule polishing should be considered when surgeons are considering whether to incorporate this into their surgical technique.

R. Tipperman, MD

Lightless cataract surgery using a near-infrared operating microscope

Kim B-H (HenAm Kim Eye Ctr, Haenam-Gun, South Korea)
J Cataract Refract Surg 32:1683-1690, 2006   1–12

Purpose.—To describe the near-infrared (NIR) operating microscopy (NIOM) system using the NIR wavelength as the illumination source and to evaluate the feasibility of this system for lightless cataract surgery.

Setting.—HenAm Kim Eye Center, Haenam-Gun, South Korea.

Methods.—In this noncomparative interventional case series, cataract surgery was performed in 4 patients with bilateral cataract using the NIOM system in 1 eye and conventional microscopy in the fellow eye. The primary components of the system include an optical filter, a stereoscopic camera, head-mounted displays, and a recording system. This system uses invisible NIR (wavelength 850 to 1300 nm) illumination to facilitate cataract surgery without light. The differences between the NIOM system and conventional microscopy during cataract surgery were evaluated.

Results.—The NIOM system provided excellent 3-dimensional viewing in real time. The image resolution was sufficient while performing all steps of cataract surgery. Immediately postoperatively and at 10 and 30 minutes and 1 hour, the visual acuity was better in the 4 eyes in which the NIOM system was used than in the 4 eyes in which conventional microscopy was used. However, using the NIOM system required good surgical skill.

Conclusions.—Lightless cataract surgery using the NIOM system seems useful for obtaining good visual acuity immediately postoperatively. The system may also reduce the incidence of light-induced retinal toxicity and the need for mydriatic administration and be a good educational tool.

▶ I thought this was a really unique and interesting article and merited inclusion in the YEAR BOOK, even though it is not likely that many surgeons will incorporate this into their surgical technique. For those surgeons who have experience with the LADARWave 6000 (Alcon, Fort Wort, Texas) platform for refractive surgery, they can see how an infrared-type viewing system can lead to excellent visualization without traditional light sources.

Theoretically, this type of system could be helpful in reducing the incidence of retinal phototoxicity. The reality, however, is that clinically significant presentations of this phenomenon are not common and, to my knowledge, there is not a commercially available version of the near-infrared light source available. Nonetheless, I believe most anterior segment surgeons will find the whole concept very thought provoking.

R. Tipperman, MD

Effect of anterior capsule polishing on the posterior capsule opacification–inhibiting properties of a sharp-edged, 3-piece, silicone intraocular lens: Three- and 5-year results of a randomized trial
Bolz M, Menapace R, Findl O, et al (Med Univ of Vienna)
J Cataract Refract Surg 32:1513-1520, 2006   1–13

Purpose.—To evaluate the long-term effects of anterior capsule polishing on regeneratory posterior capsule opacification (PCO), anterior capsule opacification (ACO), and fibrotic PCO with a silicone intraocular lens (IOL) with sharp optic edges.

Setting.—Department of Ophthalmology, Medical University of Vienna, Vienna, Austria.

Methods.—This prospective bilateral randomized patient- and examiner-masked clinical trial comprised 130 eyes of 65 patients with bilateral age-related cataract. All eyes had implantation of a 3-piece silicone IOL with a truncated, sharp-edged optic (CeeOn Edge 911A, Advanced Medical Optics). In 1 eye, the anterior capsule was extensively polished using an aspiration curette after phacoemulsification and cortex aspiration. Regenerative PCO was quantified objectively, while ACO and fibrotic PCO were graded subjectively 1, 2, 3, and 5 years postoperatively.

Results.—The mean ACO score was significantly lower in the eyes in which the anterior capsule had been polished (1 year, $P<.02$; 2 years, $P<.03$; 3 years, $P<.01$; 5 years, $P<.01$). The mean difference in regeneratory PCO and fibrotic PCO scores between the 2 groups was not statistically significant.

Conclusions.—Three years after cataract surgery, eyes in which the anterior capsule had been polished had significantly less ACO. However, polishing did not lower PCO intensity when a sharp-edged CeeOn 911A IOL was implanted in the bag. Although results indicate that anterior capsule polishing may enhance the development of regeneratory PCO, this trend did not reach statistical significance.

▶ Again, because of concerns regarding both long-term capsular stability and posterior capsule clarity, issues such as anterior capsule polishing have been studied. The belief is that by removing these cells through anterior capsule polishing it may be possible to decrease the incidence of posterior capsule opacification.

In this study, the incidence of PCO did not decrease and, in fact, there was a trend for it to increase (though not statistically significant). This has been ascribed to the fact that PCO probably occurs secondary to migration of equatorial epithelial cells that would not be removed by anterior capsular polishing. In addition, removing the anterior capsular epithelial cells decreases the ability of the anterior capsule to "shrink wrap" and adhere to the posterior capsule, which may have an inhibitory effect on posterior capsule opacification.

R. Tipperman, MD

Preoperative prediction of posterior capsule plaque in eyes with posterior subcapsular cataract
Vasavada AR, Praveen MR, Jani UD, et al (Iladevi Cataract & IOL Research Centre, Ahmedabad, India)
Indian J Ophthalmol 54:169-172, 2006   1–14

Aim.—To determine whether the plaque on the posterior capsule can be predicted preoperatively, in patients with posterior subcapsular cataract (PSC), undergoing cataract surgery.

Materials and Methods.—A prospective study of 140 consecutive eyes with PSC, who underwent cataract surgery, was conducted. The prediction of preoperative presence or absence of plaque within the PSC was noted on slit lamp examination, in dilated pupils. A single observer made the observations under oblique illumination, where the slit lamp was placed at an angle of 30° to 45°. Evaluation of the plaque through slit lamp examination was standardized in terms of illumination and magnification. The observations were recorded using a video camera (Image archiving system, Carl Zeiss, Jena Germany) attached to a slit lamp (Carl Zeiss, SL 120 Jena, Germany), keeping the illumination at 100%. The prediction of plaque was noted in terms of its presence or absence on the posterior capsule. All the patients received counseling regarding the presence of plaque. Capsule polishing of the posterior capsule in Cap Vac mode, was done in all cases. The posterior capsule was examined for presence or absence of plaque, either on the first postoperative day, or within a week, with maximal mydriasis. The observer's results were tabulated and later analyzed to judge the incidence of predictability of plaque in PSC.

Results.—The mean age of the patients was 45±6.2 years (range 32-61 years); 104 (74.3%) were males. One hundred and eight (77.1%) patients were under 50 years. The presence or absence of plaque was predicted correctly in 124 (88.6%) eyes. The prediction of plaque was incorrect in 16 (11.4%) eyes.

Conclusion.—The prediction of presence or absence of plaque was accurate in 88.6% cases. We believe that counseling patients with posterior capsule plaque before the surgery is the key to avoiding unpleasant surprises.

▶ I chose this article because I believe it is a very important topic for surgeons implanting multifocal or presbyopic lenses. Many of the patients interested in these lens technologies will be younger patients, and many of them will have posterior capsule plaque cataracts. As such, they will often have significant capsular opacification after cataract removal. We know that patients with these advanced-technology lenses are incredibly sensitive to decline in visual function with only minimal capsular opacification.

The ability to identify and predict preoperatively those patients who might have capsular opacification and require an early YAG capsulotomy can be very helpful as it will allow preoperative counseling of these issues. Otherwise, if the patient has reduced vision after surgery, they will often ascribe it to their IOL rather than the previously discussed capsular haze.

R. Tipperman, MD

Cataract Evaluations/Psychosocial Issues

Longitudinal rates of cataract surgery
Williams A, Sloan FA, Lee PP (Duke Univ, Durham, NC)
Arch Ophthalmol 124:1308-1314, 2006   1–15

Objective.—To determine the cumulative probability of cataract surgery and factors accounting for such surgery.

Methods.—Respondents to the Asset and Health Dynamics Among the Oldest Old survey, a national longitudinal panel, were interviewed in 1998, 2000, and 2002 to determine whether they had undergone cataract extraction since the previous interview (N = 8363 in 1998). Multivariate analysis was used to identify factors affecting cataract surgery rates.

Results.—The annual incidence of cataract surgery from January 1, 1995, to December 31, 2002, was 7.4%. The prevalence of unilateral pseudophakia increased from 7.6% in 1998 to 9.8% in 2002; the prevalence of bilateral pseudophakia increased from 10.5% in 1998 to 22.3% in 2002. The self-reported vision of persons undergoing cataract surgery improved related to that of others (a difference of 0.4 on a 9-point scale; P<.001). Black individuals were less likely to undergo cataract surgery than white individuals (P<.01). The highest rates of surgery were for persons who were 65 years or older in 1998. However, persons with Medicare parts A and B coverage underwent more procedures than those with primary private employer-based coverage or the uninsured.

Conclusions.—At 5.3%, the cataract surgery incidence is similar to that given in previous reports. Persons undergoing cataract surgery more often had low self-reported vision before surgery, and their vision improved on average relative to others after surgery.

▶ This report is an excellent study of the longitudinal rates of cataract surgery. General studies of population demographics demonstrate that the population pyramid is going to become heavily weighted toward older people in the US population over the next few decades as the baby boomers begin to reach age 60 years and beyond.

Even if the rate of cataract surgery remains stable because there will be a larger population of people requiring surgery (because of demographic shifts), it seems likely that the absolute number of cataract surgeries will increase. This will further financially stress a reimbursement system that, because of attempts at budget neutrality, is already struggling to keep up with the current levels of cataract surgery. Studies such as the current one will allow for increased planning and public policy measures to accommodate not only fair reimbursement for surgeons but also allow access to cataract surgery care for those patients requiring such services.

R. Tipperman, MD

Association between visual impairment and patient-reported visual disability at different stages of cataract surgery
Acosta-Rojas ER, Comas M, Sala M, et al (Municipal Inst of Med Research, Barcelona)
Ophthalmic Epidemiol 13:299-307, 2006   1–16

Purpose.—To evaluate the association between visual impairment (visual acuity, contrast sensitivity, stereopsis) and patient-reported visual disability at different stages of cataract surgery.

Methods.—A cohort of 104 patients aged 60 years and over with bilateral cataract was assessed preoperatively, after first-eye surgery (monocular pseudophakia) and after second-eye surgery (binocular pseudophakia). Partial correlation coefficients (PCC) and linear regression models were calculated.

Results.—In patients with bilateral cataracts, visual disability was associated with visual acuity (PCC = −0.30) and, to a lesser extent, with contrast sensitivity (PCC = 0.16) and stereopsis (PCC = −0.09). In monocular and binocular pseudophakia, visual disability was more strongly associated with stereopsis (PCC = −0.26 monocular and −0.51 binocular) and contrast sensitivity (PCC = 0.18 monocular and 0.34 binocular) than with visual acuity (PCC = −0.18 monocular and −0.18 binocular). Visual acuity, contrast sensitivity and stereopsis accounted for between 17% and 42% of variance in visual disability.

Conclusions.—The association of visual impairment with patient-reported visual disability differed at each stage of cataract surgery. Measuring other forms of visual impairment independently from visual acuity, such as contrast sensitivity or stereopsis, could be important in evaluating both needs and outcomes in cataract surgery. More comprehensive assessment of the impact of cataract on patients should include measurement of both visual impairment and visual disability.

▶ This article is interesting for several reasons and I chose it because, again, it appears in a journal not likely to be read by most practicing ophthalmologists. The article demonstrates what ophthalmologists have known for a long time clinically—that visual acuity measurements alone are not always good predictors of visual function. I especially found the study's findings regarding the changes in visual function when patients were unilateral pseudophakes versus bilateral pseudophakes.

This study was performed with a cohort of patients that had monofocal intraocular lens (IOL) implanted; however, the types of findings seen with unilateral versus bilateral IOL implantation mirror what is seen with multifocal IOLs. In multifocal IOL patients, it is clear that there is a significantly greater improvement in overall visual function when the second eye is implanted than would be seen with just "1 + 1 = 2." Perhaps this phenomenon has been occurring all along with monofocal lenses but was not as readily apparent. Nonetheless, it does support the observation that patients function best when bilaterally implanted with multifocal IOLs.

R. Tipperman, MD

Characterizing pseudoexfoliation syndrome through the use of ultrasound biomicroscopy

Guo S, Gewirtz M, Thaker R, et al (Univ of Medicine & Dentistry of New Jersey, Newark)

J Cataract Refract Surg 32:614-617, 2006   1–17

Purpose.—To determine the clinical utility of ultrasound biomicroscopy (UBM) in diagnosis of pseudoexfoliation (PEX) syndrome by characterizing the lens capsule and zonules before cataract surgery.

Setting.—Veterans Administration Hospital, East Orange, and University of Medicine & Dentistry of New Jersey–New Jersey Medical School, Newark, New Jersey, USA.

Methods.—Ultrasound biomicroscopy was performed on 10 patients clinically diagnosed with PEX syndrome. The clinical diagnosis was made by the presence of fibrillin deposits on the anterior lens capsule, lack of pigment at the pupillary ruff, and poor pharmacologic dilation. Five persons without PEX were used as controls. The thickness of the anterior lens capsule was measured in 5 locations in each eye: centrally and in the peripheral lens capsule superiorly, inferiorly, nasally, and temporally. Four measurements were taken from the zonule at the thickest point on each fiber. The UBM also found the presence or absence of nodular deposits on the zonules.

Results.—The anterior and peripheral lens capsule in patients with PEX was thicker than that in the control group. Additionally, patients with PEX had thicker zonules than the control group and had nodular deposits present; the control group had no deposits. These differences were all significant with a 99% confidence interval.

Conclusions.—A thicker anterior lens capsule and lens zonule nodules were associated with PEX. These abnormalities can be visualized with the UBM to confirm the diagnosis of PEX and identify patients at risk for operative complications.

▶ Many studies have documented that cataract surgery in patients with PEX has a higher rate of complications than when PXF is not present. Fortunately for most patients with this condition, the surgery is still routine and uncomplicated. Clinically, it would be incredibly helpful if there were a way to determine which PEX patients were at the highest level of risk during cataract surgery.

This article demonstrates how UBM can be used to identify and diagnose PEX syndrome. It would be interesting to observe if this approach could be quantified over time to help identify the patients at the greatest risk for complications with PEX. Clearly, clinically, the amount of PXF material present visually by slit-lamp biomicroscopy is not a good indicator; however, it might be that the parameters measured by UBM could help identify the patients at the highest level of risk during cataract surgery.

R. Tipperman, MD

Psychological distress and visual functioning in relation to vision-related disability in older individuals with cataracts
Walker JG, Anstey KJ, Lord SR (Centre for Mental Health Research, Canberra, Australia; Falls and Balance Research Group at the Prince of Wales Med Research Inst, Sydney)
Br J Health Psychol 11:303-317, 2006   1–18

Objective.—To determine whether demographic, health status and psychological functioning measures, in addition to impaired visual acuity, are related to vision-related disability.

Methods.—Participants were 105 individuals (mean age = 73.7 years) with cataracts requiring surgery and corrected visual acuity in the better eye of 6/24 to 6/36 were recruited from waiting lists at three public out-patient ophthalmology clinics. Visual disability was measured with the Visual Functioning-14 survey. Visual acuity was assessed using better and worse eye logMAR scores and the Melbourne Edge Test (MET) for edge contrast sensitivity. Data relating to demographic information, depression, anxiety and stress, health care and medication use and numbers of co-morbid conditions were obtained.

Results.—Principal component analysis revealed four meaningful factors that accounted for 75% of the variance in visual disability: recreational activities, reading and fine work, activities of daily living and driving behaviour. Multiple regression analyses determined that visual acuity variables were the only significant predictors of overall vision-related functioning and difficulties with reading and fine work. For the remaining visual disability domains, non-visual factors were also significant predictors. Difficulties with recreational activities were predicted by stress, as well as worse eye visual acuity, and difficulties with activities of daily living were associated with self-reported health status, age and depression as well as MET contrast scores. Driving behaviour was associated with sex (with fewer women driving), depression, anxiety and stress scores, and MET contrast scores.

Conclusion.—Vision-related disability is common in older individuals with cataracts. In addition to visual acuity, demographic, psychological and health status factors influence the severity of vision-related disability, affecting recreational activities, activities of daily living and driving.

▶ I chose this article for several reasons. Foremost is that it appears in a journal that is not likely to be read by most ophthalmologists, yet it is a topic that is very important. When patients are evaluated for cataract surgery we often focus on the patient's driving status and Snellen acuity. Certainly these are important parameters for many of our patients. However, what this article demonstrates is the very significant negative impact visual impairment from cataracts has on overall quality of life and activities of daily living. Functional improvement in vision would be expected to produce improvement in overall quality of life and activities of daily living.

R. Tipperman, MD

Is cataract surgery cost-effective among older patients with a low predicted probability for improvement in reported visual functioning?
Naeim A, Keeler EB, Gutierrez PR, et al (Univ of California, Los Angeles)
Med Care 44:982-989, 2006   1–19

Introduction.—Although cataract surgery has been demonstrated to be effective and cost-effective, 5% to 20% of patients do not benefit functionally from the procedure. This study examines the cost-effectiveness of cataract surgery versus watchful waiting in a subgroup of patients who had less than a 30% predicted probability of reporting improvements in visual function after surgery.

Methods.—Randomized trial (first eye surgery vs. watchful waiting) of 250 patients who based on a cataract surgery index (CSI) were felt to have less than a 30% probability of reporting improvements in visual functioning after surgery. Cost was estimated using monthly resource utilization surveys and Medicare billing and payment data. Effectiveness was evaluated at 6 months using the Activities of Daily Vision Scale (ADVS) and the Health Utilities Index, Mark 3 (HUI3).

Results.—In terms of overall utility, the incremental cost-effectiveness of surgery was Dollars 38,288/QALY. In the subgroup of patients with a CSI score > 11 (< 20% probability of improvement), the cost-effectiveness of cataract surgery was Dollars 53,500/QALY. Sensitivity analysis demonstrated that often this population of patients may not derive a utility benefit with surgery.

Conclusion.—Cataract surgery is cost-effective even in a subpopulation of patients with a lower, < 30%, predicted probability of reporting improved visual functioning after surgery. There may be a subgroup of patients, CSI > 11, for whom a strategy of watchful waiting may be equally effective and considerably less expensive.

▶ In patients with advanced cataracts and concomitant ocular disease, such as advanced ARMD or glaucoma, it can be difficult to decide whether to proceed with cataract surgery. I typically tell my patients the more important question is not whether they can have cataract surgery, but instead whether cataract surgery will yield enough improvement in visual function and overall quality of life to justify the surgery in the first place. In many instances, even when Snellen visual acuity does not improve, patients still feel that the overall visual function is improved, as is the quality of life.

This study demonstrates that for almost all patients (even when the prognosis is poor) cataract surgery can be beneficial. However, there is a subgroup with an even more limited prognosis in whom clinical observation is probably warranted. Unfortunately, these patients can be difficult to identify preoperatively since the overall improvement in quality of life may be difficult to predict.

R. Tipperman, MD

2 Refractive Surgery

Are We LASIK Surgeons or Refractive Surgeons?

by Christopher J. Rapuano, MD

A running theme at refractive surgery courses when I became involved with them in the early 1990s was that refractive surgeons should not be "one-trick ponies." That is, they should not be "radial keratotomy (RK) surgeons" or "photorefractive keratectomy (PRK) surgeons" or "laser-assisted in situ keratomileusis (LASIK) surgeons," but rather "refractive surgeons" because refractive surgery is not a one-size fits all specialty. Some procedures are better for some patients than other procedures, and the comprehensive refractive surgeon should be able to treat most patients with the best procedure for each particular patient. We have learned, sometimes the hard way, that patients with forme fruste keratoconus, or significant anterior basement membrane dystrophy, or thin corneas may not be the best candidates for LASIK. While they may not be great candidates for any refractive surgery, there may be a refractive procedure that is right for them. Unfortunately, that is where the problem lies with many of the patients I see who are interested in refractive surgery. They come into my office inquiring about LASIK and only LASIK.

Over the years, ophthalmologists have done an excellent job marketing refractive surgery. Back in the 1980s, a large percentage of people in this country knew that RK was a procedure to correct vision. Many even knew that it was developed in Russia and involved a scalpel cutting into the cornea. In fact, when laser refractive surgery came on the scene in the mid 1990s, most interested patients referred to it as RK. (It didn't help the confusion that the first excimer laser refractive surgery to gain FDA approval was PRK.) People eventually learned the difference between the "blade" procedure and the "laser" procedure, but they still aren't aware that numerous laser procedures are available. Many patients have only heard of LASIK, so they think LASIK is the only procedure to have.

It isn't surprising that LASIK is on their mind. It is the most popular refractive surgery in the world. It has been on the cover of national magazines. You can't drive down a highway in most urban areas without seeing one or more billboards advertising it. You can't read a Sunday paper in most cities without seeing several ads promoting a certain surgeon or laser center or "sale" or special financing for it. The problem is that LASIK isn't right for everyone, and yet that is what we are selling. The marketing gurus have told us that we need a "catch phrase" and "LASIK" is perfect for that. We are told promoting "refractive surgery" is either too boring or too clinical—not what patients want to hear or what they will remember. The downside of that strategy is that when I see a patient in the office who is not a good candidate for LASIK but is a good candidate for a surface ablation procedure, it is that much more difficult for me to get them to understand what I'm saying. They are so focused on "LASIK" that when I tell them LASIK may not be the best option for them, they are thrown for a loop and don't hear the rest of the discussion.

Patient mentality regarding LASIK/refractive surgery is fascinating to me. When most patients go to the dentist with a problem, they don't ask for a specific treatment plan, but rather the best solution to their problem, be it medication or surgery. The same goes for our cars. When we have a car malfunction we (at least most of us) don't tell the mechanic how to fix it, but just that we want it fixed. For some reason, many patients feel they have the expertise to decide what procedure is best for them. Certainly some of this "knowledge" comes from friends and family who have had LASIK and are happy. But much of this "LASIK is the only refractive surgery to have" attitude comes from refractive surgeons and our marketing efforts.

I believe we should remember the lessons of years ago. We should be marketing vision correction as a concept and not LASIK as a specific procedure. That may be more difficult in the short-term, but in the long-term, I believe both patients and surgeons will benefit. It will focus the patient's and the surgeon's goals, namely making patients happy by improving uncorrected vision. To do that, surgeons need to remember to address the patient's visual needs: Is reading without glasses most important to the patient? Is good uncorrected vision while playing golf or tennis critical to their happiness? Is using the computer without correction the goal? These are the crucial issues we should be discussing, not trying to convince them why one refractive surgical procedure is better for them than another. Additionally, as intraocular lenses become better and better at correcting more than sphere, they will be much easier to incorporate into a refractive practice if we market vision correction rather than a single surgical option. We should be promoting vision without crutches, not one specific procedure which isn't for everyone, and, if history teaches us anything, will likely be replaced at some point by a better procedure. Concentrating on "vision correction" rather than "LASIK" will help achieve our ultimate goal—very happy patients.

Functional Outcome and Patient Satisfaction After Artisan Phakic Intraocular Lens Implantation for the Correction of Myopia

Tahzib NG, Bootsma SJ, Eggink FAGJ, et al (Academic Hosp Maastricht, The Netherlands)
Am J Ophthalmol 142:31-39, 2006   2–1

Purpose.—To determine patient satisfaction after Artisan phakic intraocular lens (PIOL) implantation to correct myopia.

Design.—Non-comparative prospective case series.

Methods.—One hundred twenty eyes of 60 patients who had undergone Artisan PIOL implantation to correct myopia were analyzed. A validated questionnaire that consisted of 66 satisfaction items were self-administered by patients 12 months after surgery. Clinical parameters (PIOL decentration, the difference between pupil size and PIOL optical zone, and optical aberrations) were measured. Main outcome measures of satisfaction scale scores (global satisfaction, quality of uncorrected and corrected vision, night vision, glare, day and night driving) were analyzed. Correlations with clinical parameters were obtained.

Results.—After surgery, 98.3% of patients were satisfied, and 73.3% of patients considered their night vision to be the same or better; 44.1% of patients reported more bothersome glare. The night vision score correlated with spherical aberration ($r = -0.303$; $P = .020$). The glare score correlated with the difference between scotopic pupil size and PIOL optical zone ($r = -0.280$; $P = .030$) and vertical coma ($r = -0.337$; $P = .009$). The night driving score correlated with postoperative spheric equivalent ($r = 0.375$; $P = .009$), total root mean square aberrations ($r = -0.337$; $P = .017$), higher order root mean square aberrations ($r = -0.313$; $P = .027$), and vertical coma ($r = -0.297$; $P = .036$).

Conclusion.—Overall satisfaction after Artisan PIOL implantation for myopia is excellent. The quality of night vision and night driving were related to scotopic pupil size, individual higher order aberrations, and residual refractive error.

▶ What amazes me is not that 98.3% of patients (N = 60) were satisfied or very satisfied 12 months after Artisan (aka Verisyse phakic iris clip anterior chamber intraocular lens implantation). What amazes me is that almost all were satisfied, yet 26.7% considered their night vision worse or much worse than preoperatively, 32.8% and 44.1% considered daytime glare and glare from lights at night, respectively, more bothersome than preoperatively, and 39.2% had more trouble driving than preoperatively. I wish my patients who felt they had worse night vision, glare, or difficulty with night driving felt satisfied with their refractive surgery. These issues need to be addressed and improved before this lens will gain widespread acceptance, even prior to addressing long-term safety unknowns.

C. J. Rapuano, MD

Complications and Visual Outcome of LASIK Performed by Anterior Segment Fellows vs Experienced Faculty Supervisors

Al-Swailem SA, for the King Khaled Eye Specialist Hospital Excimer Laser Study Group (King Khaled Eye Specialist Hosp, Riyadh, Saudi Arabia)
Am J Ophthalmol 141:13-23, 2006   2–2

Purpose.—To determine the complication rates and visual outcome of laser-assisted in situ keratomileusis (LASIK) that is performed by anterior segment fellows and to compare their results with the results of their experienced faculty supervisors.

Design.—A single-center, retrospective, interventional, nonrandomized, comparative case series.

Methods.—Chart review of the initial 50 LASIK procedures that were performed by each of 10 anterior segment fellows and the first 50 inclusion criteria-matched, contemporaneously performed cases of four faculty members at the King Khaled Eye Specialist Hospital between March and December 2003.

Results.—There were no statistically significant differences between fellow and faculty cases with respect to complication rates and final visual outcomes. The fellows were significantly more likely to experience microkeratome-related flap complications during their first 25 cases, com-

TABLE 2.—Microkeratome-related and Postoperative Complications That Occurred in the Fellow and Faculty Supervisor LASIK Treatment Groups

Variable	Fellows (n)	Faculty Members (n)	P Value
Eyes	500	200	
Microkeratome-related flap complication			
Incomplete flap	10 (2.0%)	3 (1.5%)	
Complete flap	2 (0.4%)	0	
Button-hole flap	3 (0.6%)	1 (0.5%)	
Total	15 (3.0%)	4 (2.0%)	.61
Postoperative complication			
Striae requiring repositioning	4 (0.8%)	2 (1.0%)	
Epithelial defect >48 hours	4 (0.8%)	2 (1.0%)	
Diffuse lamellar keratitis >2+	3 (0.6%)	0	
Epithelial ingrowth	1 (0.2%)	0	
Interface debris requiring removal	2 (0.4%)	0	
Ectasia	2 (0.4%)	0	
Interface haze/scarring	1 (0.2%)	0	
Steroid induced increased intraocular pressure	0	2 (1.0%)	
Microbial keratitis	0	0	
Total	17 (3.4%)	6 (3.0%)	1.0
Loss of 2 lines of BSCVA	7 (1.4%)*	1 (0.5%)*	.45
Loss of 3 lines of BSCVA	3 (0.6%)†	0	.56
Total	10 (2.0%)	1 (0.5%)	.19

BSCVA = Best spectacle corrected visual acuity.

*All from 2020 to 2030.

†Two eyes from 2020 to 2040 because of bilateral ectasia; one eye from 2025 to 2050 because of persistent epitheliopathy.

(Reprinted by permission of the publisher from Al-Swailem, SA for the King Khaled Eye Specialist Hospital Excimer Laser Study Group: Complications and visual outcome of LASIK performed by anterior segment fellows vs experienced faculty supervisors. *Am J Ophthalmoli* 141:13-23, 2006. Copyright 2006 by Elsevier Science Inc.)

pared with their second 25 cases (4.8% vs 1.2%; $P = .03$) (Table 2). Fellows were significantly more likely to perform enhancements (8.0% vs 2.0%; $P = .0002$), after which the eyes in their group were more likely to be within 1 diopter of the intended refractive target than those in the faculty group (96.0% vs 91.0%; $P = .01$). Although not statistically significant, eyes in the fellow group were four-fold (2.0% vs 0.5%) more likely to lose two or more lines of best spectacle corrected visual acuity than those in the faculty group.

Conclusion.—To minimize the adverse impact of complications during the learning curve of novice LASIK surgeons, the introduction of this procedure in a well-structured, supervised setting (such as a subspecialty fellowship training program) is recommended.

▶ In the Cornea Service at Wills Eye Institute, most of our clinical fellows are interested in learning how to perform refractive surgery. Most did not do so as residents, and a surprising number have had little didactic teaching and are not certified for surface ablation or LASIK. For the past many years, we have had excimer laser and microkeratome certification courses for the third-year residents and the clinical fellows at Wills during the summer. Almost all interested residents and fellows get to do phototherapeutic keratectomy cases. However, the refractive cases have been much harder to come by. Before the popularity of LASIK, all fellows, and most interested residents, were able to do some photorefractive keratectomy (PRK) cases. My sense is that patients did not consider the actual surgical technique of PRK to be all that difficult and were okay having a trainee do it; this was before every consumer magazine article on refractive surgery, so it seemed, said to "make sure you go to an experienced surgeon who has done more than X cases," where X is some very high number. As a result, it has been harder and harder to get LASIK cases for the trainees to perform on. We have been moderately successful over the past several years getting patients who are affiliated with Jefferson, our parent institution, after offering them free complete refractive surgery evaluations and half-price surgery. We continue to work hard on this, and I agree with the authors that a fellowship program is the ideal place to learn how to best do refractive surgery.

C. J. Rapuano, MD

Outcome of LASIK for Myopia in Women on Hormone Replacement Therapy
O'Doherty MA, O'Doherty JV, O'Keefe M (Mater Private Hosp, Dublin; Natl Univ of Ireland, Dublin)
J Refract Surg 22:350-353, 2006   2–3

Purpose.—To investigate the effect of hormone treatment on refractive and visual outcome after LASIK in women.

Methods.—A retrospective review of the hospital notes of all women on hormone replacement therapy (HRT) and oral contraceptives at the time of

LASIK was performed. Their refractive and visual outcomes were compared with those of women not on hormone treatment.

Results.—At 6 months after LASIK, 20 (45%) HRT eyes and 61 (75%) control eyes had a visual acuity of ≥20/20. Thirty-six (82%) eyes from the HRT group and 74 (91%) eyes from the control group could see ≥20/40. A statistically significant difference was noted in both refractive and visual outcome in women taking HRT at the time of surgery in comparison to controls. Women on the oral contraceptive pill did not differ in outcome from controls.

Conclusions.—Women on HRT are at an increased risk of refractive regression after LASIK.

▶ This study is far from perfect—it is retrospective and controls were not age matched. However, it is good enough to give us pause when performing LASIK on patients using hormone replacement therapy (HRT). For unknown reasons (possibly greater dry eye, possibly different healing responses, etc), after statistically correcting for age, the authors still found greater refractive regression and worse uncorrected visual acuity in patients using HRT than controls at 2 and 6 months postoperatively. Refractive results of a younger cohort of women using oral contraceptives were not different from controls. Surgeons need to be aware of these results to give patients appropriate expectations. If it is dry eye-related, would preoperative topical cyclosporine help? (See comment, Abstract 2–20.)

C. J. Rapuano, MD

Predicting Patients' Night Vision Complaints With Wavefront Technology
Tuan K-MA, Chernyak D, Feldman ST (VISX Inc, Santa Clara, Calif; ClearView Eye and Laser Med Ctr, San Diego, Calif)
Am J Ophthalmol 141:1-6, 2006   2–4

Purpose.—To evaluate the accuracy of the diagnostic capabilities of optical metrics generated from wavefront measurements in relationship to post–laser-assisted in situ keratomileusis (LASIK) visual complaints as expressed and drawn by patients.

Design.—Retrospective analysis and observational case series.

Methods.—Patient wavefront data from an investigational device exemption study for wavefront-guided ablations were used to derive normative modulation transfer function (MTF), encircled energy (EE), and Strehl ratio. These optical metrics and their point-spread functions (PSF) were compared with data from five postoperative patients with night vision complaints. Patients were asked to draw their symptoms, which were elicited by testing with a Fenthoff muscle light, while using their best-corrected distance vision.

Results.—The MTF, EE, and Strehl ratio of most patients were markedly different from those of the averages of 208 normal myopic eyes before and after LASIK surgery. The spatial extent of the PSF correlated positively with

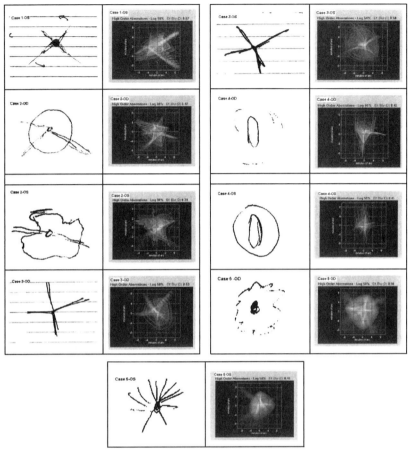

FIGURE 1.—Pictures of point spread function (PSF) drawn by patients looking at a muscle light are paired with PSF maps derived from wavefront measurements. The similarities between drawings and maps are immediately apparent. (Reprinted by permission of the publisher from Tuan K-MA, Chernyak D, Feldman ST: Predicting patients' night vision complaints with wavefront technology. *Am J Ophthalmol* 141:1-6, 2006. Copyright 2006 by Elsevier Science Inc.)

the severity of the visual complaints. Wavefront-derived PSFs were markedly similar to the patients' drawings (Fig 1).

Conclusions.—The results of this study demonstrate the diagnostic capability of the wavefront system in predicting visual symptoms and complaints of patients with high-order aberrations. Objective visual metrics from patients with night vision complaints were different from those of normal myopic eyes that had undergone LASIK procedures.

▶ When I read the title of this article, I thought it meant predicting preoperatively who would develop night vision complaints postoperatively. Not so. What the authors mean is that certain characteristics of postoperative wavefront maps correlate with patients' night vision complaints. I immediately thought "Big deal. So what?" As I read on, I realized that this finding is still quite important. If the objective wavefront data correlate well with subjective complaints (in contrast to Snellen visual acuity data), then effective treatments of the wavefront aberrations are potentially possible. While the vast majority of refractive surgery patients are very happy, a small minority are not. Not only can these patients ruin the doctor's day, but they truly have visual problems. This research is a good step in the direction of making at least some of these patients, and doctors, happy again.

C. J. Rapuano, MD

Wavefront-Guided Ablation: Evidence for Efficacy Compared to Traditional Ablation

Netto MV, Dupps W Jr, Wilson SE (Cleveland Clinic Found, Ohio; Univ of São Paulo, Brazil)
Am J Ophthalmol 141:360-368, 2006   2–5

Purpose.—To provide an evidence-based overview of wavefront-guided refractive surgery outcomes, benefits, and limitations.

Design.—Literature review.

Methods.—Review of FDA study reports and indexed, peer-reviewed literature.

Results.—More than 400 reports investigating wavefront applications in refractive surgery exist, but studies comparing the outcomes of wavefront-guided treatment with conventional treatment are few in number. Available studies do not overwhelmingly demonstrate superior visual results attributable to a wavefront-guided approach (Table).

Conclusions.—While wavefront-guided refractive surgery provides excellent results, evidence is limited that it outperforms conventional laser in situ keratomileusis that incorporates broad ablation zones, smoothing to the periphery, eye-trackers, and other technological refinements. However, it is evident that wavefront-customized ablation holds a promising future and merits ongoing investigation.

▶ The authors reviewed hundreds of peer-reviewed articles and FDA-study reports comparing results of wavefront-guided ablations versus standard ablations for LASIK and surface ablations. They were interested in finding the data to support the "conventional wisdom" that wavefront-guided excimer laser ablations are far superior to standard ablations. Interestingly, they did not find conclusive evidence to that effect. Most studies demonstrated very similar results in both groups with wavefront ablations generally having slight advantages here and there. There are several potential reasons for this finding: (1) There really is no difference in results of wavefront ablations when compared to the current (non–broad beam) conventional treatments. (2) The studies haven't been large enough or designed well enough to demonstrate real differences. (3) We aren't looking at the right outcome data (eg, we know Snellen visual acuity is a mediocre measurement of quality of vision).

TABLE.—Wavefront Platforms and FDA Approved Wavefront-Guided Results (Listed in Order of FDA Approval)

Company (Laser) Aberrometer (Principle)	Limit of Spherical Correction (FDA-Approved)	Limit of Astigmatic Correction (FDA-Approved)	Number of Eyes Included in the Trial and Mean Preop Refraction	UCVA of 20/20 and 20/40 or Better Respectively (% of Eyes at 6 Months)	SE MRx within ± 0.5 D and ± 1.0 D of Intended Correction (% of Eyes at 6 Months)	Lost ≥2 Lines of Vision (Number of Eyes)
Alcon (Ladar/Vision 4000) Ladarwave (Shack-Hartmann)	−7.00 D (−8.00 D*)	−0.50 D (−4.00 D*)	139 eyes −3.23 ± 1.31 D (SE)	79.9% (20/20) 98.6% (20/40)	74.8% 95.7%	0 eyes
VISX (VISX S4) Wavescan (Shack-Hartmann)	−6.00 D to (+3.00 D†)	−3.00 D to (+2.00 D†)	351 eyes (277 eligible) −3.32 ± 1.44 D (Sph. Myopia/n = 71 eyes) −0.68 ± 0.56 D (Myopic astigmatism/n = 206 eyes)	95.8% (20/20) 100% (20/40) 93.2% (20/20)	91.5% 98.6% 89.8%	0 eyes 1 eye at 3 months
B&L (Technolas 217z) Zywave (Shack-Hartmann)	−7.00 D	−3.00 D	340 eyes −3.17 ± 1.60 D (Sph. Myopia/n = 117 eyes) −0.71 ± 0.56 D (Myopic astigmatism/n = 223 eyes)	99.5% (20/40) 94% (20/20) 100% (20/40) 90.1% (20/20) 99.1% (20/40)	99.5% 84.6% 96.6% 71.3% 92.4%	1 eye at 3 and 6 months 3 eyes at 3 months and 1 eye at 6 months
Wavelight (Allegreto Wave) Wavelight analyzer (Tscherning)	−12.00 D‡	−6.00 D‡	Not FDA approved for wavefront-guided treatment	Not FDA approved for wavefront-guided treatment	Not FDA approved for wavefront-guided treatment	Not FDA approved for wavefront-guided treatment
NIDEK (NIDEK EC 5000CXII) OPD (Dynamic skiascopy)	Not FDA approved	Not FDA approved	Not FDA approved	Not FDA approved	Not FDA approved	Not FDA approved
Carl Zeiss - Meditec (MEL 80) WASCA/ (Shack-Hartmann)	Not FDA approved	Not FDA approved	Not FDA approved	Not FDA approved	Not FDA approved	Not FDA approved

UCVA = uncorrected visual acuity; SE = spherical equivalent; MRx = manifest refraction.
*FDA approved expanded range software (results described in the text).
†FDA recent approval (results described in the text).
‡Wavefront-guided treatment not FDA approved.
(Reprinted by permission of the publisher from Netro MV, Dupps W Jr, Wilson SE: Wavefront-guided ablation: Evidence for efficacy compared to traditional ablation. *Am J Ophthalmoli* 141:360-368, 2006. Copyright 2006 by Elsevier Science Inc.)

My own take on the matter is that I get the same sense from my results, which is that custom wavefront patients are doing a little better than conventional patients as a whole. I seem to have fewer complaints of diminished quality of vision. It may be wishful thinking. I certainly don't believe many of the laser companies' marketing efforts that claim custom treatments are head and shoulders better than conventional treatments (they have a strong financial interest in promoting wavefront treatments), and I make my patients aware of this. I do believe that we have not yet reached the full potential of wavefront treatments, and as that technology improves the superiority gap will slowly widen.

C. J. Rapuano, MD

Size of Corneal Topographic Effective Optical Zone: Comparison of Standard and Customized Myopic Laser In Situ Keratomileusis

Racine L, Wang L, Koch DD (Baylor College of Medicine, Houston)
Am J Ophthalmol 142:227–232, 2006   2–6

Purpose.—To investigate the corneal topographic effective optical zone (EOZ) in eyes after wavefront-guided myopic laser in situ keratomileusis (LASIK) and to compare them with the EOZ after standard LASIK.

Design.—Retrospective, case-control study.

Methods.—We evaluated the corneal topographic maps of 41 eyes of 25 consecutive patients who had CustomVue LASIK (CV LASIK) and 41 eyes of 23 patients who had standard LASIK with correction up to -7 diopters using the VISX Star S4 laser (VISX Inc, Santa Clara, California, USA). On the refractive map of the Humphrey Topography System, we defined the EOZ as the area outlined by a change of corneal power of 0.5 diopters from the power at the center of the pupil. We analyzed the differences in EOZs of the two ablation patterns and the correlation between EOZ and magnitude of refractive correction.

Results.—The mean postoperative EOZs were 17.9 ± 3.7 mm^2 and 11.4 ± 3.4 mm^2 after CV and standard LASIK, representing 60% and 40% of the laser-programmed optical zones, respectively (both $P < .0001$). There was no correlation between the postoperative EOZs and the magnitude of refractive correction for both ablations (all $P > .05$). In eyes with spherical correction (cylinder ≤ 0.25 diopters), CV LASIK increased the preoperative EOZ by 3.8 ± 5.6 mm^2 ($P = .018$), whereas standard LASIK decreased EOZ by 4.5 ± 5.2 mm^2 ($P = .005$).

Conclusion.—CV LASIK created larger corneal topographic EOZs than standard ablation. In eyes with spherical correction, the preoperative EOZ was expanded by CV LASIK and reduced by standard LASIK.

▶ The findings of a larger "effective optical zone" after custom wavefront LASIK versus conventional ablation with the VISX laser are consistent with the claims of better quality vision and fewer night vision symptoms with custom ablations. However, the effective optical zones were nowhere close to the laser-programmed optical zones, although custom treatments were larger (60%) than standard treatments (40%). Interestingly, they found no correlation between effective optical zone and amount of myopia treated. I believe this finding is due to the study being limited to patients with 6.5 D or less of myopia, as that was the limit of custom treatment when the study was performed. However, there is at least one downside to custom treatments—they typically require deeper ablations, theoretically increasing the risk of postoperative haze and ectasia.

C. J. Rapuano, MD

Wavefront-Guided versus Standard LASIK Enhancement for Residual Refractive Errors
Alió JL, Montés-Mico R (VISSUM Ophthalmologic Inst of Alicante, Spain; Univ Miguel Hernández, Elche, Spain)
Ophthalmology 113:191-197, 2006   2–7

Objective.—To assess efficacy, safety, predictability, stability, and changes in higher-order aberrations (HOAs) and contrast sensitivity (CS) after wavefront-guided and standard LASIK enhancement for the correction of residual refractive errors.

Design.—Prospective, randomized, comparative clinical study.

Participants.—Twenty eyes of 20 consecutive patients (spherical equivalent [SE], -2.01 ± 1.36 diopters [D]) treated with wavefront-guided Zyoptix Ablation Refinement software (ZAR) LASIK and 20 eyes of 20 consecutive patients (SE, -1.81 ± 1.21 D) treated with standard Planoscan LASIK, both for residual refractive error enhancement.

Main Outcome Measures.—Efficacy, safety, predictability, stability, HOAs, and CS were evaluated before and after enhancement at 6 months' follow-up.

Methods.—Uncorrected visual acuity (UCVA), best-corrected visual acuity (BCVA), manifest refraction, CS by means of the Functional Acuity Contrast Test, and HOAs by means of Zywave aberrometry were evaluated preoperatively and 6 months after retreatment.

Results.—At 6 months postoperatively, UCVA was 20/25 or better in 100% of the eyes. Efficacy indexes were 1.09 for ZAR patients and 0.95 for Planoscan patients. No eyes lost ≥ 1 line of BCVA; in the ZAR group, 2 eyes gained 1 line and 6 eyes gained ≥ 2 lines; in the Planoscan group, 3 eyes gained 1 line. The ZAR group showed a percentage of eyes (94.4%) within the 0.5-D range in SE higher than that shown by the Planoscan group (88.8%). After 6 months, the HOA root mean square (RMS) increased on average by a factor of 1.44 for the Planoscan group ($P = 0.003$). No change or reduction in HOA RMS was found in the ZAR group (factor of 0.96; $P>0.01$). Contrast sensitivity was reduced in the Planoscan group only at the highest spatial frequency (18 cycles per degree; $P<0.01$). There was a significant reduction of CS as a function of HOA increase for the Planoscan group

(P<0.0001). No changes were observed for the ZAR group at any spatial frequency (1.5–18 cycles per degree; P>0.01).

Conclusions.—Wavefront-guided LASIK using the ZAR algorithm is an effective and safe procedure for treatment of residual refractive errors. Wavefront-guided LASIK does not increase HOAs and does not modify CS compared with preoperative values. Wavefront-guided LASIK seems to be better than standard LASIK for retreatments.

▶ With only 20 eyes in each group it is difficult to really demonstrate anything but large differences, so it isn't surprising that there are few important statistically significant differences in this study. Having said that, total HOAs were unchanged in the wavefront group and increased by 44% in the standard ablation group. Spherical aberration increased by 61% in the wavefront group and by 125% in the standard ablation group. Coma-like aberrations were unchanged in the wavefront ablation group and increased by 51% in the standard ablation group.

Overall, the impression is that wavefront LASIK re-treatments seemed somewhat better than standard ablation LASIK re-treatments. Interestingly, the HOAs did not decrease from preoperatively in the wavefront group, however, they did not increase to the same degree as in the standard ablation group. These findings are similar to what has been reported in primary treatments. As technology improves, one hope is that HOAs will actually decrease with wavefront treatments.

C. J. Rapuano, MD

Surgical Monovision and Monovision Reversal in LASIK
Reilly CD, Lee WB, Alvarenga L, et al (Univ of California, Sacramento)
Cornea 25:136-138, 2006   2–8

Purpose.—This study was designed to assess the success of surgical monovision in presbyopic patients.

Methods.—A university refractive surgery center retrospective chart review of 82 patients who elected to undergo surgical monovision with laser in situ keratomileusis (LASIK) between January 2000 and January 2003 was conducted. Specific factors included for analysis included preoperative and postoperative defocus spherical equivalent, whether the patient underwent enhancements, whether the patient underwent a preoperative monovision trial with contact lens, and whether the patient underwent monovision reversal.

Results.—Eighty-two patients who underwent LASIK for monovision were analyzed. Mean preoperative spherical equivalent in the distance-corrected eye was −4.07 (standard deviation (SD), 2.49); for the eye corrected for near vision, mean preoperative spherical equivalent was −4.10 (SD, 2.56). Postoperative spherical equivalent in the distance eyes was −0.01 (SD, 0.38) and in the near eyes −1.24 (SD, 0.91). There were 6 enhancements in the near eyes (7%) and 17 enhancements in the distance vision eyes (21%). This difference was statistically significant ($P = 0.007$). Thirty patients underwent a contact lens trial of monovision before LASIK, and none of those patients elected monovision reversal. There were 52 patients who did not undergo a contact lens monovision trial before LASIK monovision, and 2 of these patients underwent monovision reversal. Monovision success in this population was 97.6%.

Conclusion.—Surgical monovision can help presbyopic patients achieve their goal of reduced dependence on spectacles. A trial of monovision contact lenses or spectacles may be important in helping surgeons select patients for successful surgical monovision.

▶ A few points should be emphasized regarding this study.

(1) While the authors' "success" with monovision was quite high (98%), that was only in the patients who decided to undergo monovision correction. Since they only had 82 monovision patients in 3 years, I presume the vast majority of their patients decided not to undergo monovision correction.

(2) While only 2 of 52 patients who did not undergo a contact lens trial of monovision preoperatively elected to have their monovision reversed, none of the 30 patients who had a contact lens trial did so. I agree with the authors that a contact lens trial is useful in most patients considering monovision, and certainly in all patients with doubts regarding it.

(3) The refractive results in the distance eye need to be "perfect." They had a 21% enhancement rate in distance eyes (compared with 7% for near eyes). Twenty-one percent is a very high enhancement rate given that the mean amount of myopic correction was approximately −4 D. Be prepared for more enhancements in monovision patients.

(4) The study looked at relatively short-term results, 6 months to a few years. Patients are very likely to need extra power in their reading eye as they age, making them less spectacle independent and potentially less happy over time. Hopefully by then new technology (perhaps multifocal lenses or multifocal ablations), will solve the presbyopia problem.

C. J. Rapuano, MD

Evidence for Delayed Presbyopia after Photorefractive Keratectomy for Myopia

Artola A, Patel S, Schimchak P, et al (Vissum, Inst of Ophthalmology, Spain; Univ Miguel Hernández, Alicante, Spain)
Ophthalmology 113:735-741, 2006   2–9

Purpose.—To evaluate uncorrected near visual acuity (NVA), accommodation, corneal aberrations, and the optical quality of the retinal image in presbyopic eyes after photorefractive keratectomy (PRK).

Design.—Nonrandomized comparative retrospective study.

Participants.—Ten post-PRK patients and 10 normal patients.

Methods.—Twenty eyes (10 right and 10 left after PRK for myopia, minimum of 10 years after the operation; group A) were compared with 20 eyes

(10 right and 10 left age- and gender-matched normal controls; group B). All subjects were over 40 years of age.

Main Outcome Measures.—With best distance correction, NVA was measured at 40 cm (Jaeger, J series), and the range of accommodation (diopters [D]) was measured subjectively (negative relative amplitude and positive relative amplitude). The modulation transfer function (MTF) and corneal aberrations such as comalike, spherical (SAs), and higher order (HOAs) were measured with a Hartmann-Shack aberrometer. From the MTF curves, the spatial frequencies corresponding to contrast values of 0.1 and 0.5 were noted.

Results.—Mean ages (± standard deviations [SDs]) were 46.3 years (4.7) for group A and 47.6 years (4.9) for group B ($P>0.05$). Near acuity was J1 or better in 12 of 20 post-PRK and 4 of 20 control eyes. Mean accommodations (± SDs) were 3.2 D (1.14) for right group A eyes and 2.1 D (0.94) for right group B eyes ($P = 0.0152$), and 3.4 D (0.99) for left A eyes and 2.3 D (1.02) for left B eyes ($P = 0.0168$). Total HOA indexes (± SDs) were 1.449 (0.409) for right group A eyes and 0.824 (0.241) for right group B eyes ($P = 0.008$), and 1.464 (0.388) for left A eyes and 1.067 (0.542) for left B eyes ($P = 0.0752$). Pooling the data from post-PRK and control eyes, a significant correlation was found between near acuity and SA (right eyes, $r = -0.535$, $P = 0.015$; left eyes, $r = -0.493$, $P = 0.027$). Significant associations were found between accommodation, near acuity, HOA, and comalike aberration for right eyes only. Mean spatial frequencies (± SDs) corresponding to contrast values of 0.1 for right and left eyes were 14.96 (5.71) for right group A eyes and 22.02 (6.85) for right group B eyes ($P = 0.074$), and 15.11 (7.80) for left

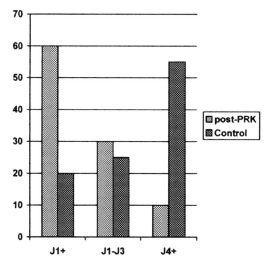

FIGURE 1.—Percentage frequency distribution of near acuities (Jaeger J series) in the 20 post–photorefractive keratectomy (post-PRK) eyes and 20 control eyes investigated. A highly favorable near acuity is noted by J1+. An acceptable near acuity lies between J1 and J3. Near acuity of J4 or greater is unfavorable. (Reprinted from Artola A, Patel S, Schimchak P, et al: Evidence for delayed presbyopia after photorefractive keratectomy for myopia. *Ophthalmology* 113:735-741, 2006. Copyright 2006, with permission from Elsevier Science.)

A eyes and 21.41 (9.00) for left B eyes ($P = 0.271$). Mean spatial frequencies (± SDs) corresponding to contrast values of 0.5 for right and left eyes were 2.86 (0.63) for right group A eyes and 3.21 (0.35) for right group B eyes ($P = 0.596$), and 2.76 (0.98) for left A eyes and 3.22 (0.27) for left B eyes ($P = 0.194$) (Fig 1).

Conclusions.—Compared with normal eyes, in previously myopic eyes treated with first-generation PRK lasers there is a tendency for (1) the optical quality of the retinal image to be reduced at low contrast, (2) the aberrations attributed to the corneal surface to increase, and (3) both measured subjective accommodation and near acuity to be greater than expected. We postulate that the corneal aberrations induced by PRK for myopia may reduce the quality of the retinal image for distance but enhance near acuity by way of a multifocal effect that can delay the onset of age-related near vision symptoms.

▶ Those of us who started performing PRK in the early and mid 1990s with broad beam VISX and Summit excimer lasers often had patients over 40 to 45 years old with unexpectedly good uncorrected near vision. That is, the distance correction was essentially "plano" and yet the patients saw well at near. I tell these patients they are fortunate, but eventually they will need reading glasses. I almost had a problem when a 50-year-old patient of mine who saw essentially 20/20 and J1+ without glasses after PRK referred a friend of similar age who also expected similar excellent distance and near results. She could not understand why I couldn't tell her she would likely get the same results as her friend.

This study confirms the fact that many patients who underwent PRK with the early broad-beam lasers had delayed presbyopia at a slight cost to the quality of their distance vision. The good news is that studies are ongoing to purposely create a multifocal ablation to achieve excellent uncorrected distance and near vision. The bad news is that there has been great effort, first with scanning laser technology and now with wavefront treatments, to reduce aberrations; consequently, I believe uncorrected distance visual acuity has improved, but uncorrected near visual acuity has worsened. We are still learning from the multifocal intraocular lens experience. I am not convinced that it is possible to achieve excellent quality distance and excellent quality near vision through one lens or one cornea. I hope in the future I can be convinced.

C. J. Rapuano, MD

Correction of Presbyopia by Technovision Central Multifocal LASIK (PresbyLASIK)

Alió JL, Chaubard JJ, Caliz A, et al (Miguel Hernández Univ, Alicante, Spain; Vissum-Instituto Oftalmologico de Alicante, Spain; Vision Future, Nice, France)
J Refract Surg 22:453-460, 2006   2–10

Purpose.—To investigate central multifocal presbyLASIK based on the creation of a central hyperpositive area.

Methods.—Twenty-five patients (50 eyes) underwent presbyLASIK in an open-label, prospective, non-comparative pilot study. Mean patient age was 58 years (range: 51 to 68 years), mean preoperative spherical equivalent refraction was +1.6 ± 0.63 diopters (D) (range: +0.50 to +3.00 D), and mean spectacle near addition was +2.27 ± 0.37 D (range: +1.75 to +3.00 D). The ablation pattern was performed with proprietary software from Technovision using an H. Eye Tech. excimer laser platform.

Results.—Mean postoperative spherical equivalent refraction was −0.37 ± 0.55 D (range: −1.50 to +1.00 D) and mean spectacle near addition was +1.72 ± 0.34 D (range: +1.25 to +2.25 D). After 6 months, 16 (64%) patients achieved a distance uncorrected visual acuity (UCVA) of ≥20/20 and 18 (72%) patients achieved a near UCVA of ≥20/40. Seven (28%) patients lost a maximum of 2 lines of best spectacle-corrected visual acuity (BSCVA) The safety index for distance was 0.98 binocular and for near was 0.99 binocular. After 6 months, no significant change was noted in contrast sensitivity at 1.5 cycles/degree. A significant mean reduction was found at spatial frequencies of 3, 6, 12, and 18 cycles/degree (*P*<.001). There was a significant change in corneal aberrations after surgery. The coefficients for coma increased and the coefficients for spherical aberrations decreased. A significant decrease was noted in point spread function values (*P*=.0018).

Conclusions.—Central presbyLASIK may be used to provide improvement in functional near vision in patients with presbyopia associated with low and moderate hyperopia. However, factors involved in the loss of BSCVA in some cases and loss in vision quality should be further clarified prior to its general use.

▶ It was shown years ago that post–radial keratotomy (RK) patients often had reduced need for reading glasses. As discussed in the comment for Abstract 2–9, similar findings have been observed in post-PRK patients. This effect is thought to result from a multifocal cornea. In this paper the authors try to consistently create a multifocal cornea with the excimer laser. They created a +1.50 power zone in the central 3.0 mm of the cornea to give good uncorrected near and good uncorrected distance vision in a group of hyperopes. While reasonably successful, there was a moderate loss of best corrected vision and a moderate decrease in quality of vision in some patients. The authors noted a tradeoff between uncorrected distance and near vision—the better near vision, the worse the distance vision, and vice versa. Interestingly, they measured preoperative pupil size in light and dark conditions, but they did not correlate visual acuity results with pupil size—future studies need to track this. While I am still skeptical about the success of this technology, this study is a step in the right direction.

C. J. Rapuano, MD

Topography-Guided Surface Ablation for Forme Fruste Keratoconus
Koller T, Iseli HP, Donitzky C, et al (Institut für Refraktive und Ophthalmochirurgie, Zurich; Wavelight Laser Technologie AG, Erlangen, Germany; Aristotle Univ of Thessaloniki, Greece)
Ophthalmology 113:2198-2202, 2006   2–11

Purpose.—To evaluate the efficacy of customized surface ablation in cases of forme fruste keratoconus.

Design.—Prospective noncomparative case series.

Participants.—Eleven eyes of 8 contact lens-intolerant patients with forme fruste keratoconus treated at the Institute of Refractive and Ophthalmic Surgery and the University Eye Clinic Zurich.

Intervention.—Topography-guided customized surface ablation by means of a scanning spot excimer laser.

Main Outcome Measures.—Visual acuity, refraction, quality of vision (ghosting), corneal topography including the Zernike parameter Z3.

Results.—Statistically significant reduction of manifest refractive error, corneal irregularity, and ghosting. The spherical equivalent was reduced by -2.8 ± 0.62 diopters (D) ($P = 0.0007$), the cylinder by 1.34 ± 0.18 D ($P = 0.015$), Z3 was reduced by 41% ($P<0.001$), and all patients had less ghosting compared to their preoperative status. No eye lost ≥ 1 lines in best spectacle-corrected visual acuity; however, 7 of 11 eyes gained ≥ 1 line (Table 2).

TABLE 2.—Postoperative Data

Patient	Eye	$BSCVA_{pre}$	$BSCVA_{post}$	Refraction$_{post}$	Ghosting	Follow-up (mos)
1	Right	20/30	20/25	Plano	+	12
	Left	20/30	20/30	Plano	+	18
2	Right	20/30	20/20	+0.5 cyl −2.0/160	0	9
	Left	20/25	20/20	+1.0 cyl −2.5/150	+	10
3	Left	20/25	20/25	−1.25 sph	0	9
4	Right	20/60	20/40	+0.25 cyl −0.75/45	0	12
5	Left	20/80	20/30	+1.5 cyl −1.5/100	0	18
6	Right	20/16	20/12	+0.25 cyl −0.5/90	0	18
7	Right	20/30	20/25	+0.25 cyl −1.0/97	0	24
	Left	20/20	20/20	+0.25 cyl −0.75/116	0	25
8	Right	20/16	20/16	Plano	0	12

cyl = cylinder; $BSCVA_{pre/post}$ = best spectacle-corrected visual acuity preoperatively or postoperatively; sph = sphere.
(Reprinted from Koller T, Iseli HP, Donitzky C, et al: Topography-guided surface ablation for forme fruste keratoconus. *Ophthalmology* 113:2198-2202, 2006. Copyright 2006, with permission from Elsevier Science.)

Conclusion.—Topography-guided surface ablation is a promising option to rehabilitate vision in contact lens-intolerant patients with forme fruste keratoconus.

▶ While LASIK is now considered contraindicated in keratoconus and forme fruste keratoconus, surface ablations are still in a gray area for these conditions. While most surgeons probably wouldn't treat frank keratoconus with a surface ablation procedure, many will treat forme fruste keratoconus. Differentiating these two entities is not always easy. The authors of this study defined forme fruste keratoconus as (1) no change in manifest refraction over 3 to 5 years or longer, (2) no change in corneal topography over 2 years or more, and (3) age 40 years or older. Exclusion criteria for their study included keratometry readings ≥49 D, minimal central corneal thickness less than 500 μm, and a predicted residual stromal thickness less than 450 μm. Interestingly, 3 of their 8 patients were between 28 and 38 years of age.

Standard surface ablations have been shown to be safe and effective, at least in the short term, in eyes with forme fruste keratoconus. However, given that these corneas have irregular astigmatism, a customized type of ablation seems as if it would yield better clinical results than a standard ablation. Customized ablations can be topography-guided, wavefront aberrometry–guided, or a combination of both. These authors used a topography-guided ablation in this study. With between 9 and 25 months of follow-up, they found excellent visual results. No eyes lost any lines of best corrected vision, and 3 eyes gained 2 or more lines of best corrected vision. Myopia and astigmatism decreased significantly and "ghosting" was reduced in all eyes. These are encouraging results. Whether wavefront aberrometry–guided ablations would be better or worse than topography-guided ablations remains to be seen; however, since the vast majority of the optical imperfection in these eyes is related to the cornea, including topographic data in the ablation profile seems like a good idea. One other consideration is that custom ablations tend to remove more tissue than standard ablations. This may not be ideal in corneas with questionable mechanical stability.

C. J. Rapuano, MD

Customized transepithelial photorefractive keratectomy for iatrogenic ametropia after penetrating or deep lamellar keratoplasty
Pedrotti E, Sbabo A, Marchini G (Univ of Verona, Italy)
J Cataract Refract Surg 32:1288-1291, 2006   2–12

Purpose.—To evaluate the safety and efficacy of customized transepithelial photorefractive keratectomy (PRK) for the correction of iatrogenic ametropia after penetrating keratoplasty (PKP) or deep lamellar keratoplasty.

Setting.—Eye Clinic, Department of Neurological and Visual Sciences, University of Verona, Verona, Italy.

TABLE 1.—Summary of the Preoperative and Postoperative Patient Data

Case	Age (Y)/Sex	Indication for Graft	Graft to CTPK (Mo)	Before CTPK			After CTPK		
				UCVA	BSCVA	Refraction	UCVA	BSCVA	Refraction
1	30/M	Keratoconus	21	20/100	20/20	-6.00×180	20/20	20/20	Plano
2	59/M	Keratoconus	36	20/200	20/20	$-4.00 - 3.00 \times 107$	20/32	20/20	-2.50
3	31/M	Keratoconus	48	CF	20/20	-8.00×50	20/20	20/20	Plano
4	41/M	Keratoconus	102	20/200	20/20	-5.00×90	20/20	20/20	Plano
5	37/M	Perforating trauma	31	20/40	20/20	$+1.00 - 2.00 \times 100$	20/20	20/20	Plano
6	31/M	Keratoconus	21	20/200	20/20	$-4.25 - 6.00 \times 180$	20/63	20/20	-2.00×90
7	45/F	Keratoconus	17	20/200	20/25	$-2.50 - 6.00 \times 60$	20/25	20/20	-1.00
8	37/M	Keratoconus	18	20/32	20/25	$-0.75 - 2.75 \times 20$	20/25	20/20	-1.50×100
9	42/F	Keratoconus	19	20/63	20/20	$+1.00 + 4.00 \times 170$	20/20	20/20	Plano

BSCVA = best spectacle corrected visual acuity; CF = counting fingers (at 1 meter); CTPK = customized transepithelial photorefractive keratectomy; UCVA = uncorrected visual acuity.

(Reprinted by permission of the publisher from Pedrotti E, Shabo A, Marchini G: Customized transepithelial photorefractive keratectomy for iatrogenic ametropia after penetrating or deep lamellar keratoplasty. *J Cataract Refract Surg* 32:1288-1291, 2006. Copyright 2006 by Elsevier Science Inc.)

Methods.—This study comprised 9 patients who had irregular astigmatism from 2.0 to 8.0 diopters (D) after PKP or deep lamellar keratoplasty. The ametropia was corrected with customized transepithelial PRK and the Corneal Interactive Programmed Topographic Ablation (CIPTA) software program (LIGI). Complete ophthalmic examinations were performed before and after surgery.

Results.—The mean age of the patients was 39.2 years (range 31 to 59 years). All patients gained at least 2 Snellen lines of uncorrected visual acuity; 2 patients had an increase of at least 5 lines, and 3 patients had an increase of 8 lines. The mean refractive spherical equivalent changed from -2.98 D ± 3.11 (SD) (range -7.25 to $+3.00$ D) before PRK to -0.58 ± 0.84 D (range 0 to -2.50 D) at the last follow-up visit. One patient presented with grade 1 haze that did not improve with topical steroid therapy. No patient lost best spectacle-corrected visual acuity.

Conclusion.—Customized transepithelial PRK with the CIPTA software was a safe and effective treatment for irregular astigmatism after PKP or deep lamellar keratoplasty (Table 1).

▶ While most corneal transplantation patients get very good vision without correction or with glasses, there are certainly those who do not. These grafts often look absolutely beautiful and yet have high degrees of ametropia and/or irregular astigmatism. Rigid gas-permeable contact lenses can often correct the problem, but many patients are contact lens intolerant. When PRK was used in corneal transplants in the past, it was thought to cause significant corneal scarring. LASIK can be successful, but there is a greatly increased risk of flap complications and I always worry about the PK wound.

The authors report very good results with a custom surface ablation using Orbscan topographic data and the patients manifest refraction and a flying spot laser in a transepithelial fashion. No mitomycin-C was used. With 1 year of follow-up, uncorrected vision and manifest refraction improved dramatically with no loss of best-corrected vision. Seven of 9 eyes had 20/25 or better uncorrected vision; the last two eyes were 20/32 and 20/63, both correcting to 20/20. This system is not currently available in the United States. I hope to see equally encouraging results for custom ablation platforms that we have available to us currently.

C. J. Rapuano, MD

Risk Factors for Corneal Ectasia after LASIK
Tabbara KF, Kotb AA (Eye Ctr and Eye Found for Research in Ophthalmology, Riyadh, Saudi Arabia; Johns Hopkins Univ, Baltimore, Md)
Ophthalmology 113:1618-1622, 2006   2–13

Purpose.—To establish a grading system that helps identify high-risk individuals who may experience corneal ectasia after LASIK.

Design.—Retrospective, comparative, interventional case series.

TABLE 1.—Preoperative Grading System for the Detection of Patients Who Are at Risk of Corneal Ectasia after LASIK in the Correction of Myopia (Spherical Equivalent, −4.00 to −8.00 D)

	Grade 1	Grade 2	Grade 3
Keratometry (D)	>45	45-47	>47
Oblique cylinder (D)	<0.5	0.5-1.5	>1.5
Pachymetry (µm)	>520	500-520	<500
Posterior surface elevation (µm)	<30	30-40	>40
Difference between inferior and superior corneal diopteric power	<1.0	1.0-1.4	>1.4
Posterior BSF/anterior BSF	<1.20	1.20-1.27	>1.27

BSF = best sphere fit; D = diopters.
(Reprinted from Tabbara KF, Kotb AA: Risk factors for corneal ectasia after LASIK. *Ophthalmology* 113:1618-1622, 2006. Copyright 2006, with permission from Elsevier Science.)

Participants.—One hundred forty-eight consecutive patients (148 eyes) were included in this study. Thirty-seven patients who underwent LASIK at other refractive centers experienced corneal ectasia in 1 eye after LASIK. One hundred eleven eyes of 111 patients who underwent successful LASIK during the same period were age and gender matched and served as controls.

Intervention.—All patients underwent preoperative and postoperative topographic analysis of the cornea. The follow-up period in both groups of patients ranged from 2 to 5 years, with a mean follow-up of 3.6 years. All patients underwent LASIK for myopia (spherical equivalent, −4.00 to −8.00 diopters).

Main Outcome Measures.—Corneal keratometry, oblique cylinder, pachymetry, posterior surface elevation, difference between the inferior and superior corneal diopteric power, and posterior best sphere fit (BSF) over anterior BSF were given a grade of 1 to 3 each. An ectasia grading system was established, and the cumulative risk score was assessed.

Results.—Patients who had a grade of 7 or less showed no evidence of corneal ectasia, whereas 16 (59%) of 27 patients who had a grade of 8 to 12 had corneal ectasia. Twenty-one (100%) of 21 patients with a grade of more than 12 had corneal ectasia after LASIK ($P<0.0001$) (Table 1).

Conclusions.—A risk score may help in the prediction of patients who are at risk of experiencing corneal ectasia after LASIK. A prospective clinical study is needed to assess the validity of these risk factors.

► The authors identified 37 eyes with ectasia after LASIK and matched them with 111 eyes that did not develop ectasia to quantify risk factors for this condition. They set up three grades of risk—low, moderate, and high—for six parameters from Orbscan imaging, ranging from K (corneal diopteric power) readings to pachymetry to posterior corneal elevation. Not surprisingly, the more high-risk characteristics the eye had, the greater the chance they were in the ectasia group. All the data were generated from Orbscan II studies. Whether similar parameters will hold true for newer imaging systems, such as optical coherence tomography and Scheimpflug photography, remains to be seen. I agree with the authors that this type of grading system does not substitute for a comprehensive examination including other risk factors such as young patient age and family history of keratoconus.

C. J. Rapuano, MD

Corneal Ectasia After Laser In Situ Keratomileusis in Patients Without Apparent Preoperative Risk Factors
Klein SR, Epstein RJ, Randleman JB, et al (Rush Univ, Chicago; Emory Univ, Atlanta, Ga)
Cornea 25:388-403, 2006   2–14

Purpose.—To evaluate patients who developed ectasia with no apparent preoperative risk factors.

Methods.—Potential cases of patients who developed ectasia without apparent risk factors were identified by contacting participants in the Kera-Net (n = 580), ASCRS-Net (n = 450), and ISRS/AAO ISRS-Net (n = 525) internet bulletin boards from April to October 2003. Cases were included if ectasia developed after laser in situ keratomileusis in the absence of apparent preoperative risk factors. Reported cases were excluded for the following reasons: (1) calculated residual stromal bed less than 250 µm, (2) preoperative central pachymetry less than 500 µm, (3) any keratometry reading greater than 47.2 diopters (D), (4) a calculated inferior-superior value greater than 1.4, (5) more than 2 retreatments, (6) attempted initial correction greater than -12.00 D, (7) an Orbscan II "posterior float" (if obtained) greater than 50 µm, and (8) surgical/flap complications.

Results.—A total of 27 eyes of 25 patients were submitted for consideration. Eight eyes (8 patients) met our inclusion criteria. Mean age was 27.7 years (range, 18–41 years). Preoperative manifest refraction spherical equivalent was -4.61 D (range, -2.00 to -8.00 D); steepest keratometric reading was 43.86 D (range, 42.50–46.40 D); keratometric astigmatism was 0.93 D (range, 0.25–1.90 D); and preoperative central pachymetry was 537 µm (range, 505–560 µm). The mean calculated ablation depth was 82.8 µm (range, 21–125.4 µm), and mean calculated residual stromal bed was 299.5 µm (range, 254–373 µm). Mean time to recognition of ectasia onset was 14.2 months (range, 3–27 months) postoperatively. At the time of ectasia diagnosis, the mean manifest refraction spherical equivalent was -1.23 D (range, $+0.125$ to -3.00) with a mean of 2.72 D (range, 0.75–4.00 D) of astigmatism.

Conclusions.—Ectasia can occur after an otherwise uncomplicated laser in situ keratomileusis procedure, even in the absence of apparent preoperative risk factors.

▶ Scary stuff! The last thing we want to do is take someone who sees well with glasses or contacts and convert them to someone who needs a rigid gas permeable contact lens or a corneal transplant to see well. For LASIK, once the flap is made without complications, and the first week or two go by without infection, the vast majority of patients will do well and be happy. The long-term worry with LASIK is ectasia. We have greatly tightened our exclusion criteria over the years. Minimal residual bed thickness has gone from 225 to 250 μm, and for some surgeons from 275 to 300 μm. Treatments over −10.00 to −12.00 D are less and less common. Even mild irregular inferior steepening is now a huge red flag. I certainly believe these steps have reduced the number of cases of ectasia after LASIK in recent years.

For this reason, this study disturbs me. The authors collected 8 eyes of 8 patients with ectasia after LASIK with no apparent risk factors. Other than the fact that these 8 patients were younger than other series of LASIK patients, they weren't that different. The bottom line is that anyone can develop ectasia after LASIK. For that matter, anyone can develop ectasia after surface ablation, but also anyone can develop keratoconus without refractive surgery. The surgeon's job is to reduce the risk to an acceptable level for the surgeon and the patient. If the acceptable range is zero, then either the surgeon should not do refractive surgery or the patient should not have refractive surgery. I am hopeful that new technology, perhaps corneal interferometry or hysteresis measurements, will help identify patients at increased likelihood of developing ectasia after refractive surgery so we can further reduce the risk of this dreaded complication.

C. J. Rapuano, MD

Comparison of Single-Segment and Double-Segment Intacs for Keratoconus and Post-LASIK Ectasia
Sharma M, Boxer Wachler BS (Boxer Wachler Vision Inst, Beverly Hills, Calif; Univ of California, Irvine)
Am J Ophthalmol 141:891-895, 2006   2–15

Purpose.—To evaluate the efficacy of single-segment Intacs and compare with double-segment Intacs in subjects with post-LASIK ectasia and keratoconus.

Design.—Retrospective comparative analysis.

Methods.—SETTING: Boxer Wachler Vision Institute, Beverly Hills, California, USA. STUDY POPULATION: Thirty-seven eyes of 28 patients with keratoconus and post-LASIK ectasia classified into two groups: single-segment group (17 eyes, 11 patients) and double-segment group (20 eyes, 17 patients). Both groups were matched for age, visual acuity (uncorrected, UCVA; best spectacle-corrected, BSCVA), refractive error (sphere, cylinder, spherical equivalent), and keratometry (K) value (flat, steep, average) by *t* test for equality of means. INTERVENTION: Single- or double-segment Intacs procedure with axis of incision for insertion in the steep axis of manifest refraction. MAIN OUTCOME MEASURE: Improvement of acuity, refractive error, K values, and inferior-superior (I-S) ratio.

TABLE 3.—Comparison of LogMAR and Snellen Acuities in Single-Segment and Double-Segment Intacs Groups

| | Preoperative-Postoperative Change | | |
| | Single-Segment | Double-Segment | |
Variable	Group	Group	P Value*
UCVA			
logMAR mean ± SD	0.89 ± 0.75	0.24 ± 0.54	<.01
Snellen	9 lines	2.5 lines	
BSCVA			
logMAR mean ± SD	0.24 ± 0.17	0.07 ± 0.17	<.01
Snellen	2.5 lines	<1 line	

BSCVA = best spectacle-corrected visual acuity; UCVA = uncorrected visual acuity.
*Change in single-segment vs double-segment group.
(Reprinted by permission of the publisher from Sharma M, Boxer Wachler BS: Comparison of single-segment and double-segment Intacs for keratoconus and post-LASIK ectasia. *Am J Ophthalmol* 141:891-895, 2006. Copyright 2006 by Elsevier Science Inc.)

Results.—There was more improvement in UCVA in the single-segment group (nine lines) than the double-segment group (2.5 lines), $P < .01$; in BSCVA in the single-segment group (2.5 lines) than the double-segment group (<1 line), $P < .01$; in steep K values in the single-segment group (2.76 diopters ± 2.68) than the double-segment group (0.93 diopters ± 2.01), $P = .02$; and in I-S ratio in the single-segment group (9.51 ± 7.49) than the double-segment group (4.22 ± 4.82), $P = .01$; and greater cylinder decrease after Holladay vector analysis in the single-segment group (5.69 diopters ± 3.10) than the double-segment group (1.58 diopters ± 3.09), $P < .01$ (Table 3).

Conclusions.—Single-segment Intacs improved both UCVA and BSCVA by differential flattening of inferior meridian and steepening of superior meridian as reflected by change in I-S ratio.

▶ Intacs were first introduced in the 1990's and approved by the Food and Drug Administration (FDA) in 1999 to treat low degrees of myopia (−1.00 to −3.00 D). While the FDA study results for visual acuity and complication data were quite good, the real-life results were disappointing and it was a commercial failure. The technology was eventually bought by Addition Technology and they received FDA approval through an HDE (Humanitarian Device Exemption) for the treatment of a mild to moderate keratoconus in 2004.

Initially, the Intacs segments were used in the same manner as for myopia —namely, two at a time. When some patients noted no significant improvement with two Intacs, the superior segment was removed and often the visual acuity improved significantly. That led some surgeons to place only one Intacs segment inferiorly. This study retrospectively evaluated single-segment versus double-segment Intacs for classic inferior steepening due to keratoconus and post-LASIK ectasia and found better results for the single-segment group. The authors now use single-segment Intacs in corneas with classic inferior keratoconus, but still use paired Intacs segments for central cones.

C. J. Rapuano, MD

Long-term Follow-up of Intacs for Post-LASIK Corneal Ectasia

Kymionis GD, Tsiklis NS, Pallikaris AI, et al (Univ of Crete, Greece)
Ophthalmology 113:1909-1917, 2006   2–16

Objective.—To report long-term follow-up of Intacs microthin prescription inserts for the management of post-LASIK corneal ectasia.

Design.—Long-term (5 years), retrospective, nonrandomized study.

Participants.—Eight eyes of 5 patients with post-LASIK corneal ectasia (3 men and 2 women) ages 31 to 54 years (mean age±standard deviation [SD], 41.60±9.24 years) who had completed 5 years of follow-up (mean follow-up ± SD, 60.1±4.9 months; range, 57–68 months).

Intervention.—Two Intacs segments, inserted in the usual fashion, were used for low myopia correction (1 each nasally and temporally), with thickness based on the residual refraction of the patients.

Main Outcome Measures.—Manifest refraction, uncorrected and best spectacle-corrected visual acuity, patient satisfaction, topography, and confocal microscopy analysis.

Results.—No intraoperative or late postoperative complications occurred in this series of patients. At 5 years, the SE error was statistically significantly reduced (pre-Intacs mean±SD, $-5.47±2.66$ diopters [D]; range, -11.50 to -3.00 D) to $-2.56±3.44$ D (range, -9.50 to 1.5 D; $P = 0.01$). At the end of the first postoperative year, refractive stability was obtained and remained stable during the follow-up period with no significant changes between the interval meantime ($P>0.05$). Pre-Intacs uncorrected visual acuity was 20/100 or worse in all eyes (range, counting fingers–20/100), whereas at the last follow-up examination, 6 (75%) of 8 eyes had uncorrected visual acuity of 20/40 or better (range, counting fingers–20/25). Two eyes (25%) maintained the pre-Intacs best spectacle-corrected visual acuity, whereas the rest of the eyes (6 eyes; 75%) experienced a gain of 1 or 2 lines. At the end of the first postoperative year, uncorrected and best-spectacle corrected visual acuity and topographic stability were obtained and were shown to have remained stable during the follow-up period with no significant changes between the interval meantime. Lamellar channel deposits were observed in confocal microscopy at or adjacent to the intrastromal ring segment (Fig 3).

Conclusions.—Refractive stability was maintained for up to 5 years in the treatment of post-LASIK corneal ectasia after Intacs implantation. There was no evidence of progressive time-dependent corneal ectasia, late regression, or sight-threatening complications in this study.

▶ While Intacs for low myopia did not turn out to be a huge success, Intacs are finding a place in ophthalmology in the treatment of keratoconus (see Abstract 2–15) and post-LASIK ectasia. It is unclear whether the exact same mechanisms are at work in keratoconus and post-LASIK ectasia. Keratoconus may be primarily related to a genetic corneal abnormality, whereas post-LASIK ectasia may be primarily related to a mechanical weakening of normal corneal tissue due to the refractive surgery. Consequently, it is also unclear whether the long-

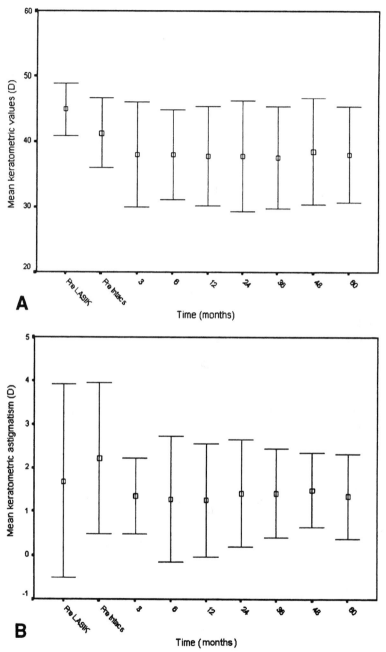

FIGURE 3.—Graphs showing the (**A**) mean keratometric values and (**B**) topographic astigmatism after Intacs implnatation during the 5-year follow-up. D = diopters. (Reprinted from Kymionis GD, Tsiklis NS, Pallikaris AI, et al: Long-term follow-up of intacs for post-LASIK corneal ectasia. *Opthalmology* 113:1909-1917, 2006. Copyright 2006, with permission from Elsevier Science.)

term results of Intacs for keratoconus should be comparable to Intacs for post-LASIK ectasia.

These authors obtained follow-up data from patients who underwent two segment Intacs placements using a mechanical separator 5 years prior. Their previously published 1-year results on 14 patients were quite good. At 5 years, they were only able to examine 5 of the original 14 patients. However, all 5 had stable results from the 1-year visit. Uncorrected vision, best-corrected vision, refraction, keratometry readings, and corneal topography were all essentially unchanged from 1 to 5 years (see Fig 3). It certainly is not intuitive that results of Intacs should be stable in these eyes. I could easily see how mechanical "weakening" of the cornea could progress over time, even with Intacs in place. I could also see how the Intacs channels could remodel over time, inducing less and less corneal curvature change. It is encouraging to see such stable results at 5 years in 5 patients. The next step is more follow-up time in more patients.

C. J. Rapuano, MD

Prospective Randomized Double-Masked Trial to Evaluate Perioperative Pain Profile in Different Stages of Simultaneous Bilateral LASIK
Cheng ACK, Young AL, Law RWK, et al (Chinese Univ of Hong Kong)
Cornea 25:919-922, 2006   2–17

Purpose.—To evaluate the perioperative pain profile in simultaneous bilateral LASIK.

Methods.—Fifty consecutive Chinese patients undergoing simultaneous bilateral LASIK were randomly allocated to have either the right or left eye operated first. The pain scores for each eye at speculum placement, microkeratome cut, laser ablation, and at 15, 30, and 45 minutes after the procedure were recorded. In addition, an overall score for the whole operation was evaluated immediately after the procedure for each eye. Comparisons between eyes and among different stages of the procedures were analyzed.

Results.—The second eye was significantly more painful than the first eye at the stage of speculum placement and microkeratome pass ($P < 0.001$). Laser ablation was the least painful stage for both eyes. There were no statistical differences in pain scores for the postoperative period.

Conclusion.—Higher pain scores were associated with the stages involving eyelid manipulation. In patients with small palpebral fissures where stretching of the eyelid structures are anticipated, supplementary anesthesia for the lid region should be considered when required

▶ None of these results are surprising to me, but it is interesting to see them scientifically verified. The most uncomfortable (actually painful) parts of LASIK are (1) placement of the eyelid speculum, and (2) passage of the microkeratome. The second eye is typically more uncomfortable than the first eye.

Immediately before surgery, I sit down with my patients and run through each step of the LASIK procedure. I describe the eyelid "holder" (not "speculum"—who wants a speculum in their eye?), and explain how that is the most uncomfortable part of the surgery. I explain that when I turn the suction ring on there will be a "pressure sensation, like someone pressing a thumb on their eye," while I make the flap. I stay away from the word "pain," but still want them to know what they will be going through and that I understand it is not a perfectly comfortable procedure. My impression is that this discussion helps the vast majority of patients get through the surgery without significant "painful" symptoms.

C. J. Rapuano, MD

Comparison of Corneal Sensitivity and Tear Function Following Epi-LASIK or Laser in Situ Keratomileusis for Myopia
Kalyvianaki MI, Katsanevaki VJ, Kavroulaki DS, et al (Univ of Crete, Greece; Univ Hosp of Heraklion, Crete, Greece; Univ Hosp of Alexandroupolis, Thrace, Greece; et al)
Am J Ophthalmol 142:669-671, 2006   2–18

Purpose.—To compare the effect of Epi-LASIK or Laser In Situ Keratomileusis (LASIK) on corneal sensitivity and tear function.

Design.—Prospective, non-randomized comparative clinical trial.

Methods.—Seventy-nine eyes (Group A) underwent Epi-LASIK and 61 eyes underwent LASIK (Group B) for the treatment of myopia. Matching parameters between the groups were age and attempted correction. Corneal sensitivity, tear break-up time (BUT), and Schirmer test II were evaluated before and at one, three, and six months after the procedure.

Results.—Corneal sensitivity and BUT were decreased at one month in Group A ($P < .001$) to be restored by the third month ($P = .71$ and $P = .58$, respectively). In Group B, corneal sensitivity and BUT were reduced postoperatively ($P < .001$). There was a significant difference in corneal sensitivity between the two groups at all postoperative intervals. Schirmer test II was not significantly decreased postoperatively in Group A. In Group B, it was decreased at one and three months and restored by the sixth month (Table 1).

Conclusion.—Epi-LASIK-treated eyes had faster rehabilitation of corneal sensitivity and tear function than LASIK-treated eyes. Several studies have evaluated corneal sensitivity, tear break up time and Schirmer's scores after a variety of different refractive surgery procedures. This study compared LASIK versus Epi-LASIK, where an epithelial flap is created with an epitome. Epi-LASIK is gaining popularity as a surface ablation procedure because of the potential advantages of less discomfort and faster healing time compared to photorefractive keratectomy and laser subepithelial keratectomy (LASEK)

▶ The authors found corneal sensation was decreased at 1 month, but recovered by 3 months in the Epi-LASIK group; the corneal sensation was decreased for at least 6 months in the LASIK group (see Table 1). Schirmer's results were not affected by Epi-LASIK, but were significantly decreased at 1 and 3 months and recovered at 6 months in the LASIK group.

TABLE 1.—Mean Corneal Sensitivity of Epi-LASIK (A) and LASIK (B) Groups During Follow-up

	Preop	1 Month	3 Months	6 Months
Group A	5.70 (range 5 to 6)	5.16 (range 3 to 6) ($P < .001$)	5.69 (range 4 to 6) ($P = .71$)	5.77 (range 5 to 6) ($P = .01$)
Group B	5.74 (range 5 to 6)	4.75 (range 1.5 to 6) ($P < .001$)	5.34 (range 4 to 6) ($P < .001$)	5.49 (range 3.5 to 6) ($P = .008$)
P	.68	.002	<.001	0.032

P values in parentheses represent statistical significance of corneal sensitivity changes at each postoperative interval as compared with preoperative values (Wilcoxon signed ranked test). *P*: power of statistical differences between the two groups at each postoperative interval (Mann-Whitney test).

Preop = preoperative; Group A = Epi-LASIK-treated eyes; Group B = LASIK-treated eyes.

(Reprinted by permission of the publisher from Kalyvianaki MI, Katsanevaki VJ, Kavroulaki DS, et al: Comparison of corneal sensitivity and tear function following Epi-LASIK or laser in situ keratomileusis for myopia. *Am J Ophthalmol* 142:669-671, 2006. Copyright 2006 by Elsevier Science Inc.)

In this study, the epithelial layer was replaced at the end of the Epi-LASIK procedure. Many surgeons now feel their results are better if they discard the epithelial flap. It would be interesting to repeat this study comparing retaining versus discarding the epithelial flap. Overall, these results reinforce the current belief that dry eye symptoms may well be worse after LASIK than Epi-LASIK.

C. J. Rapuano, MD

The Incidence and Risk Factors for Developing Dry Eye After Myopic LASIK

De Paiva CS, Chen Z, Koch DD, et al (Baylor College of Medicine, Houston)
Am J Ophthalmol 141:438-445, 2006   2–19

Purpose.—To determine the incidence of dry eye and its risk factors after myopic laser-assisted in situ keratomileusis (LASIK).

Design.—Single-center, prospective randomized clinical trial of 35 adult patients, aged 24 to 54 years, with myopia undergoing LASIK.

Methods.—SETTING AND STUDY POPULATION: Participants were randomized to undergo LASIK with a superior or a nasal hinge flap. They were evaluated at 1 week and 1, 3, and 6 months after surgery. INTERVENTION: Bilateral LASIK with either a superior-hinge Hansatome microkeratome (n = 17) or a nasal-hinge Amadeus microkeratome (n = 18). MAIN OUTCOME MEASURES: The criterion for dry eye was a total corneal fluorescein

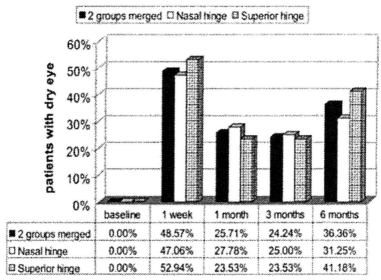

	baseline	1 week	1 month	3 months	6 months
■ 2 groups merged	0.00%	48.57%	25.71%	24.24%	36.36%
▢ Nasal hinge	0.00%	47.06%	27.78%	25.00%	31.25%
▨ Superior hinge	0.00%	52.94%	23.53%	23.53%	41.18%

FIGURE 2.—Comparison of dry eye incidence in patients allocated to receive either nasal-hinge or superior-hinge LASIK surgery, according to time. (Reprinted by permission of the publisher from De Paiva CS, Chen Z, Koch DD, et al: The incidence and risk factors for developing dry eye after myopic LASIK. *Am J Ophthalmol* 141:438-445, 2006. Copyright 2006 by Elsevier Science Inc.)

staining score ≥3. Visual acuity, ocular surface parameters, and corneal sensitivity were also analyzed. Cox proportional-hazard regression was used to assess rate ratios (RRs) with 95% confidence intervals.

Results.—The incidence of dry eye in the nasal- and superior-hinge group was eight (47.06%) of 17 and nine (52.94%) of 17 at 1 week, seven (38.89%) of 18 and seven (41.18%) of 17 at 1 month, four (25%) of 16 and three (17.65%) of 17 at 3 months, and two (12.50%) of 16 and six (35.29%) of 17 at 6 months, respectively (Fig 2). Dry eye was associated with level of preoperative myopia (RR 0.88/each diopter, *P* = .04), laser-calculated ablation depth (RR 1.01/µm, *P* = 0.01), and combined ablation depth and flap thickness (RR 1.01/µm, *P* = 0.01).

Conclusions.—Dry eye occurs commonly after LASIK surgery in patients with no history of dry eye. The risk of developing dry eye is correlated with the degree of preoperative myopia and the depth of laser treatment.

▶ In this study, patients with no evidence of dry eye syndrome were randomized to receive either superior-hinge or nasal-hinge LASIK. The degree of preoperative myopia was not controlled for. In a large enough study, the amount of preoperative myopia would be expected to equalize between the two groups. Unfortunately, in this study the mean spherical equivalent was statistically higher (−4.90 D) for the superior-hinge group than for the nasal-hinge group (−3.03 D, *P* = 0.01).

Consequently, the ablation depth in the superior-hinge group was statistically significantly greater than in the nasal hinge group (75 µm vs 53 µm; *P* = 0.03). It is difficult for me to understand how to completely separate the results of nasal hinge vs. superior hinge when the ablation depths are so different in the 2 groups. For example, uncorrected visual acuity was statistically significantly better in the nasal-hinge group than in the superior hinge group at 1 week and 3 months postoperatively. Was this really due to the hinge location? I think it is much more likely to be related to the greater degree of myopia treated in the superior-hinge group.

I thought the most interesting finding was that about 50% of eyes in both groups had significant superficial punctate keratopathy (their definition of dry eye syndrome) at 1 week, about 25% at 1 and 3 months, and 35% at 6 months. Thirty-five percent is certainly much higher than I expected at 6 months. The chance of dry eye was directly related to the amount of myopia treated, with a 1% greater risk for every 1 µm increase in ablation depth. Interestingly, there were no differences between men and women.

I tell all my patients, whether they have preoperative dry eye syndrome or not, that they can develop dry eyes after LASIK. The dry eyes may last for months or, occasionally, forever. I also tell patients that surface ablations tend to induce fewer dry eye symptoms than LASIK and let them add that to their decision process.

C. J. Rapuano, MD

Safety and efficacy of cyclosporine 0.05% drops versus unpreserved artificial tears in dry-eye patients having laser in situ keratomileusis

Salib GM, McDonald MB, Smolek M (Los Angeles; Tulane Univ, New Orleans, La; Louisiana State Univ, New Orleans)

J Cataract Refract Surg 32:772-778, 2006   2–20

Purpose.—To evaluate dry-eye signs, symptoms, and refractive outcomes in patients with dry-eye disease having laser in situ keratomileusis (LASIK).

Methods.—In this randomized parallel double-masked prospective clinical trial, 42 eyes of 21 myopic patients (mean spherical equivalent −4.3 diopters [D], range − 1.00 to − 10.63 D) with dry-eye disease were treated with unpreserved artificial tears or cyclosporine 0.05% ophthalmic emulsion twice a day beginning 1 month before LASIK. Treatment with the study drug was discontinued for 48 hours post surgery and then resumed for 3 additional months. Both groups used additional artificial tears as needed. Study visits occurred pretreatment (baseline), before surgery, and at 1 week and 1, 3, 6, and 12 months after surgery.

Results.—Statistically significant increases from baseline were found in Schirmer scores for artificial tears at 1 month (P = .036) and for cyclosporine 0.05% before surgery and 1 week, 1 month, and 6 months after surgery ($P<.018$). There were no significant differences from baseline or between groups in responses to the Ocular Surface Disease Index questionnaire or best corrected visual acuity (BCVA), nor were there significant between-group differences in superficial punctate keratitis or uncorrected visual acuity. Mean refractive spherical equivalent in cyclosporine-treated eyes was significantly closer to the intended target at 3 and 6 months after surgery than in artificial-tears–treated eyes (P = .007). A greater percentage of cyclosporine eyes was within ±0.5 D of the refractive target 3 months after surgery than artificial tears eyes (P = .015).

Conclusion.—Successful outcomes after LASIK were achieved for dry-eye disease patients. Treatment with cyclosporine 0.05% provided greater refractive predictability 3 and 6 months after surgery than unpreserved artificial tears.

▶ This is an often-quoted study at refractive surgery and dry eye meetings. The findings are interesting. No significant difference was found between the artificial tear and the cyclosporine group in uncorrected visual acuity, best corrected visual acuity, superficial punctate keratopathy, and dry eye symptoms between groups; however, there were better refractive results at 3 and 6 months in the cyclosporine group. The artificial tear group started with somewhat more myopia than the cyclosporine group (spherical equivalent −4.66 vs −3.94). Was this a factor in the better refractive results? We'll never know.

There are several schools of thought regarding dry eyes and LASIK. One is to avoid LASIK altogether and do a surface ablation, which induces fewer dry eye symptoms. Another option is to do LASIK. If dry eye symptoms develop, then treat the patient postoperatively. A third option is to treat patients who have dry eyes with cyclosporine 0.05% for 2 to 12 weeks before LASIK and 4 months after LASIK. And lastly, some surgeons treat all patients before LASIK with cyclosporine 0.05%. Personally, I try to avoid LASIK in patients with significant dry eye syndrome and consider surface ablation or, occasionally, no refractive surgery at all. In mild to moderate dry eye patients, I often start cyclosporine 0.05% drops 4 to 6 weeks preoperatively and reevaluate the patient to make sure the dry signs and symptoms have improved prior to proceeding with surgery. I tell all my patients (surface ablation and LASIK, preoperative dry eye or not) that they are likely to develop dry eye symptoms after surgery, which typically last for weeks, sometimes for months, and occasionally forever.

C. J. Rapuano, MD

Inadvertent stromal dissection during mechanical separation of the corneal epithelium using an epikeratome
Kim J-H, Oh C-H, Song J-S, et al (Korea Univ, Seoul; KEPCO Med Found, Seoul, Korea)
J Cataract Refract Surg 32:1759-1763, 2006   2–21

Epithelial flap complications occurred in 2 patients during epithelial separation using a Centurion SES epikeratome (Norwood Eye Care) in epi-laser in situ keratomileusis (LASIK). The complications consisted of stromal dissection at the margin of the pupil and an epithelial free cap including the superficial stroma. The epithelial flaps were repositioned without laser ablation. Three months postoperatively, the best corrected visual acuity in both patients was 20/20 and neither complained of visual discomfort. Slitlamp biomicroscopic examination showed that both corneas were completely healed with trace opacity, and topographic examinations revealed that irregularities in the stromal cutting sites were decreased. The patients had successful photorefractive keratectomy after complete healing of the dissected stroma. Stromal dissection during mechanical separation of the epithelium with an epikeratome is a potential complication of the epi-LASIK procedure, but proper management can result in good recovery without severe visual impairment.

▶ This group of surgeons in Korea had 2 partial stromal dissections with the Centurion SES epikeratome during their first 91 epi-LASIK cases. They were managed appropriately with replacement of the stromal portion and epithelial flap and no excimer laser treatment. Both patients underwent mechanical scraping photorefractive keratectomy 8 months later with excellent results. Not the end of the world, but it just goes to show you, nothing is as safe as it is promoted to be.

C. J. Rapuano, MD

Infectious Keratitis after Photorefractive Keratectomy in the United States Army and Navy

Wroblewski KJ, Pasternak JF, Bower KS, et al (Kimbrough Army Health Clinic, Fort Meade, Md; Natl Naval Med Ctr, Bethesda, Md; Walter Reed Army Med Ctr, Washington, DC; et al)
Ophthalmology 113:520-525, 2006   2–22

Purpose.—To review the incidence, culture results, clinical course, management, and visual outcomes of infectious keratitis after photorefractive keratectomy (PRK) at 6 Army and Navy refractive surgery centers.

Design.—Retrospective study.

Participants.—Twelve thousand six hundred sixty-eight Navy and Army sailors and service members.

Methods.—Army and Navy refractive surgery data banks were searched for cases of infectious keratitis. A retrospective chart review and query of the surgeons involved in the care of those patients thus identified provided data regarding preoperative preparation, perioperative medications, treatment, culture results, clinical course, and final visual acuity.

Results.—Between January 1995 and May 2004, we performed a total of 25 337 PRK procedures at the 6 institutions. Culture proven or clinically suspected infectious keratitis developed in 5 eyes of 5 patients (Table 1). All patients received topical antibiotics perioperatively. All cases presented 2 to 7 days postoperatively. Cultures from 4 cases grew *Staphylococcus*, including 2 methicillin-resistant *S. aureus* (MRSA). One case of presumed infectious keratitis was culture negative. There were no reported cases of mycobacterial or fungal keratitis. In addition, we identified 26 eyes with corneal infiltrates in the first postoperative week that were felt to be sterile, and which resolved upon removal of the bandage contact lens and increasing antibiotic coverage.

Conclusions.—Infectious keratitis is a rare but potentially vision-threatening complication after PRK. It is often caused by gram-positive organisms, including MRSA. Early diagnosis, appropriate laboratory testing, and aggressive antimicrobial therapy can result in good outcomes.

▶ Five cases of clinically proven or highly suspected cases of infectious keratitis after PRK in over 25,000 eyes—less than 1 in 5000—is quite low. That's great news. The flip side is that if there had been more cases, then perhaps the authors would have been able to elucidate predisposing factors for corneal infections. Are certain prophylactic antibiotics better than others? Is one nonsteroidal drop more associated with infection than another? Are postoperative topical anesthetics a risk factor for infection (2 of the 5 cases used postoperative topical anesthesia)? I guess we should just be happy that the infection rate is so low.

C. J. Rapuano, MD

TABLE 1.—Summary of Cases of Infectious Keratitis After Photorefractive Keratectomy at 6 Army and Navy Refractive Surgery Centers Between 1994 and May 2004

Patient	Day of Presentation	Antibiotic	Culture	Follow-up (mos)	Final UCVA	Final BSCVA	Postoperative Anesthetic*	Postoperative NSAIDs
1	6	Ofloxacin	MRSA	5	$20/30^{-1}$	20/30	No	Acular†
2	2	Polytrim‡	*Staphylococcus aureus*	3	20/25	NA	Tetracaine	Acular†
3	3	Levofloxacin	MRSA	7	20/16	20/16	Tetracaine	Acular†
4	7	Ofloxacin	Negative	12	20/20	20/15	No	Voltaren§
5	3	Ofloxacin	Coagulase (−) *Staphylococcus*	12	20/20	20/20	No	Voltaren§

Abbreviations: BSCVA = best spectacle-corrected visual acuity; *MRSA* = methicillin-resistant *Staphylococcus aureus*; *NA* = not available; *NSAID* = nonsteroidal anti-inflammatory drug; *UCVA* = uncorrected visual acuity.

*Nonpreserved tetracaine hydrochloride 0.5% (Alcon Laboratories, Ft. Worth, TX).
†Ketorolac tromethamine (Allergan, Irvine, CA).
‡Trimethoprim sulfatepolymyxin b sulfate combination (Allergan).
§Diclofenac sodium 0.1% ophthalmic solution (Novartis Ophthalmics, Duluth, GA).
(Reprinted from Wroblewski KJ, Pasternak JF, Bower KS, et al: Infectious keratitis after photorefractive keratectomy in the United States Army and Navy. *Ophthalmology* 113:520-525, 2006. Copyright 2006, with permission from Elsevier Science.)

Corneal Keratocyte Deficits After Photorefractive Keratectomy and Laser In Situ Keratomileusis

Erie JC, Patel SV, McLaren JW, et al (Mayo Clinic, Rochester, Minn)

Am J Ophthalmol 141:799-809, 2006   2–23

Purpose.—To measure changes in keratocyte density up to five years after photorefractive keratectomy (PRK) and laser in situ keratomileusis (LASIK).

Design.—Prospective, nonrandomized clinical trial.

Methods.—Eighteen eyes of 12 patients received PRK to correct a mean refractive error of -3.73 ± 1.30 diopters, and 17 eyes of 11 patients received LASIK to correct a mean refractive error of -6.56 ± 2.44 diopters. Corneas were examined by using confocal microscopy before and six months, one year, two years, three years, and five years after the procedures. Keratocyte densities were determined in five stromal layers in PRK patients and in six stromal layers in LASIK patients. Differences between preoperative and postoperative cell densities were compared by using paired t tests with Bonferroni correction for five comparisons.

Results.—After PRK, keratocyte density in the anterior stroma decreased by 40%, 42%, 45%, and 47% at six months, two years, three years, and five years, respectively ($P < .001$). At five years, keratocyte density decreased by 20% to 24% in the posterior stroma ($P < .05$). After LASIK, keratocyte density in the stromal flap decreased by 22% at six months ($P < .02$) and 37% at five years ($P < .001$). Keratocyte density in the anterior retroablation zone decreased by 18% ($P < .001$) at one year and 42% ($P < .001$) at five years. At five years, keratocyte density decreased by 19% to 22% ($P < .05$) in the posterior stroma.

Conclusions.—Keratocyte density decreases for at least five years in the anterior stroma after PRK and in the stromal flap and the retroablation zone after LASIK.

▶ Bill Bourne's group at the Mayo Clinic has done excellent work over many years looking longitudinally at corneal cells. They have some of the best data that exist on changes in endothelial cell density in normal corneas over time and in corneal transplants over decades.

This study extended their previous work looking at keratocyte density after PRK and LASIK out to 5 years. The authors found much greater cell loss than expected after both PRK and LASIK as compared with normal corneas. "Normal," probably age-related, keratocyte loss is 0.45% per year. From 6 months to 5 years, they found keratocyte cell loss of 3.2% per year for PRK and 4.2% per year for LASIK. While these numbers may seem ominous, we don't know what they mean. Even with this amount of cell loss, all their patients had clear corneas and excellent vision. Relatively small, but longer-term (>10 years) studies on PRK patients do not report significant long-term complications. Refractive surgeons who have performed many thousands of PRK and LASIK cases with much longer than 5-year follow-up have also not reported any long-term adverse effects to corneal clarity. As the authors note, these findings warrant continued monitoring, and hopefully they won't come back to haunt us.

C. J. Rapuano, MD

Presence of mitomycin-C in the anterior chamber after photorefractive keratectomy
Torres RM, Merayo-Lloves J, Daya SM, et al (Universidad de Valladolid, Spain; Queen Victoria Hosp, East Grinstead W, England)
J Cataract Refract Surg 32:67-71, 2006   2–24

Purpose.—To assess the presence of mitomycin-C (MMC) in hen aqueous humor after photorefractive keratectomy (PRK).

Setting.—Instituto Universitario de Oftalmobiología Aplicada, Faculty of Medicine, University of Valladolid, and Department of Analytical Chemistry, Faculty of Sciences, University of Valladolid, Valladolid, Spain.

Methods.—Mitomycin-C 0.02% was applied topically for 2 minutes to a right hen's eye after PRK (Group A) and to the left eye with intact epithelium (Group B). At different time points (10, 30, 60, 360, and 720 minutes), aqueous humor was extracted and high-performance liquid chromatography was performed to detect and quantify MMC levels.

Results.—The mean maximum drug concentration of MMC measured in the aqueous humor was 187.250 µg/L ± 4.349 (SD) in Group A and 93.000 ± 4.899 µg/L in Group B, both detected 10 minutes after topical application (Fig 1). Statistically significant differences were found between Groups A

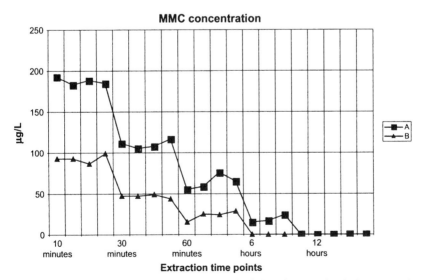

FIGURE 1.—Mitomycin-C concentrations detected by high-performance liquid chromatography (HPLC) in aqueous humor at different time points. (Reprinted by permission of the publisher from Torres RM, Merayo-Lloves J, Daya SM, et al: Presence of mitomycin-C in the anterior chamber after photorefractive keratectomy. *J Cataract Refract Surg* 32:67-71, 2006. Copyright 2006 by Elsevier Science.)

and B at 10, 30, and 60 minutes, with decreasing MMC levels in both groups but a higher concentration in Group A. After 360 minutes, MMC levels were undetectable in Group B and after 720 minutes in Group A.

Conclusions.—Mitomycin-C was detectable in the aqueous humor of the hen eye after topical application in PRK-treated eyes and in eyes with intact epithelium. The presence of MMC is of concern as it may lead to ocular toxicity in the long term.

▶ The history of the use of MMC in corneal surgery is very interesting. I believe it was first used to prevent recurrent pterygia several decades ago, initially as a postoperative drop given for a few weeks and later applied intraoperatively. It is used frequently in glaucoma surgery to prevent scarring. It is also used as a drop 4 times a day for various periods of time for conjunctival and corneal malignancies. In the refractive surgery arena, MMC was initially used to treat subepithelial fibrosis/corneal haze after refractive surgery, such as radial keratotomy and photorefractive keratectomy. Initial doses were in the 0.02% for 2 minutes range, although some surgeons now use lower doses and a shorter duration of application. It has similarly been used to prevent recurrences of Salzmann's nodular degeneration, corneal dystrophies, and corneal scars after phototherapeutic keratectomy. In all these conditions, existing corneal pathology is being treated, so surgeons and patients are generally willing to take some risk. Furthermore, the number of patients in these groups is rather small.

The bigger issue is the use of prophylactic MMC to prevent corneal haze after surface ablations. These eyes have no existing haze, and most are at low risk of developing haze, even without MMC. The problem is that when haze does develop, it can severely affect the visual outcome and is not easy to treat. MMC works well to significantly reduce the risk of haze after excimer laser surface ablations, although it does not eliminate the risk. Initial prophylactic MMC doses were in the same range as above. Most surgeons have since decreased the duration of application to 1 minute or less; some also use lower concentrations than 0.02%. In addition, many surgeons only apply MMC in eyes considered at higher risk for postoperative haze, such as high myopia treatments—for example, over −5 D or over 75-μm depth ablations. I currently use 0.02% MMC for 12 seconds in eyes being treated for over −5.0 to −6.0 D, with appropriate informed consent. Informed consent is a key issue. I explain to patients that MMC is effective in reducing the risk of haze and appears safe in the short- and medium-term (5-10 years), but we do not know the long-term risks (>10 years). My patients sign a special MMC informed consent documenting our discussion.

This article highlights just one of many potential issues related to MMC. The authors found MMC in the aqueous after photorefractive keratectomy on hen corneas using a 2-minute application of MMC 0.02%. They also found MMC (albeit less) in the aqueous after a 2-minute application of MMC 0.02% on hen corneas with intact epithelium. Continued research should give us a better understanding of the long-term effects of this potent medication.

C. J. Rapuano, MD

Intraoperative Mitomycin and Corneal Endothelium After Photorefractive Keratectomy

Morales AJ, Zadok D, Mora-Retana R, et al (Codet-Aris Vision Inst, Tijuana, Mexico; Tel Aviv Univ, Israel)
Am J Ophthalmol 142:400-404, 2006

2-25

Purpose.—To determine whether there is an increased risk to the corneal endothelium when mitomycin C (MMC) is administered after photorefractive keratectomy (PRK).

Design.—Prospective, randomized, double-blind, placebo-controlled crossover trial.

Methods.—Corneal endothelium was analyzed preoperatively and postoperatively in 18 eyes of nine patients who were administered either MMC- or balanced salt solution (BSS)–supplemented PRK at Codet Aris Vision, Tijuana, Mexico. After laser ablation, one eye was randomly assigned to intraoperative topical MMC 0.02% treatment for 30 seconds, and the fellow eye (the control eye) was treated in a standard fashion with topical BSS. Preoperative pachymetry and endothelial cell count were performed and compared with postoperative measurements after one month and three months. Main outcome measure studied was endothelial cell loss.

Results.—There was no significant difference in the preoperative endothelial cell count between the 2 groups: MMC group 2835 ± 395, control group 2779 ± 492, $P = .62$. In the control group, at one month and three months the difference in the endothelial cell count was not statistically significant ($P = .27, P = .14$, respectively). However, in the MMC group the endothelial cell loss was statistically significant: at one month $14.7 \pm 5.1\%$, and at three months $18.2 \pm 9.0\%$ ($P = .0006, P = .002$, respectively).

Conclusions.—The use of intraoperative topical MMC 0.02% for 30 seconds after PRK may affect the endothelial cell count.

▶ Double scary. While this study had only 9 patients, with one eye treated with MMC and the other eye treated with BSS, the authors found a statistically significant decrease in endothelial cell counts in the MMC-treated eye at 1 month (14.7%) and 3 months (18.2%) after PRK. It is also noteworthy that the authors used the standard MMC concentration (0.02% = 0.2 mg/mL) for 30 seconds. While many refractive surgeons started off several years ago using MMC for 1 to 2 minutes, most have decreased the application time to 12 seconds or less. Is 12 seconds any safer than 30 seconds? I hope so, but we won't know until a large (ideally larger than 9 patients) study addresses the question. In the meantime, appropriate informed consent is critical.

C. J. Rapuano, MD

Cellular effects of mitomycin-C on human corneas after photorefractive keratectomy

Rajan MS, O'Brart DPS, Patmore A, et al (St Thomas' Hosp, London)
J Cataract Refract Surg 32:1741-1747, 2006   2–26

Purpose.—To investigate the effects of mitomycin-C (MMC) on epithelial and keratocyte cell kinetics after photorefractive keratectomy (PRK) using an in vitro human cornea model.

Setting.—Department of Academic Ophthalmology, Rayne Institute, St. Thomas' Hospital, London, United Kingdom.

Methods.—Twenty-four human eye-bank corneas were placed in a specially designed acrylic corneal holder and cultured using the air-interface organ culture technique for up to 4 weeks. The corneas were divided into 3 groups. Group 1 consisted of 8 human corneas that had -9.00 diopter (D) myopic PRK without MMC application. Group 2 consisted of 8 corneas that had -9.00 D PRK with MMC (0.2 µg/mL) application for 1 minute on the stromal surface after ablation. Group 3 consisted of 8 corneas that had -9.00 D PRK with 2-minute exposure to MMC (0.2 µg/mL). Temporal events in epithelial and keratocyte cell kinetics were evaluated using digital imaging, confocal microscopy, and light microscopy.

Results.—Epithelial latency was significantly delayed with MMC application in Groups 2 and 3 ($P<.001$). Epithelial migration was delayed in Group 3 (2-minute exposure) compared to migration in Group 2 ($P<.04$), with a consequent delay in epithelial closure ($P<.001$). Group 3 corneas had poorly differentiated epithelium that was significantly thinner than in Groups 1 and 2 ($P<.0001$). A significant delay in keratocyte regeneration occurred after MMC application ($P<.0005$). At 4 weeks, the anterior stromal cell density was significantly lower in Group 3 than Group 2 ($P<.001$). There were no significant differences in the mid- and posterior stromal keratocyte density between the groups.

Conclusions.—Results suggest that epithelial healing after MMC is characterized by prolonged latency and decreased migration rate dependent on exposure time. Mitomycin C application did not result in increased loss of keratocytes, but it significantly delayed keratocyte repopulation in the anterior stroma. The use of MMC 0.2 µg/mL for 1 minute resulted in optimum modulation of healing characterized by reduced keratocyte activation with normal epithelial differentiation.

▶ This study used a novel technique of an in vitro corneal model using human eye bank corneas to evaluate the effects of MMC after excimer laser ablation for high myopia at 4 weeks. How applicable this model really is to real life remains to be seen. However, the rabbit model, one of the most commonly used for in vitro corneal studies, is far from perfect.

The authors found significant deleterious effects of a 2-minute exposure of MMC 0.02% (0.2 mg/ml), but not a 1-minute exposure, on the epithelium. I find this result interesting, as I used MMC for 2 minutes in many of my photo-therapeutic keratectomy cases — I now use it for 1 minute — and never thought there was a difference between the MMC-treated eyes and non–MMC-treated eyes in terms of reepithelialisation. It is worth mentioning that for certain refractive surface ablation patients I apply MMC for only 12 seconds.

The good news from this study is that at 4 weeks, the authors noted no difference in the endothelial cells and corneal thickness between the non-MMC and MMC groups. Whether this experimental model proves to be accurate is still up in the air. If so, I wonder whether studies can be extended longer than 4 weeks.

C. J. Rapuano, MD

Time to Resolution of Corneal Edema After Long-Term Contact Lens Wear

Nourouzi H, Rajavi J, Okhovatpour MA (Shahid Beheshti Univ of Med Sciences, Tehran, Iran)
Am J Ophthalmol 142:671-673, 2006   2–27

Purpose.—To evaluate corneal thickness changes after soft contact lens (SCL) removal in laser in situ keratomileusis (LASIK) candidates.

Design.—Observational case series.

Methods.—A total of 100 eyes daily wearing SCL for at least six months were evaluated. The central corneal thickness (CCT) was measured by pachymetry immediately after lens removal and then repeated daily until it became stable.

Results.—CCT immediately after lens removal was 557.4 ± 32 μm, and when edema completely resolved was 521.8 ± 25 μm. Corneal edema required two to 15 days after discontinuation of SCL wear to resolve. Corneal

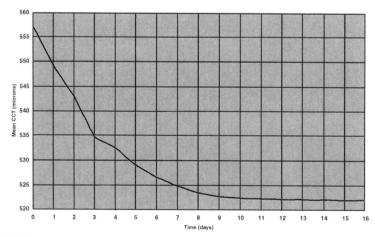

FIGURE 1.—Mean central corneal thickness (CCT) changes after soft contact lens (SCL) removal. Nine days after lens removal, reduction of mean CCT was less than 1 μm and after 15 days it was ceased. (Reprinted from permission of the publisher from Nourouzi H, Rajavi J, Okhovatpour MA: Time to resolution of corneal edema after long-term contact lens wear. *Am J Ophthalmol* 142:671-673, 2006. Copyright 2006 by Elsevier Science Inc.)

thickness stabilized in 74% of patients within the first week and in 26% of patients during the second week (Fig 1). Older patients and more primary corneal edema needed longer time to recover ($P < .0001$).

Conclusion.—Discontinuing SCL wear at least 15 days before kerato-refractive surgery is recommended to achieve accurate pachymetry.

▶ This focused study evaluated US pachymetry in patients who wore SCLs every day for at least the previous 6 months to determine the change in CCT once the contacts were removed. Seventy-four percent had induced corneal edema, which resolved by 7 days, 97% had resolution by 10 days, and 100% had resolution by 15 days. This confirms many excimer laser manufacturers' guidelines, and also my personal guidelines, which is to have patients out of their SCLs for at least 2 weeks before their refractive surgery evaluation and also before their surgery.

C. J. Rapuano, MD

3 Glaucoma

What to do with new measures of IOP

by Jonathan S. Myers, MD

The last five years have shown a surprising amount of research on tonometry. The findings of the Ocular Hypertension Treatment Study (OHTS) correlating the risk of the development of glaucoma to the thickness of the cornea reinvigorated interest in methods of intraocular pressure (IOP) measurement.[1] Additional reports showed possible increased risk of progressive disease with greater IOP variability.[2]

The Proview Home Tonometer was released to aid in patient measurement of IOP when not in the office, and showed disappointing results with high variability compared to Goldmann Applanation Tonometry.[3,4] Dynamic Contour Tonometry promised measurement less dependent on corneal thickness, and to some extent may be delivering, but is affected by corneal curvature.[5] Rebound Tonometry, an innovative approach, appears also to be affected by the properties of the cornea and shows a fair degree of variability in comparison to Goldmann measurements.[6]

What if we had a new method of measuring intraocular pressure that was completely devoid of influence from the cornea? This would certainly be a step forward in removing one more confounder from the complicating morass of glaucoma diagnosis and management, wouldn't it? Perhaps. First, the OHTS investigators found corneal thickness to be independently associated with the risk of glaucoma even after its affect on the IOP was accounted for, so corneal thickness would still be of interest.

Secondly, consider that every major study upon which we base our understanding of glaucoma and upon which we base our treatment of glaucoma (eg, OHTS, Early Manifest Glaucoma Trial (EMGT), Collaborative Initial Glaucoma Treatment Study (CIGTS), Advanced Glaucoma Intervention Study (AGIS), Collaborative Normal-Tension Glaucoma Study (CNTGS)) used Goldmann applanation tonometery. Any new method of tonometry, even if a more valid method that differs significantly from Goldmann tonometry, will then need to be studied and correlated to glaucoma diagnosis and therapeutic outcomes. The findings of those major studies will not be able to be applied directly to that new measure of IOP. For example, if different patients measure different pressures with the new technique, then old findings such as a 10% increase in risk for every 1 mm Hg increase in intraocular pressure with Goldmann tonometry seen in OHTS and EMGT, will not necessarily be true with the new measurement, as perhaps some of the higher/lower risk patients may measure higher/lower pressures with the new instrument.

A similar issue is involved in 24 hour IOP measurements and supine IOP. Recent studies have reported differences in 24 hour IOP variability with different medications and higher supine pressures.[7,8] Consider a case in which a clinician uses a goal pressure of 17 mm Hg for a patient with open-angle glaucoma with characteristics similar to those of subjects in AGIS based on that study's finding that the risk of progression was lower in subjects whose IOP was consistently less than 18 mm Hg. If the clinician then learns that the patient's overnight IOP hits 20, or is 20 in the supine position, should the clinician advance therapy? The AGIS investigators never measured IOP in either scenario, and so there is no applicable data to guide the clinician as to whether this finding is of clinical significance. Common sense would suggest that lower IOP is better, up to a point, but it is also possible that many of the patients in the stable AGIS group with pressures less than 18 mm Hg during office hours also had pressures of 20 mm Hg at night or in the supine position.

Simply stated, any new measure must be validated by studies correlating it to diagnosis and outcomes. New innovations are crucial to progress in the management of glaucoma, and must be welcomed and encouraged. However, when it comes to the current treatment of our patients, some patience is needed for research to deliver the information necessary to understand how new innovations are best applied to patient care, be they IOP measurement devices or new surgical techniques.

References

1. Gordon MO, Beiser JA, Brandt JD, et al: The Ocular Hypertension Treatment Study: Baseline factors that predict the onset of primary open-angle glaucoma. *Arch Ophthalmol* 120:714-720, 2002.
2. Asrani S, Zeimer R, Wilensky J, et al: Large diurnal fluctuations in intraocular pressure are an independent risk factor in patients with glaucoma. *J Glaucoma* 9:134-142, 2000.
3. Li J, Herndon LW, Asrani SG, et al: Clinical comparison of the Proview eye pressure monitor with the Goldmann applanation tonometer and the Tonopen. *Arch Ophthalmal* 122:1117-1121, 2004.
4. Alvarez TL, Gollance SA, Thomas GA, et al: The Proview phosphene tonometer fails to measure ocular pressure accurately in clinical practice. *Ophthalmology* 111:1077-1085, 2004.
5. Francis BA, Hsieh A, Lai M-Y, et al: Effects of corneal thickness, corneal curvature, and intraocular pressure level on goldmann applanation tonometry and dynamic contour tonometry. *Ophthalmology* 114:20-26, 2007.
6. Martinez-de-la-Casa JM, Garcia-Feijoo J, Castillo A, et al: Reproducibility and clinical evaluation of rebound tonometry. *Invest Ophthalmol Vis Sci* 46:4578-4580, 2005.
7. Mosaed S, Liu JH, Weinreb RN. Correlation between office and peak nocturnal intraocular pressures in healthy subjects and glaucoma patients. *Am J Ophthalmol* 139:320-324, 2005.

8. Liu JH, Kripke DF, Weinreb RN. Comparison of the nocturnal effects of once-daily timolol and latanoprost on intraocular pressure. *Am J Ophthalmol* 138:389-395, 2004.

A multicenter, retrospective pilot study of resource use and associated with severity of disease in glaucoma

Lee PP, Walt JG, Doyle JJ, et al (Duke Univ Med Ctr, Durham, NC)
Arch Ophthalmol 124:12-19, 2006
3–1

Objective.—To examine resource consumption and the direct costs of treating glaucoma at different disease severity levels.

Design.—Observational, retrospective cohort study based on medical record review.

Participants.—One hundred fifty-one records of patients with primary open-angle or normal-tension glaucoma, glaucoma suspect, or ocular hypertension (age ≥18 years) were randomly selected from 12 sites in the United States and stratified according to severity based on *International Classification of Diseases, Ninth Revision, Clinical Modification* codes. Patients had to have been followed up for a minimum of 5 years. Patients with concomitant ocular disease likely to affect glaucoma treatment-related resource consumption were excluded.

Methods.—Glaucoma severity was assessed and assigned using a 6-stage glaucoma staging system, modified from the Bascom Palmer (Hodapp-Anderson-Parrish) system. Clinical and resource use data were collected from the medical record review. Resource consumption for low-vision care and vision rehabilitation was estimated for patients with end-stage disease based on specialist surveys. For each stage of disease, publicly available economic data were then applied to assign resource valuation and estimate patient-level direct costs from the payer perspective.

Main Outcome Measures.—Average annual resource use and estimated total annual direct cost of treatment were calculated at the patient level and stratified by stage of disease. Direct costs by specific resource types, including ophthalmology visits, glaucoma surgeries, medications, visual field examinations, and other glaucoma services, were also assessed.

Results.—Direct ophthalmology-related resource use, including ophthalmology visits, glaucoma surgeries, and medication use, increased as disease severity worsened. Average direct cost of treatment ranged from $623 per patient per year for glaucoma suspects or patients with early-stage disease to $2511 per patient per year for patients with end-stage disease. Medication costs composed the largest proportion of total direct cost for all stages of disease (range, 24%-61%).

Conclusions.—The study results suggest that resource use and direct cost of glaucoma management increase with worsening disease severity. Based on these findings, a glaucoma treatment that delays the progression of disease could have the potential to significantly reduce the health economic burden of this chronic disease over many years.

Management of Ocular Hypertension: A Cost-effectiveness Approach From the Ocular Hypertension Treatment Study

Kymes SM, and Ocular Hypertension Treatment Study Group (OHTS) (Washington Univ, St Louis; et al)

Am J Ophthalmol 141:997-1008, 2006   3–2

Purpose.—The Ocular Hypertension Treatment Study (OHTS) demonstrated that medical treatment of people with intraocular pressure (IOP) of ≥24 mm Hg reduces the risk of the development of primary open-angle glaucoma (POAG) by 60%. There is no consensus on which people with ocular hypertension would benefit from treatment.

Design.—Cost-utility analysis with the use of a Markov model.

Methods.—We modeled a hypothetic cohort of people with IOP of ≥24 mm Hg. A hypothetical cohort of people with IOP of ≥24 mm Hg was modeled. Four treatment thresholds were considered: (1) Treat no one; (2) treat people with a ≥5% annual risk of the development of POAG; (3) treat people with a ≥2% annual risk of the development of POAG, and (4) treat everyone. The incremental cost-effectiveness ratio was evaluated.

Results.—The incremental cost-effectiveness ratios for treatment of people with ocular hypertension were $3670 per quality adjusted life-year (QALY) for the Treat ≥5% threshold and $42,430/QALY for the Treat ≥2% threshold. "Treat everyone" cost more and was less effective than other options. Assuming a cost-effectiveness threshold of $50,000 to $100,000/QALY, the Treat ≥2% threshold would result in the most net health benefit. The decision was sensitive to the incidence of POAG without treatment, treatment effectiveness, and the utility loss because of POAG.

Conclusion.—Although the treatment of individual patients is largely dependent on their attitude toward the risk of disease progression and blindness, the treatment of those patients with IOP of ≥24 mm Hg and a ≥2% annual risk of the development of glaucoma is likely to be cost-effective. Delay of treatment for all people with ocular hypertension until glaucoma-related symptoms are present appears to be unnecessarily conservative (Table 3).

▶ These 2 studies (Abstracts 3–1 and 3–2) create cost models for glaucoma treatment and the burdens of ocular hypertension, respectively. They use entirely different methods to derive cost considerations for these conditions.

The study by Lee et al (Abstract 3–1) looks retrospectively at care provided to patients with glaucoma, and also at the severity of the glaucoma. The study finds that the cost of treatment increases with the severity of disease, suggesting yet another reason why delaying disease progression will save money, in addition to reducing human suffering and the indirect costs of lost productivity, etc.

The study by Kymes et al (Abstract 3–2) takes a very different approach and is based on QALYs. Simply put, QALYs are the years of life that a person would be willing to sacrifice to avoid a condition. For example, a person who is blind and 55 years of age might be willing to die 10 years earlier in exchange for 10

TABLE 3.—Comparison of the Cost-effectiveness of Strategies for Treatment of Persons With Ocular Hypertension

Strategy	Total Cost ($)	Total Effectiveness (QALYs)*	Incremental Cost ($)	Incremental Effectiveness (QALYs)*	Incremental Cost-effectiveness Ratio (Cost ($)/QALYs)*
Treat no one	4006	13.5370			
Treat ≥5% annual risk of development of primary open-angle glaucoma	4086	13.5588	80	0.0218	3670
Treat ≥2% annual risk of development of primary open-angle glaucoma	5308	13.5876	1222	0.0288	42430
Treat all persons with ocular hypertension	11245	13.5870	5937	−0.0006	Dominated

*QALYs = Quality adjusted life-years.
(Reprinted by permission of the publisher from Kymes SM, and Ocular Hypertension Treatment Study Group [OHTS]: Management of ocular hypertension: A cost-effectiveness approach from the Ocular Hypertension Treatment Study. *Am J Ophthalmol* 141:997-1008, 2006. Copyright 2006 by Elsevier Science Inc.)

years of restored sight. This would be equivalent to 10 QALYs for the condition of blindness. Although this may seem very subjective to those not familiar with this incipient field, this measure has been shown in studies to be valid and reproducible across populations of patients.

The authors create a Markov model based on the likelihood of progression with and without treatment from the OHTS data, the costs of treatment, and the QALY data for each stage of glaucoma severity, including blindness. From this, the cost per QALY is derived for treatment of patients, depending on the threshold risk to treat (eg, the risk of glaucoma progression at which the decision to treat is made). For treatment at an annual threshold risk of 5% or greater and 2% or greater, the costs are $3670 and $42,430 per QALY, respectively. Compared with most conditions, these figures are acceptable costs for industrialized nations. Many other medical and surgical conditions have much higher costs per QALY.

Economics has been described as the study of how societies make decisions given limited resources and unlimited wants. As health care costs continue to escalate, treatment decisions will involve not just the patient and clinician, but the choices of society, as guidelines and frameworks for approved treatment are developed from studies like these. Clinicians need to be aware of this burgeoning field and should be actively involved in making sure that these studies ask the right questions for our patients.

J. S. Myers, MD

Patients' and Physicians' Perceptions of the Travoprost Dosing Aid: An Open-Label, Multicenter Study of Adherence with Prostaglandin Analogue Therapy for Open-Angle Glaucoma or Ocular Hypertension
Flowers B, for the Travatan™ Dosing Aid Study Group (Ophthalmology Associates, Fort Worth, Tex; et al)
Clin Ther 28:1803-1811, 2006   3–3

Objective.—This study describes patients' and physicians' perceptions of issues related to dosing adherence with topical therapies for lowering intraocular pressure before and after use of the travoprost dosing aid (Travatan™ Dosing Aid, Alcon Research Ltd., Fort Worth, Texas).

Methods.—The study had an open-label, multicenter, single-treatment-arm design that included sequential patients with open-angle glaucoma (with or without pigment dispersion or pseudoexfoliation component) or ocular hypertension who were taking any prostaglandin analogue monotherapy. Ten participating physicians were chosen on the basis of factors such as their experience, qualifications, and previous clinical study participation. The study consisted of 2 visits: screening and week 4. Patients were asked to complete a survey about their medication adherence before study entry at the screening visit and at study exit during the week-4 visit. In addition, each physician was asked to complete an entry and exit survey on each patient as well as a survey to provide feedback on the travoprost dosing aid.

Results.—Of the 87 enrolled patients, 6 did not complete the exit survey; therefore, 81 patients were included in the intent-to-treat analysis. Mean (SD) age at enrollment was 65.4 (11.6) years; 61.7% (50/81) of the patients were women and 60.5% (49/81) were white. Most patients (96.3% [78/81]) had open-angle glaucoma. Participating physicians perceived that problems involving dosing and adherence were reduced after patients used the dosing aid. Physicians indicated that they would recommend continued use of the travoprost dosing aid for 91.3% (73/80) of patients. All 10 participating physicians said that they would recommend the dosing aid to patients in the future. Of the 81 patients, the majority (68.8% [55/80]) indicated that they would like to continue using the travoprost dosing aid. For 67.5% (54/80) of patients, dosing adherence as recorded by the travoprost dosing aid was >70%. The dosing lever (39.7% [31/78]) and the visual alarm (29.5% [23/78]) were the 2 most favored features of the dosing aid reported by all evaluable patients. The majority of patients (58.8% [47/80]) indicated that they were "relieved" or "very relieved" that the doctor was able to monitor when they dosed their medication; few (7.5% [6/80]) were "concerned" or "very concerned" that the doctor was able to monitor their dosing.

Conclusions.—The travoprost dosing aid was perceived to be effective in reminding this group of patients to take their medication as prescribed. In this study, the device was well accepted by both patients and physicians.

▶ The travoprost dosing aid is a device which cradles a bottle of travoprost, while at the same time providing an alarm to remind patients to use the drop, and a small computer chip to monitor and record medication use. In this 1-month study, 81 patients receiving monotherapy with travoprost and 10 physicians were surveyed regarding the use of an adherence and monitoring aid. About two thirds of the patients were interested in continuing with the device. Only 8% of the patients were concerned that their doctor was monitoring their dosing. The physicians wished to continue with the device in more than 90% of the enrolled patients. Dosing adherence was measured by the device at greater than 70%.

L. J. Katz, MD

24-Hour Control With a Latanoprost-Timolol Fixed Combination vs Timolol Alone
Konstas AGP, Lake S, Economou AI, et al (AHEPA Hosp, Thessaloniki, Greece)
Arch Ophthalmol 124:1553-1557, 2006   3–4

Objective.—To evaluate 24-hour intraocular pressure (IOP) control with an evening-dosed latanoprost-timolol maleate fixed combination vs timolol alone in patients with primary open-angle glaucoma.

Methods.—After a medicine-free period, qualified patients were randomized to either placebo dosed in the morning with a latanoprost-timolol fixed combination dosed in the evening or timolol alone dosed twice daily for 8 weeks. Patients were then switched to the opposite treatment for 8 weeks. At baseline and at the end of each treatment period, patients underwent IOP measurements.

Results.—34 patients were enrolled. Both treatments reduced the IOP from untreated baseline at each time point and for the 24-hour curve ($P<.001$). When treatments were compared, the latanoprost-timolol fixed combination decreased the IOP more than timolol alone at each time point and for the 24-hour curve (2.9 mm Hg), and provided a lower absolute IOP at each time point ($P<.001$) and for the range (fluctuation) in IOP ($P = .003$) and for the 24-hour curve. Several adverse effects were observed more often with the latanoprost-timolol fixed combination, including ocular stinging ($P = .05$), conjunctival hyperemia ($P = .02$), and ocular itching ($P = .04$).

Conclusion.—The evening-dosed latanoprost-timolol fixed combination may provide better IOP control than timolol alone over 24 hours and may demonstrate a narrower range of IOP fluctuation in patients with primary open-angle glaucoma.

Twice-Daily 0.2% Brimonidine–0.5% Timolol Fixed-Combination Therapy vs Monotherapy With Timolol or Brimonidine in Patients With Glaucoma or Ocular Hypertension: A 12-Month Randomized Trial

Sherwood MB, Craven ER, Chou C, et al (Univ of Florida College of Medicine, Gainesville)

Arch Ophthalmol 124:1230-1238, 2006   3–5

Objective.—To evaluate the intraocular pressure (IOP)–lowering efficacy and safety of a fixed combination of 0.2% brimonidine tartrate and 0.5% timolol maleate (fixed brimonidine-timolol) compared with the component medications.

Methods.—In 2 identical, 12-month, randomized, double-masked multi-center trials, patients with ocular hypertension or glaucoma were treated with fixed brimonidine-timolol twice daily (n = 385), 0.2% brimonidine tartrate 3 times daily (n = 382), or 0.5% timolol maleate twice daily (n = 392).

Main Outcomes Measures.—Mean change from baseline IOP and incidence of adverse events.

Results.—The mean decrease from baseline IOP during 12-month follow-up was 4.4 to 7.6 mm Hg with fixed brimonidine-timolol, 2.7 to 5.5 mm Hg with brimonidine, and 3.9 to 6.2 mm Hg with timolol. Mean IOP reductions were significantly greater with fixed brimonidine-timolol compared with timolol at all measurements ($P\leq.002$) and brimonidine at 8 AM, 10 AM, and 3 PM ($P<.001$) but not at 5 PM. The incidence of treatment-related adverse events in the fixed-combination group was lower than that in the brimonidine group ($P = .006$) but higher than that in the timolol group ($P<.001$). The rate of discontinuation for adverse events was 14.3% with the fixed combination, 30.6% with brimonidine, and 5.1% with timolol.

Conclusions.—Twice-daily fixed brimonidine-timolol therapy provides sustained IOP lowering superior to monotherapy with either thrice-daily brimonidine or twice-daily timolol and is better tolerated than brimonidine but less well tolerated than timolol.

Application to Clinical Practice.—Fixed brimonidine-timolol is an effective and convenient IOP-lowering therapy.

▶ In recognition of the need for multiple drugs to achieve the desired target intraocular pressure range and the reduction in adherence with multiple bottle therapy, there is a great deal of interest in fixed-combination glaucoma medications. Konstas et al (Abstract 3–4) demonstrated consistently lower IOP with the fixed combination of latanoprost-timolol versus timolol, although there were more ocular side effects with the fixed combination (stinging, hyperemia, itching).

Sherwood and coauthors (Abstract 3–5) did a 1-year comparison of the fixed combination brimonidine-timolol versus brimonidine or timolol alone. The fixed combination was able to keep the IOP <18 in two thirds of the eyes compared with only one fourth with brimonidine and one third with timolol. Fewer ocular side effects were noted with the fixed combination compared with brimonidine alone, suggesting a "protective" effect of timolol.

L. J. Katz, MD

Topical β-Blockers Are Not Associated with an Increased Risk of Treatment for Depression

Kaiserman I, Kaiserman N, Elhayany A, et al (Barzilai Med Ctr, Ashkelon, Israel; Hadassah Med Ctr, Jerusalem; Clalit Health Services, Central District, Rehovot, Israel; et al)
Ophthalmology 113:1077-1080, 2006   3–6

Purpose.—To investigate the effect of topical β-blockers on the prevalence of depression among glaucoma patients.

Design.—Retrospective observational population-based cohort study.

Participants.—We reviewed the electronic medical records of all the members in a district of the largest health maintenance organization in Israel (Central District of Clalit Health Services) who were older than 20 years (317 469 members).

Methods.—We documented all antiglaucoma prescriptions (n = 274 023) and all antidepressant prescriptions (n = 16 948) filled by glaucoma patients in the district between January 1, 2001 and December 31, 2003. We included only those patients who filled at least 6 consecutive antiglaucoma prescriptions at least once every 2 months (n = 6597; 5846 [88.6%] were treated with topical β-blockers). Depressed patients were defined as patients that filled at least four prescriptions for antidepressants during the study period (n= 810, 12.3% of all glaucoma patients).

Main Outcome Measure.—Relationship of topical β-blocker use and prevalence of depression among glaucoma patients.

Results.—No significant demographic differences were noted between glaucoma patients treated and not treated with topical β-blockers. Of those treated and not treated with β-blockers, 12.2% (12.7% after age-adjustment) and 12.7%, respectively, were also receiving drug therapy for depression ($P = 0.7$, chi-square test). With stratification by age, treatment with topical β-blockers did not influence the prevalence of depression in any age group. Logistic regression analysis revealed a significant effect of age, place of birth, and gender on the prevalence of depression, but the prevalence of use of topical β-blockers had no significant effect.

Conclusions.—Use of topical β-blockers by glaucoma patients does not appear to increase the risk of depression in this population.

Open-Angle Glaucoma and Cardiovascular Mortality: The Blue Mountains Eye Study

Lee AJ, Wang JJ, Kifley A, et al (Univ of Sydney, Westmead, Australia)
Ophthalmology 113:1069-1076, 2006   3–7

Purpose.—To evaluate the association between open-angle glaucoma (termed *glaucoma*) and 9-year mortality in an older population-based cohort.

Design.—Population-based cohort.

Participants.—Three thousand six hundred fifty-four persons aged 49 to 97 years (82.4% of the eligible population), residents of the Blue Mountains, west of Sydney, Australia.

Methods.—At baseline (1992–1994), glaucoma was diagnosed from congruous typical glaucomatous visual field changes (full-threshold fields) and optic disc cupping (stereo-optic disc photography). Demographic information from baseline participants was matched with the Australian National Death Index data (December 2001) to obtain the number and causes of deaths. Cox proportional hazards regression analysis, controlling for age, male gender, diabetes, hypertension, heart disease, stroke, use of oral β-blockers, current smoking history, alcohol use, myopia, and nuclear cataract were performed to assess hazard ratios for cardiovascular mortality. Adjustments for all-cause mortality also included history of cancer.

Main Outcome Measures.—Cardiovascular and all-cause mortality.

Results.—At baseline, glaucoma was diagnosed in 108 participants (3.0%). Of 873 deaths (23.9%) before January, 2002, 312 people (8.5%) died of cardiovascular events. The age-standardized all-cause mortality was 24.3% in persons with and 23.8% in those without glaucoma, whereas cardiovascular mortality was 14.6% in persons with and 8.4% in those without glaucoma. After multivariate adjustment, those with glaucoma had a nonsignificant increased risk of cardiovascular death (relative risk [RR], 1.46; 95% confidence interval [CI], 0.95–2.23). Increased cardiovascular mortality was observed mainly in glaucoma patients aged <75 years (RR, 2.78; 95% CI, 1.20–6.47). Further stratified analyses showed that cardiovascular mortality was higher among those with previously diagnosed glaucoma (RR, 1.85; 95% CI, 1.12–3.04) (Table 4), particularly in those also treated with topical timolol (RR, 2.14; 95% CI, 1.18–3.89).

TABLE 4.—Final Multivariate Model of Risk Factors Associated With Cardiovascular Mortality (n = 312)

Variable	Number at Risk (%)	Number (%) With Cardiovascular Mortality	Relative Risk (95% Confidence Interval)	P Value
Age				
Gender (male)	1582 (43.3)	162 (51.9)	1.92 (1.51-2.44)	<0.0001
Diabetes	284 (7.8)	42 (13.6)	1.64 (1.17-2.29)	0.004
Hypertension	1669 (46.0)	186 (61.2)	1.42 (1.11-1.82)	0.005
Heart disease*	590 (16.2)	113 (36.2)	2.15 (1.67-2.77)	<0.0001
Stroke	193 (5.3)	47 (15.1)	1.95 (1.40-2.71)	<0.0001
Use of oral β-blockers	700 (19.2)	63 (9.0)	0.67 (0.50-0.91)	0.01
Current smoking history	544 (14.9)	49 (15.8)	1.89 (1.36-2.62)	0.0001
Current alcohol use	2330 (63.8)	163 (52.2)	0.69 (0.54-0.88)	0.003
Myopia	501 (13.7)	62 (12.4)	1.36 (1.00-1.84)	0.049
Nuclear cataract grade				
Moderate	449 (12.3)	71 (15.8)	1.08 (0.81-1.45)	0.6
Severe	18 (0.5)	9 (50.0)	2.67 (1.23-5.78)	0.01
Glaucoma				
Newly diagnosed	53 (1.5)	8 (2.6)	0.94 (0.44-2.02)	0.9
Previously diagnosed	55 (1.5)	18 (32.7)	1.85 (1.12-3.04)	0.02

*Includes history of heart attack or angina.
(Reprinted from *Ophthalmology*, 113, Lee AJ, Wang JJ, Kifley A, et al: Open-angle glaucoma and cardiovascular mortality: The Blue Mountains Eye Study, pp 1069-1076, Copyright 2006, with permission from Elsevier Science.)

Conclusions.—Findings from the Blue Mountains Eye Study demonstrate an increased cardiovascular mortality in persons with previously diagnosed glaucoma. There was a suggestion of higher cardiovascular mortality in glaucoma patients using topical timolol that merits further study.

Scientific Challenges in Postmarketing Surveillance of Ocular Adverse Drug Reactions

Fraunfelder FW, Fraunfelder FT (Oregon Health and Science Univ, Portland)
Am J Ophthalmol 143:145-149, 2007   3–8

Purpose.—To highlight the challenges of postmarketing surveillance for drug-related adverse events in the practice of ophthalmology.

Design.—A retrospective review of the medical literature and postmarketing surveillance databases.

Methods.—MEDLINE literature review of sildenafil-associated or amiodarone-associated optic neuropathy and chloramphenicol-associated blood dyscrasias.

Results.—Sildenafil, amiodarone, and chloramphenicol may all cause adverse ocular events; however, the data are not conclusive.

Conclusions.—Reports in peer-reviewed medical journals may be proven incorrect over time. For drug-induced adverse ocular events, there is little true science after the drug reaches the marketplace, so the percentage of incorrect conclusions may be high. Clinicians should be wary of reports of adverse ocular effects until data are confirmed by multiple authors over the long-term. Even so, spontaneous reports from postmarketing surveil-

TABLE 2.—WHO Definitions: Causality Assessment of Suspected Adverse Reactions

Certain: A clinical event, including a laboratory test abnormality occurring in a plausible time relationship to drug administration, and which cannot be explained by concurrent disease or other drugs or chemicals. The response to withdrawal of the drug (dechallenge) should be clinically plausible. The event must be definitive pharmacologically or phenomenologically, using a satisfactory rechallenge procedure if necessary.

Probable/Likely: A clinical event, including a laboratory test abnormality, with a reasonable time sequence to administration of the drug, unlikely to be attributed to concurrent disease or other drugs or chemicals, and which follows a clinically reasonable response on withdrawal (dechallenge). Rechallenge information is not required to fulfill this definition.

Possible: A clinical event, including laboratory test abnormality, with a reasonable time sequence to administration of the drug, but which could also be explained by concurrent disease or other drugs or chemicals. Information on drug withdrawal may be lacking or unclear.

Unlikely: A clinical event, including laboratory test abnormality, with a termporal relationship to drug administration, which makes a causal relationship improbable, and in which other drugs, chemicals or underlying disease provide plausible explanations.

Conditional/Unclassified: A clinical event, including a laboratory test abnormality, reported as an adverse reaction, about which more data is essential for a proper assessment or the additional data are under examination.

Unassessible/Unclassifiable: A report suggesting an adverse reaction which cannot be judged because information is insufficient or contradictory, and which cannot be supplemented or verified.

WHO = world health organizations.

(Reprinted by permission of the publisher from Fraunfelder FW, Fraunfelder FT: Scientific challenges in postmarketing surveillance of ocular adverse drug reactions. *Am J Ophthalmol* 143:145-149, 2007. Copyright 2007 by Elsevier Science Inc.)

lance databases may be the first and only signal of an adverse ocular event (Table 2).

▶ The systemic side effects of topical β-blockers have been well recognized, especially with regard to bronchospasm and bradyarrhythmias. However, Kaiserman et al (Abstract 3–6) evaluated the relationship between topical β-blockers and depression in Israel. The prevalence of antidepressive medical therapy was 12%, whether or not topical β-blockers were used to treat glaucoma. This seems to contradict previous reports connecting topical β-blockers with depression.

In a study from Australia, Lee and coworkers (Abstract 3–7) have suggested an association of a higher cardiovascular mortality with chronic glaucoma therapy, especially for those receiving topical β-blockers.

A cautionary note was expressed by Fraunfelder and Fraunfelder (Abstract 3–8) that side effects published after the release of new medications may prove to be incorrect. They recommend that clinicians should be skeptical of side effects reported in a single report. The authors suggest that confirmation by additional studies would make any association of a drug and a side effect more likely.

L. J. Katz, MD

Effect of Corneal Thickness on Dynamic Contour, Rebound, and Goldmann Tonometry

Martinez-de-la-Casa JM, Garcia-Feijoo J, Vico E, et al (Universidad Complutense, Madrid)
Ophthalmology 113:2156-2162, 2006   3–9

Purpose.—To identify correlations among intraocular pressure (IOP) measurements obtained using the rebound tonometer (RBT), the dynamic contour tonometer (DCT), and the Goldmann applanation tonometer (GAT). The effects of corneal thickness on the measures obtained using each of the 3 tonometers also were examined.

Design.—Cross-sectional study.

Participants.—One hundred forty-six eyes of 90 patients with ocular hypertension or glaucoma.

Methods.—Intraocular pressure measurements were obtained in all patients using RBT, DCT, and GAT. Central corneal thickness was determined

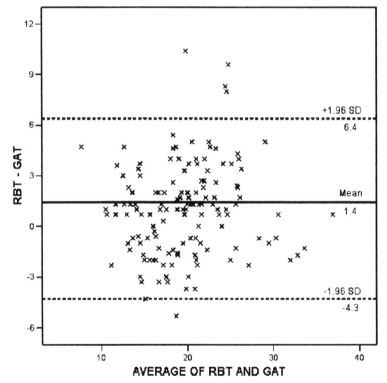

FIGURE 4.—Bland–Altman plot showing the rebound tonometer (RBT) readings minus Goldmann applanation tonometer (GAT) readings (millimeters of mercury) versus the mean of both (slope = 0.056, P = 0.218). (Reprinted from Martinez-de-la-Casa JM, Garcia-Feijoo J, Vico E, et al: Effect of corneal thickness on dynamic contour, rebound, and Goldmann tonometry. *Ophthalmology* 113:2156-2162, 2006. Copyright 2006, with permission from Elsevier Science.)

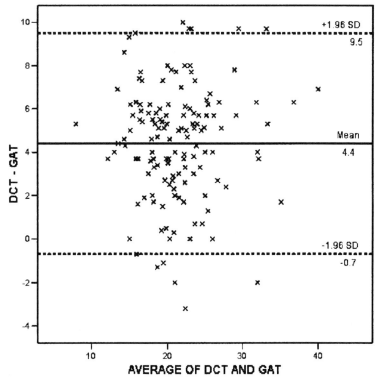

FIGURE 5.—Bland–Altman plot showing the dynamic contour tonometer (DCT) readings minus Goldmann applanation tonometer (GAT) readings (millimeters of mercury) versus the mean of both (slope = 0.016, $P = 0.717$). (Reprinted from Martinez-de-la-Casa JM, Garcia-Feijoo J, Vico E, et al: Effect of corneal thickness on dynamic contour, rebound, and Goldmann tonometry. *Ophthalmology* 113:2156-2162, 2006. Copyright 2006, with permission from Elsevier Science.)

by ultrasound pachymetry. Patients were divided randomly into 6 groups to vary the order in which the tonometers were used. All IOP measurements were made by the same examiner, who was masked to the readings obtained.

Main Outcome Measures.—Intraocular pressure and central corneal thickness.

Results.—There was good correlation between IOP readings obtained using the RBT and GAT ($r = 0.864$; $P<0.0001$), between DCT and GAT ($r = 0.871$; $P<0.0001$), and between RBT and DCT ($r = 0.804$; $P<0.0001$). Rebound tonometer and DCT readings consistently were higher than GAT measurements (RBT-GAT median difference, 1.4±2.7 mmHg; DCT-GAT median difference, 4.4±2.6 mmHg) (Figs 4 and 5). A Bland–Altman plot indicated that the 95% limits of agreement between RBT and GAT were −4.3 to 6.4 mmHg (slope = 0.056; $P = 0.218$), those between DCT and GAT were −0.7 to 9.5 mmHg (slope = 0.016; $P = 0.717$), and those between RBT and DCT were −3.1 to 9.8 mmHg (slope = −0.041; $P = 0.457$). Using

RBT, the point that best discriminated between patients with an IOP 21 mmHg or less and more than 21 mmHg as determined by GAT was >23.3 mmHg (sensitivity, 66.7%; specificity, 92.1%); using DCT, this point was >22.7 mmHg (sensitivity, 95.6%; specificity, 71.3%). In terms of pachymetry, GAT and RBT behaved similarly. Using these instruments, differences of approximately 3 mmHg were detected between the groups of patients with the thinnest (<531 μm) and thickest (>565 μm) corneas, whereas a significantly lower difference (0.5 mmHg) was noted for the DCT.

Conclusions.—Measurements obtained both with the RBT and DCT show excellent correlation with those provided by applanation tonometry. Both tonometers tend to overestimate the IOP measured with the GAT, particularly the DCT. This last tonometer seems to be less affected by the corneal thickness.

Comparison of Dynamic Contour Tonometry and Goldmann Applanation Tonometry in Glaucoma Patients and Healthy Subjects

Barleon L, Hoffmann EM, Berres M, et al (Univ of Mainz, Germany; RheinAhrCampus Remagen, Koblenz, Germany)
Am J Ophthalmol 142:583-590, 2006   3–10

Purpose.—To investigate the agreement in the measurement of intraocular pressure (IOP) obtained by dynamic contour tonometry PASCAL (DCT-PASCAL) and Goldmann applanation tonometry (GAT) in glaucoma eyes and healthy eyes with different central corneal thickness (CCT).

Design.—Prospective cross-sectional study.

Methods.—In a randomized order, three consecutive IOP measurements were performed on 197 eyes of 107 subjects by one examiner using both DCT-PASCAL and GAT on all eyes. Furthermore, ultrasonic pachymetry was performed. The Spearman correlation coefficient (r) was determined to compare IOP readings between DCT-PASCAL and GAT. Regression-based Bland and Altman analysis was used to evaluate agreement between the instruments.

Results.—Mean IOP values obtained by both instruments were significantly correlated in healthy and glaucoma eyes (all healthy eyes [n = 66]: r = 0.8, P < .001, all glaucoma eyes [n = 131]: r = 0.96, P < .001). Neither GAT nor DCT-PASCAL showed a significant correlation with CCT (GAT: all eyes: r = 0.009, P = .9, DCT-PASCAL: all eyes: r = −0.05, P = .5). Bland and Altman analysis revealed the existence of proportional bias. Thus, 95% limits of agreement between the instruments varied with the actual IOP measurement (Fig 3).

Conclusions.—DCT-PASCAL and GAT revealed a strong correlation in IOP measurements between glaucoma and healthy eyes. However, the analysis of agreement indicated some discrepancies between the instruments. Measurements with both GAT and DCT-PASCAL were not correlated with central corneal thickness.

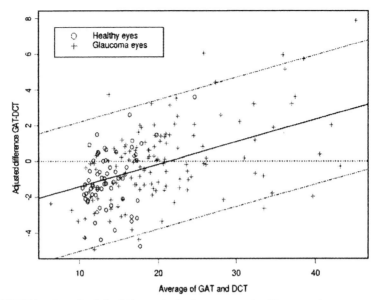

FIGURE 3.—Generalized Bland-Altman plot for the agreement of Goldmann Applanation Tonometry (GAT) and Dynamic Contour Tonometry PASCAL (DCT-PASCAL), including correlated measurements from both eyes and adjustment for central corneal thickness (CCT). The difference between GAT and DCT-PASCAL, adjusted for CCT, was regressed on the average of the two methods (solid line). The 95% limits of agreement for each comparison (mean difference ±1.96 × SD, dashed lines) are shown. (Reprinted by permission of the publisher from Barleon L, Hoffmann EM, Berres M, et al: Comparison of dynamic contour tonometry and Goldmann applanation tonometry in glaucoma patients and healthy subjects. *Am J Ophthalmol* 142:583-590, 2006. Copyright 2006 by Elsevier Science Inc.)

▶ Newer types of tonometry have recently been promoted, prompted in part by concerns over the effect of CCT on measured IOP. DCT has a large concave tip that cradles the corneal surface, allowing an integrated digital sensor to passively measure the IOP through the cornea without indentation. RBT involves a magnetized probe that is brought against the cornea, with derivation of the IOP from the measured deceleration as the probe hits the globe.

These 2 studies (Abstracts 3–10 and 3–9) investigate tonometry from different angles. The study by Martinez-de-la-Casa et al (Abstract 3–10) finds that RBT and DCT tend to give higher measured pressures than GAT, and possibly that the DCT is less influenced by CCT. It is notable that the deviation from GAT is significant (average 1.4 ± 2.7 mm Hg higher for RBT and 4.4 ± 2.6 mm Hg higher for DCT vs GAT).

The study by Barleon et al (Abstract 3–10) also finds that DCT measures higher pressures for patients, although a bit less so than the first study, and the relationship varies with IOP. Interestingly, this study did not find a correlation between measured IOP and CCT, which has been shown in many other studies.

What is the clinician to make of these studies? First, different instruments measure different pressures. Second, no instrument is clearly "correct" or independent of confounders such as IOP. Since all our clinical studies to date are based on GAT, and our treatment guidelines are based on these studies, treatment should, in almost all cases, be based on GAT measurements until further studies are available, except in those cases in which GAT cannot be accurately measured.

J. S. Myers, MD

Compromised Autoregulatory Control of Ocular Hemodynamics in Glaucoma Patients after Postural Change
Galambos P, Vafiadis J, Vilchez SE, et al (Univ Med Ctr Hamburg-Eppendorf, Germany; Centro Oftalmológico del Noroeste, Los Mochis, Mexico)
Ophthalmology 113:1832-1836, 2006   3–11

Purpose.—The autoregulatory control of retrobulbar blood flow in response to postural challenge was investigated in normal-tension glaucoma (NTG) patients in comparison with primary open-angle glaucoma (POAG) patients and healthy volunteers.

Design.—Prospective cohort study.

Participants and Controls.—Twenty POAG patients, 20 NTG patients, and 20 control subjects.

Methods.—Peak systolic velocity (PSV), end diastolic velocity (EDV), and resistivity index (RI) in the short posterior ciliary artery (SPCA), central retinal artery (CRA) and ophthalmic artery (OA) were recorded after a change from sitting upright to a supine body position using color Doppler imaging.

Main Outcome Measures.—Peak systolic velocity, EDV, and RI.

Results.—Ten minutes after postural change to a supine position, blood flow velocities in the SPCA remained unchanged in controls, whereas a significant increase of PSV and EDV was found in both glaucoma groups. The RI in the SPCA was significantly lowered in the NTG group. Recordings for the OA and CRA showed a significant increase in EDV and significant decrease in RI in all 3 groups; a significant increase in PSV in the CRA was detected only in the NTG group (Fig 1).

Conclusions.—The unaltered flow velocities in the SPCA of healthy controls may indicate tight autoregulatory control, whereas the flow velocities in the CRA and OA appeared to follow alterations in hydrostatic pressure. In contrast, NTG and POAG patients demonstrated an insufficient compensatory response to postural change, leading to accelerated flow in the SPCA. This compromised autoregulatory control could represent another contributing factor in the pathogenesis of glaucoma.

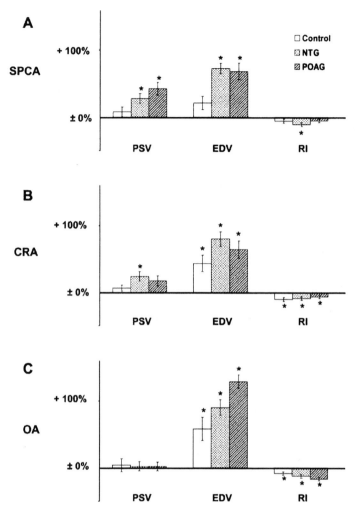

FIGURE 1.—Relative changes of the color Doppler imaging parameters after postural change from sitting to a supine body position in the (**A**) short posterior ciliary artery (SPCA), (**B**) central retinal artery (CRA), and (**C**) ophthalmic artery (OA). The ordinate represents the relative differences between the supine and upright positions. *Statistical significance ($P<0.05$). EDV = end diastolic velocity; NTG = normal-tension glaucoma; POAG = primary open-angle glaucoma; PSV = peak systolic velocity; RI = resistivity index. (Reprinted from *Ophthalmology*, 113, Galambos P, Vafiadis J, Vilchez SE, et al, Compromised autoregulatory control of ocular hemodynamics in glaucoma patients after postural change, pp 1832-1836, Copyright 2006, with permission from Elsevier Science.)

Relationship Between Central Corneal Thickness and Changes of Optic Nerve Head Topography and Blood Flow After Intraocular Pressure Reduction in Open-angle Glaucoma and Ocular Hypertension

Lesk MR, Hafez AS, Descovich D (Univ of Montreal, Quebec)

Arch Ophthalmol 124:1568-1572, 2006   3–12

Objectives.—To investigate changes in optic nerve head topography and blood flow after therapeutic intraocular pressure reduction and to correlate them with central corneal thickness.

Methods.—Sixteen patients with open-angle glaucoma and 16 patients with ocular hypertension underwent Heidelberg retina tomography and scanning laser Doppler flowmetry in 1 eye before and at least 2 months after a mean 35% sustained therapeutic reduction in intraocular pressure. Patients were assigned to a thin or thick group based on their median central corneal thickness.

Results.—Compared with 16 patients with thick corneas (mean SD central corneal thickness, 587±31 µm), the 16 patients with thin corneas (518±32 µm) had greater reductions in mean (36±32 vs 4±36 µm, $P=.003$) and in maximum cup depth (73±107 vs 4±89 µm, $P=.02$). These changes were not statistically significantly different between the patients with open-angle glaucoma and those with ocular hypertension. Smaller mean±SD improvements in neuroretinal rim blood flow were seen in patients with thinner corneas compared with those with thicker corneas (35±80 vs 110±111 arbitrary units, $P=.04$).

Conclusion.—Patients with open-angle glaucoma and ocular hypertension with thinner corneas show significantly greater shallowing of the cup, a surrogate marker for lamina cribrosa displacement (compliance), and smaller improvements of neuroretinal rim blood flow after intraocular pressure reduction.

▶ These articles (Abstracts 3–11 and 3–12) show, once again, that the retrobulbar and intraocular hemodynamics are altered in individuals with ocular hypertension, primary open-angle, and normal-tension glaucoma. The first article (Abstract 3–11) finds that autoregulatory responses to a postural change are reduced in glaucoma patients. Both glaucoma groups included in the study had significant damage (average cup-to-disc ratio 0.75 for POAG, 0.85 for NTG; the visual field mean deviation was not given). Thus, the article does not address whether the vascular issues led to the optic neuropathy or followed it. This chicken versus egg issue has remained for decades in the pressure versus ischemia pathogenesis debate for glaucoma.

The second article (Abstract 3–12) looks at changes in optic nerve head tomography and scanning laser Doppler flowmetry after a 35% reduction in intraocular pressure. Interestingly, the patients with thinner corneas showed greater movement of the bottom of the cup and lesser improvements in optic nerve head blood flow after pressure reduction. This suggests the possibility that greater deformation of the lamina cribrosa and greater compromise of blood flow with elevated pressure may be more common in eyes with thinner corneas, and that these could be the links between the non-pressure-related increase in glaucoma risk and reduced central corneal thickness.

The detailed findings in these reports are critical to researchers in the field. For clinicians, the message remains that the pathophysiology of glaucoma remains poorly understood. However, we should be attuned to vascular issues in our patients, such as the association with migraine and other vasospastic phenomena, and the possible further compromise that very high or low blood pressure may present to an already challenged vasculature.

J. S. Myers, MD

Comparison of the Moorfields Classification Using Confocal Scanning Laser Ophthalmoscopy and Subjective Optic Disc Classification in Detecting Glaucoma in Blacks and Whites
Girkin CA, DeLeon-Ortega JE, Xie A, et al (Univ of Alabama at Birmingham)
Ophthalmology 113:2144-2149, 2006   3–13

Objective.—To compare the diagnostic accuracy of the Moorfields regression classification (MRC) and subjective optic disc evaluation in discriminating early to moderate glaucomatous from nonglaucomatous eyes.

Design.—Cross-sectional observational study.

Participants.—Two hundred thirty-three patients with glaucoma and 216 normal subjects were included in the analysis. Racial groups were defined by self-description.

Methods.—All subjects underwent confocal scanning laser ophthalmoscopy, stereophotography, and standard perimetry. Glaucoma was defined by visual field defect alone and confirmed with a second visual field test. Stereo photographs were graded as either normal or glaucomatous appearing in a masked fashion by 2 independent graders and adjudicated by a third grader in cases of disagreement. Mean disc area was compared between patients correctly and incorrectly diagnosed with either technique.

Main Outcome Measures.—Sensitivity and specificity of MRC and subjective evaluation of stereophotographs in the detection of glaucomatous visual field loss.

Results.—With the MRC, the sensitivity and specificity were higher using the 95% cutoff than using the 99.9% cutoff. Classification based on subjective photo assessment had a greater agreement with the diagnosis of glaucoma than the MRC for blacks (MRC, sensitivity = 62.5%, specificity = 93.2%; Photo, sensitivity = 76.5%, specificity = 91.5%) and whites (MRC, sensitivity = 67.0%, specificity = 92.2%; photo, sensitivity = 78.4%, specificity = 91.9%) (Table 5). Disc area was significantly larger in patients incorrectly diagnosed with the MRC ($P = 0.0289$).

Conclusions.—Subjective optic disc grading by glaucoma specialists outperformed the MRC with the HRT II in both black and white subjects. Both subjective and objective diagnostic methods were associated with similar sensitivity and specificity between racial groups. The MRC was more likely to provide an incorrect diagnosis in subjects with larger optic discs.

TABLE 5.—Comparison of the Sensitivity and Specificity to Detect Glaucoma Using the Best Parameter of the Moorfields Regression Classification (MRC-Result) and Subjective Stereo Photo Results

	Subjective Stereo Photograph	MRC-result 95% CI Cutoff
Overall group		
Sensitivity*	77.3% (77.7%)	64.4% (66.1%)
Specificity	91.7%	93.1%
Black group		
Sensitivity*	76.5% (77.2%)	62.5% (64.7%)
Specificity	91.5%	93.2%
White group		
Sensitivity*	78.4% (78.4%)	67.0% (69.1%)
Specificity	91.9%	92.9%

*Sensitivity adjusted for age at the same level of specificity in parenthesis.
(Reprinted from *Ophthalmology*, 113, Girkin CA, DeLeon-Ortega JE, Xie A, et al, Comparison of the Moorfields classification using confocal scanning laser ophthalmoscopy and subjective optic disc classification in detecting glaucoma in blacks and whites, pp 2144-2149, copyright 2006 with permission from Elsevier Science.)

▶ This large study comparing the Heidelberg retina tomograph II (HRT II) to expert evaluation of the nerve for the diagnosis of glaucoma shows moderately good results for both. The patients had early to moderate glaucoma, with a mean deviation of field testing of −4 dB for the glaucoma group. The sensitivities and specificities of the HRT II MRC (about 65% and 93%, respectively) were slightly less than those for expert stereo disc photo interpretation (about 75% and 92%, respectively).

This shows that careful evaluation of the optic nerve is still a valid and necessary part of the glaucoma evaluation. Although we may not all be up to the standards of the experts in this study in terms of our ability to evaluate stereo disc photographs, stereoptic evaluation of the optic nerve remains useful and important for our patients. Aside from judging the contour of the cup and disc, meticulous examination will also reveal disc hemorrhages, nerve fiber layer defects, and pallor that may be crucial to the diagnosis and management of the patient—all of which the HRT II was not designed to detect.

J. S. Myers, MD

Baseline Optical Coherence Tomography Predicts the Development of Glaucomatous Change in Glaucoma Suspects
Lalezary M, Medeiros FA, Weinreb RN, et al (Univ of California, San Diego, La Jolla)
Am J Ophthalmol 142:576-582, 2006   3–14

Purpose.—To assess whether baseline retinal nerve fiber layer (RNFL) measurements obtained with optical coherence tomography (OCT2; Carl Zeiss Meditec, Dublin, California, USA) are predictive of the development of glaucomatous change.

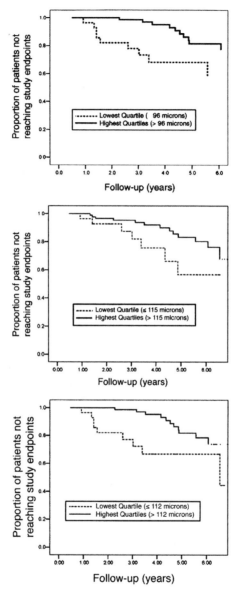

FIGURE 1.—Kaplan-Meier survival curves for the subjects with retinal nerve fiber layer (RNFL) measurement (**Top**) average thickness, (**Middle**) superior thickness, (**Bottom**) inferior thickness in the lowest quartile (1/4) (*dashed line*) compared with the subjects with thicker measurements in the upper three quartiles (3/4) (*continuous line*). Study endpoint was defined as development of glaucomatous visual field damage in three or more consecutive tests and/or progressive glaucomatous optic neuropathy (GON) on stereophotograph assessment. (Reprinted by permission of the publisher from Lalezary M, Medeiros FA, Weinreb RN, et al: Baseline optical coherence tomography predicts the development of glaucomatous change in glaucoma suspects. *Am J Ophthalmol* 142:576-582, 2006. Copyright 2006 by Elsevier Science Inc.)

Design.—Cohort study.

Methods.—Participants were recruited from the University of California, San Diego (UCSD) longitudinal Diagnostic Innovations in Glaucoma Study (DIGS). One eye was studied from each of 114 glaucoma suspects with normal standard automated perimetry (SAP) and OCT RNFL imaging at baseline. The cohort was divided into two groups based on the development of glaucomatous change (repeatable abnormal visual fields and/or a change in the stereophotographic appearance of the optic disk). Cox proportional hazards models were used to determine the predictive ability of OCT RNFL thickness measurements.

Results.—Over a 4.2-year average follow-up period, 23 eyes (20%) developed glaucomatous changes and 91 (80%) did not. At baseline, thinner RNFL measurements, higher SAP pattern standard deviation (PSD), "glaucoma" stereophotograph assessment, and thinner central corneal thickness (CCT) were associated with the study endpoints in univariate analysis. After adjusting for age, intraocular pressure (IOP), CCT, and PSD in multivariate models, a 10 μm thinner average, superior and inferior RNFL at baseline was predictive of glaucomatous change [hazard ratio (95% CI); 1.51 (1.11 to 2.12), 1.57 (1.17 to 2.18), and 1.49, (1.19 to 1.91), respectively]. Results were consistent when stereophotographic assessment was included in multivariate analysis.

Conclusions.—Thinner OCT RNFL measurements at baseline were associated with development of glaucomatous change in glaucoma suspect eyes. RNFL thinning was an independent predictor of the glaucomatous change, even when adjusting for stereophotograph assessment, age, IOP, CCT, and PSD (Fig 1).

▶ This study reports that baseline OCT measurements of glaucoma suspects are correlated to the risk of developing glaucomatous field loss or photographic disc change. Specifically, for every 10 μm thinner RNFL (average, superior or inferior) at baseline, the relative risk was about 1.5 for developing glaucoma after adjusting for age, IOP, CCT, and PSD.

These findings are consistent with prior excellent work by this group and others showing that the more abnormal the OCT, the more likely that the subject has glaucoma. However, this is the first report showing that more suspicious nerves by OCT are at increased likelihood of developing glaucomatous change in the future. These findings are very analogous to those reported by this group for HRT (Heidelberg retina tomograph) in the Ocular Hypertension Treatment Study.[1]

It should be noted, however, that these important findings do not report a cutoff value or classification of those who will develop glaucoma versus those who will remain stable. This report shows instead that the relative risk of progression is increased for every 10 μm of RNFL thinning. This suggests that patients with thinner RNFLs should be monitored more closely, and that the increased risk should possibly be considered in the discussion regarding treatment versus observation. However, clinical observation and judgment remain central to this process.

J. S. Myers, MD

Reference

1. Zangwill LM, Weinreb RN, Beiser JA, et al: Baseline topographic optic disk measurements are associated with the development of primary open-angle glaucoma: The Confocal Scanning Laser Opthalmoscopy Ancillary Study to the Ocular Hypertension Treatment Study. *Arch Ophthalmol* 123:1188-1197, 2005.

Measurements of Optic Disk Size With HRT II, Stratus OCT, and Funduscopy Are Not Interchangeable

Barkana Y, Harizman N, Gerber Y, et al (New York Eye and Ear Infirmary; Manhattan Eye, Ear, and Throat Hosp, New York; New York Univ; et al)
Am J Ophthalmol 142:375-380, 2006   3–15

Purpose.—To assess the interchangeability of optic disk size measurements using slit-lamp funduscopy, optical coherence tomography (OCT-3), and confocal scanning laser ophthalmoscopy (HRT-II) in clinical practice.

Design.—Prospective nonrandomized clinical study.

Methods.—Measurements of vertical disk diameter (VDD) were obtained with the three methods. Disk area was obtained from OCT and HRT printouts. True agreement between methods in measuring VDD was assessed using Bland-Altman graphs and 95% limits of agreement (LoA). Disks were classified as small, average, or large, and agreement between methods in this classification was assessed using κ statistics.

Results.—Forty-eight patients were enrolled (mean age 53.4 ± 14.3 years). VDD (mean ± SD) was 1.58 ± 0.15, 1.70 ± 0.22, and 1.90 ± 0.24 mm

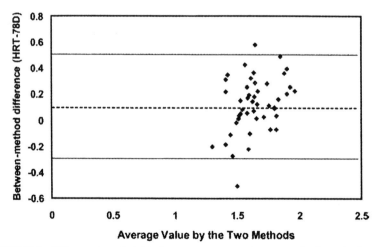

FIGURE 3.—Differences in vertical disk diameter measurements between confocal scanning laser ophthalmoscopy (HRT-II) and slit-lamp ophthalmoscopy with a 78 diopters lens. The mean difference is represented by the dotted line and the 95% confidence limits by the solid lines. (Reprinted by permission of the publisher from Barkana Y, Harizman N, Gerber Y, et al: Measurements of optic disk size with HRT II, Stratus OCT, and funduscopy are not interchangeable. *Am J Ophthalmol* 142:375-380, 2006. Copyright 2006 by Elsevier Science Inc.)

with funduscopy, HRT, and OCT, respectively. Very large LoA were observed: −0.29 to 0.70 mm for OCT and HRT, −0.07 to 0.71 mm for OCT and funduscopy, and −0.29 to 0.53 mm for HRT and funduscopy (Fig 3). There was poor agreement ($\kappa < 0.4$) in classification of disk size as small, average, or large whether disk diameter or area was compared and using two definitions of disk size.

Conclusions.—We observed a large range of differences in estimating disk size with HRT, OCT, and funduscopy. This precludes interchangeable use of these measurements in clinical practice, and does not allow simple conversion formulas to be proposed. In addition, there is poor agreement between these methods in classifying disk size as small, average, or large. At present, estimation of both absolute and relative disk size can only be defined separately for each measurement modality.

▶ In order to understand whether an optic nerve is abnormal, it helps to know what is normal. When it comes to glaucoma, one of the traditional "normal" ways to describe the nerve is the cup-to-disc ratio. However, the cup-to-disc ratio suffers from 2 flaws that limit its usefulness: 1) it does not describe the structure of interest (the neuroretinal rim); and 2) it fails to account for the effect of disc size. The fact that large nerves have large cups and small nerves have small cups is an underappreciated fact. Without knowing the nerve size, one can't understand what the expected amount of "cupping" should be. Therefore, it is important to be able to measure the nerve size. This can be done at the slit lamp or by an automated imaging device.

In this article, the authors have compared 3 techniques—a 78-D lens, the HRT II, and the OCT—and found that they all differ. While the authors seem to find their results unfortunate, I'm not sure they should be surprised. The authors found that the average VDD measured 1.58 mm (78-D lens), 1.7 mm (HRT II), and 1.9 mm (OCT). While these may seem different, there are 2 reasons to think that perhaps they are not so different. The main issue is that the authors failed to multiply their 78-D lens measurements by the magnification artifact induced by the lens. The magnification artifact is essentially the reciprocal of the laser spot size magnification specified for each lens; for the Volk 78-D lens the magnification artifact is 1.1. Thus, 1.58 mm × 1.1 is 1.74 mm—essentially the same as the HRT. This makes sense, since the HRT is not influenced by magnification artifacts.

The second point is that the OCT doesn't measure disc diameter, the OCT measures the retinal pigment epithelium (RPE) border. The RPE border is usually located next to the scleral canal, but not always. Since the authors made a point to measure disc diameter inside the scleral canal, it makes sense that the OCT would give larger disc size measurements.

My interpretation of this article is that the authors have helped to broaden the understanding of the importance of disc size, but that their conclusions are unnecessarily glum. I would argue that they have demonstrated that discs can be measured effectively using different methods.

J. D. Henderer, MD

Influence of Disease Severity and Optic Disc Size on the Diagnostic Performance of Imaging Instruments in Glaucoma

Medeiros FA, Zangwill LM, Bowd C, et al (Univ of California, San Diego)
Invest Ophthalmol Vis Sci 47:1008-1015, 2006   3–16

Purpose.—To evaluate the influence of disease severity and optic disc size on the diagnostic accuracy of three imaging technologies for structural assessment in glaucoma: confocal scanning laser ophthalmoscopy, scanning laser polarimetry, and optical coherence tomography.

Methods.—One hundred five patients with glaucoma and 61 normal subjects were recruited from the Diagnostic Innovations in Glaucoma Study (DIGS). All individuals underwent imaging with the GDx Variable Corneal and Lens Compensator (VCC; Carl Zeiss Meditec, Inc., Dublin, CA), the Heidelberg Retina Tomograph II (HRT II; Heidelberg Engineering, GmbH, Dossenheim, Germany), and the Stratus OCT (Stratus OCT; Carl-Zeiss Meditec, Inc.) within a 6-month period. Severity of disease was based on the AGIS (Advanced Glaucoma Intervention Study) visual field score. To evaluate the influence of severity of glaucoma and optic disc size on the diagnostic accuracy of the imaging instruments, the sensitivities of the tests were fitted as a function of the AGIS score and disc area, by using logistic marginal regression models.

Results.—The severity of visual field loss had a significant influence on the sensitivity of all imaging instruments. More severe disease was associated with increased sensitivity. This influence was similar among the three instruments. With regard to optic disc area, larger optic discs were associated with decreased sensitivity for the Stratus OCT parameter Average Thickness and the GDx VCC parameter Nerve Fiber Indicator, whereas small optic discs were associated with increased sensitivity. For the HRT II parameter Moorfields regression analysis classification, an inverse effect was observed..

Conclusion.—The diagnostic performances of the GDx VCC, HRT II, and Stratus OCT were significantly influenced by the severity of the disease and optic disc size. These covariates should be taken into account when comparing the performances of these tests for glaucoma diagnosis.

▶ Physicians would like to have access to a medical test that is always accurate—unfortunately, such a test does not exist. At the most basic level, in order to be considered useful, medical tests need to be able to identify diseased individuals (sensitivity) and exclude normal individuals (specificity). Even tests that are very good at these 2 tasks often have trouble when placed in unfavorable circumstances; this commonly occurs when testing for an uncommon disease. Given a condition with a low prevalence (such as glaucoma), even a test with high sensitivity will return a substantial number of false positives (people misidentified as diseased).

Other confounding variables may influence the performance of a test. The authors have investigated 2 such confounding variables on the ability of 3 commonly used optic nerve imaging devices to correctly identify glaucoma. It turns out that these 2 variables, optic nerve size and disease severity, do, in fact, influence the outcome. All 3 machines are better at identifying advanced disease as opposed to early disease. The sensitivity of the OCT and GDx was reduced by large optic nerves, while the sensitivity of the HRT was lower when confronted with small nerves. This makes some sense. Since there is no gold standard test for glaucoma, the optic nerve imaging tests rely on a computer programmer to tell the machine whether abnormal results are "disease." The programmer, in turn, relies upon the glaucoma specialist to tell him what is "disease." Since it is easier to tell when advanced disease is present as opposed to when early disease is present, it is not surprising that the machines are more accurate when looking at advanced disease. Another way to reflect on this is to consider that, at the extremes, there is less overlap between normal and abnormal, making correct classification more likely.

This is, of course, the exact opposite of how the machines are marketed. The machines are sold principally to assist doctors in identifying early disease (since advanced disease is obvious and no machine is needed). However, this is precisely the situation where the machines perform their worst. Add optic nerve size as another influential variable and it is clear that physicians have to be very careful when interpreting test results.

J. D. Henderer, MD

In Vivo Imaging and Counting of Rat Retinal Ganglion Cells Using a Scanning Laser Ophthalmoscope

Higashide T, Kawaguchi I, Ohkubo S, et al (Kanazawa Univ Graduate School of Med Science, Japan)
Invest Ophthalmol Vis Sci 47:2943-2950, 2006   3–17

Purpose.—To determine whether a scanning laser ophthalmoscope (SLO) is useful for in vivo imaging and counting of rat retinal ganglion cells (RGCs).

Methods.—RGCs of Brown Norway rats were retrogradely labeled bilaterally with the fluorescent dye 4-(4-(dihexadecylamino)styryl)-N-methylpyridinium iodine (DiA). The unilateral optic nerve was crushed intraorbitally with a clip. RGCs were imaged in vivo with an SLO with an argon blue laser (488 nm) and optical filter sets for fluorescein angiography, before and 1, 2, and 4 weeks after the crush. An image overlay analysis was performed to check cell positions in the SLO images over time. Lectin histochemical analysis was performed to determine the relationship of microglia to the newly emerged DiA fluorescence detected by image overlay analysis after the optic nerve crush.

Results.—Fluorescent RGCs were visible in vivo with an SLO. RGC survival decreased gradually after the crush. In the retina after the optic nerve crush, newly emerged DiA fluorescence detected by image overlay analysis corresponded to fluorescent cells morphologically different from RGCs in the retinal flatmount and was colocalized mostly with lectin-stained microglial processes. RGC counts by SLO were comparable to those in retinal flatmounts.

Conclusions.—The SLO is useful for in vivo imaging of rat RGCs and therefore may be a valuable tool for monitoring RGC changes over time in various rat models of RGC damage.

▶ If glaucoma is a disease of ganglion cell death, it stands to reason that the best way to monitor, and possibly to diagnose, this disease would be to count the number of ganglion cells. If there is a change that exceeds normal age-related cell death, then disease is likely to be progressing.

No technology currently exists that allows in vivo human ganglion cell counts, but two possible angles are being developed. One would be to count the number of cells undergoing apoptotic cell death and another would be to actually count the number of ganglion cells.

This article describes an attempt to count the ganglion cells in a rat model of glaucoma using the scanning laser ophthalmoscope. This wasn't as simple as pointing the camera at the retina. The rats were pretreated with fluorescent dye to stain the ganglion cells, a specially designed contact lens was placed on the cornea, and an argon blue laser was used to image the retina. One of the rat's eyes was subjected to optic nerve crush to trigger cell retinal ganglion cell death. The number of cells counted by SLO was compared with counting the cells on postmortem retinal flatmounts. Since the cells counts were very similar, the authors concluded the SLO could successfully be used to count the labeled ganglion cells. They discovered that other cell types also became labeled after optic nerve crush, and some elaborate techniques were needed to separate nonganglion cells. They also reported problems with image quality as a result of issues related to focusing.

Overall, the authors were able to demonstrate the concept that SLO can be used to count ganglion cells. A great deal of work is needed before this can be adapted to humans, but the proof of concept reported in this study means that one day glaucoma may be monitored by counting ganglion cells.

J. D. Henderer, MD

The Relationship between Retinal Ganglion Cell Function and Retinal Nerve Fiber Thickness in Early Glaucoma
Ventura LM, Sorokac N, De Los Santos R, et al (Univ of Miami, Fla)
Invest Ophthalmol Vis Sci 47:3904-3911, 2006   3–18

Purpose.—To compare relative reduction of retinal ganglion cell (RGC) function and retinal nerve fiber layer (RNFL) thickness in early glaucoma by means of steady-state pattern electroretinogram (PERG) and optical coherence tomography (OCT), respectively.

Methods.—Eighty-four persons with suspected glaucoma due to disc abnormalities (GS: mean age 56.6 ± 13.8 years, standard automated perimetry [SAP] mean deviation [MD] -0.58 ± 1.34 dB) and 34 patients with early manifest glaucoma (EMG, mean age 65.9 ± 10.7 years, SAP MD -2.7 ± 4.5

dB) were tested with PERG and OCT. Both GS and EMG patients had small refractive errors, corrected visual acuity ≥20/25, and no systemic or retinal disease other than glaucoma.

Results.—MDs from age-predicted normal values were larger for PERG amplitude (GS: −1.113 dB; EMG: −2.352 dB) compared with the PERG-matched RNFL thickness (GS: −0.217 dB; EMG: −0.725 dB). Deviations exceeding the lower 95% tolerance intervals of the normal population were more frequent for PERG amplitude (GS: 26%; EMG: 56%) than PERG-matched RNFL thickness (GS: 6%; EMG: 29%).

Conclusions.—In early glaucoma, reduction in RGC electrical activity exceeds the proportion expected from lost RGC axons, suggesting that a population of viable RGCs in the central retina is dysfunctional. By combining PERG and OCT it is, in principle, possible to obtain unique information on reduced responsiveness of viable RGCs.

▶ Everyone knows that visual fields are an imperfect way to measure ganglion cell function, and yet the only reason we treat glaucoma is to prevent field loss. Therefore, field testing remains an important tool to manage patients with glaucoma. Limitations, such as field tests sampling only a small portion of the retina and relying on good test-taking techniques, are perhaps unavoidable if we want relatively quick tests. What is perhaps more troubling is that conventional perimetry seems to be relatively insensitive in early glaucoma. Why? Ventura et al set out to investigate this question. They knew that the principal hypothesis is that the field may be insensitive because there are many more ganglion cells in the retina than are actually needed for good vision. Therefore, the death of even a substantial number would not be detected by a field test. However, experimental glaucoma models seem to indicate that, on occasion, field defects occur before ganglion cell loss. Could this be due to a phase of ganglion cell dysfunction that precedes cell death? Such a phase might be missed not only by field tests, but also by optic nerve imaging tests that are based on in vivo "tissue sampling." If so, could a different measure of ganglion cell function be used that would detect cell disease and not just cell death?

The PERG seems to be just such a test since it appears to detect ganglion cell dysfunction. If damaged ganglion cells precede dead ganglion cells, then the PERG should be abnormal before evidence of cell loss. And this is what the authors showed in a population of glaucoma suspects and early glaucoma patients. Both PERG and RNFL thickness as measured by OCT were reduced with more advanced disease, but there appeared to be only a weak correlation. This suggests that there are damaged cells that are not dead. The practical implication is 2-fold. First, damaged cells might be rescued by treatment. Two groups have shown that intraocular pressure reduction can result in improved contrast sensitivity and color vision. Second, measurement of damaged cell function could be used as a biologic marker to help better monitor the rate of glaucoma damage and its treatment. The authors should be congratulated for pushing the boundary of the structure-function relationship.

J. D. Henderer, MD

Prediction of future scotoma on conventional automated static perimetry using frequency doubling technology perimetry

Kogure S, Toda Y, Tsukahara S (Univ of Yamanashi, Japan)

Br J Ophthalmol 90:347-352, 2006   3–19

Aim.—To see if scotoma detected with frequency doubling technology (FDT) is confirmed by Humphrey field analyser (HFA) 3 years later.

Methods.—Subjects were first examined with the screening C-20-1 program of FDT. The visual field was examined annually for 4 years using HFA program C30-2. The central 58 test points in HFA were assigned to one of the 17 clusters corresponding to FDT test points. Each cluster was represented as the lowest probability symbol of total deviation (TD) of the HFA test points included in the cluster. Clusters were graded normal, suspected scotoma, and scotoma depending on probability of TD—5% or more, 5%–1%, less than 1%, respectively. Relative risk (RR) of abnormality on FDT for future scotoma on HFA was estimated.

Results.—80 eyes of 42 patients were followed up for 4 years. While 4.0% of normal clusters of HFA with normal FDT results developed into scotoma cluster, 20.8% of normal clusters with abnormal FDT results developed into scotoma cluster with HFA at the third year. RR for future scotoma was 5.24 (95% CI, 2.75 to 10.0, $p<0.05$).

Conclusion.—An abnormal result in FDT shows a high risk of future scotoma on HFA after 3 years even if the original HFA perimetry showed normal results.

▶ Ophthalmologists are on a quest to find evidence of earlier and earlier glaucoma damage because it appears that early treatment helps prevent visual disability and is less costly (as noted in other articles in this chapter). Specialized visual field testing has been hypothesized to be able to identify field defects earlier than conventional perimetry (standard achromatic perimetry [SAP]). Short wavelength automated perimetry is one such test and, more recently, FDT has been used in this capacity. Not only does FDT examine the M ganglion cells that may be damaged earlier in glaucoma, but it is small and portable, making it an attractive field test for glaucoma screening.

But does FDT detect disease earlier than SAP? The authors assembled a cohort of patients with glaucoma who underwent a screening version of the FDT and conventional SAP over a 4-year period. They compared similar regions of the field with both tests and sought to determine how many abnormal baseline FDT test locations also became abnormal SAP test locations. Interestingly, at the outset of the study, more test locations were called "abnormal" by SAP testing than FDT. In the 53 test locations identified as abnormal by FDT, 11 (20%) subsequently became abnormal by SAP. Only 4% of normal SAP points became abnormal, leading them to conclude that there was a 5-fold increase in the risk of SAP locations becoming abnormal if preceded by an abnormal FDT.

The authors did not mention whether they repeated the FDT to be sure it was reliable. They also did not mention whether the normal FDT points that had a corresponding abnormal baseline SAP point became abnormal over time. They note, but don't comment on, that more than 50% of baseline FDT abnormalities never developed an SAP defect. This, of course, reduces the positive predictive value of an abnormal FDT and the specificity of the FDT. They did note that the FDT was not very sensitive when examining the central 10° of fixation, while the test was more sensitive in the 10° to 20° from fixation range.

This is an admirable study as it aspired to the best study design incorporating both longitudinal follow-up with location analysis to be sure that abnormal test points correlated. This lends support to the notion that FDT can detect some field defects before SAP, but it is possible that FDT may also be recording a large number of false-positives. Only further follow-up will permit this determination.

J. D. Henderer, MD

Diagnostic Sensitivity of Fast Blue–Yellow and Standard Automated Perimetry in Early Glaucoma: A Comparison between Different Test Programs
Bengtsson B, Heijl A (Lund Univ, Malmö, Sweden)
Ophthalmology 113:1092-1097, 2006   3–20

Purpose.—To compare the ability of Fast Swedish interactive threshold algorithm (SITA) short-wavelength automated perimetry (SWAP), lengthier full-threshold SWAP, and standard automated perimetry (SAP) using the SITA Fast program to detect early glaucomatous visual field loss.

Design.—Cross-sectional prospective study of perimetric diagnostic sensitivity as defined by reference limits determined in the same healthy participants for all 3 test programs.

Participants.—One hundred one patients with ocular hypertension, or suspect or early manifest glaucoma.

Methods.—One eye of each patient was tested with 2 blue–yellow perimetric programs: the SITA and full-threshold SWAP and the SAP SITA Fast program.

TABLE 1.—Mean Individual Differences in Number of Significantly Depressed between the 3 Different Test Programs

	Full-Threshold SWAP – SITA SWAP	Full-Threshold SWAP – SITA Fast SAP	SITA SWAP – SITA Fast SAP
$P<5\%$ limit	0.05 ($P = 0.91^*$)	1.09 ($P = 0.08^*$)	1.04 ($P = 0.07^*$)
$P<2\%$ limit	0.15 ($P = 0.71^*$)	1.09 ($P = 0.06^*$)	0.94 ($P = 0.05^*$)

SAP = Standard automated perimetry; SITA = Swedish interactive threshold algorithm; SWAP = short wavelength automated perimetry.
*Only probability values < 0.017 should be considered as significant according to the Bonferroni correction for multiple comparisons.
(Reprinted from *Ophthalmology*, vol 113, Bengtsson B, Heijl A: Diagnostic sensitivity of fast blue-yellow and standard automated perimetry in early glaucoma: A comparison between different test programs, pp 1092-1097, 2006, copyright 2006, with permission from Elsevier Science.)

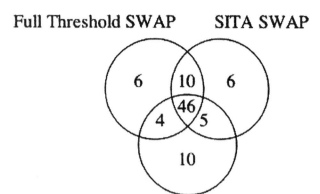

FIGURE 2.—Venn diagram showing number of eyes with clusters of at least 3 significantly depressed test point locations for each test program. SAP = Standard automated perimetry; SITA = Swedish interactive threshold algorithm; SWAP = short-wavelength automated perimetry. (Reprinted from *Ophthalmology*, vol 113, Bengtsson B, Heijl A: Diagnostic sensitivity of fast blue-yellow and standard automated perimetry in early glaucoma: A comparison between different test programs, pp 1092-1097, copyright 2006, with permission from Elsevier Science.)

Main Outcome Measures.—Glaucomatous visual field loss, defined as number of significantly depressed test point locations or the number of clusters of such test points.

Results.—No significant difference in number of significantly depressed test point locations between the 3 programs could be detected, neither at the $P<5\%$ limit nor at the $P<2\%$ limit. The difference in number of points depressed below the fifth percentile was 0.5 between full-threshold SWAP and SITA SWAP, 1.09 between full-threshold SWAP and SAP, and 1.04 between SITA SWAP and SAP. The number of eyes showing clusters of significantly depressed points also was similar with the 3 test programs: full-threshold SWAP identified clusters in 66 eyes, SITA SWAP identified clusters in 67 eyes, and SITA Fast SAP identified clusters in 65 eyes. Average test time was 12.0 minutes using full-threshold SWAP, 4.1 minutes with SITA SWAP, and 3.5 with SITA Fast.

Conclusions.—The SITA SWAP identified at least as much glaucomatous visual field loss as the older full-threshold SWAP, although test time was considerably reduced. Conventional SAP using SITA Fast was not significantly less sensitive than either of the 2 SWAP programs (Table 1, Fig 2).

▶ SWAP (blue on yellow) has been shown in many studies to detect early glaucoma earlier than SAP (white on white). However, SWAP testing is difficult and prolonged, even in younger patients without significant nuclear sclerosis.

Applying the SITA approach to SWAP has been suggested to shorten the test, and recently SITA SWAP has become available. In this study of 101 patients who were glaucoma suspects or had early disease, SWAP, SITA SWAP, and SITA Fast SAP are compared.

Given that abnormal points are more common in the more challenging SWAP test, the authors require clusters of abnormality for each test to be called abnormal with regard to glaucoma. Using this reasonable and clinically useful criterion, they found that all 3 tests were fairly equivalent (Fig 2).

Given that SWAP is a more difficult test and is not suitable for patients with significant nuclear sclerosis, the findings argue against the widespread incorporation of SWAP in clinical practice. However, with time, more studies on the new SITA SWAP should be forthcoming to confirm or refute the findings of this large and well-designed trial.

J. S. Myers, MD

Improved automated perimetry performance following exposure to Mozart
Fiorelli VM, Kasahara N, Cohen R, et al (Santa Casa of Sao Paulo, Brazil)
Br J Ophthalmol 90:543-545, 2006   3–21

Aim.—To evaluate the performance on automated perimetry (AP) after listening to a Mozart sonata in normal subjects naive to AP.

Methods.—60 naive normal subjects underwent AP (SITA 24-2). The study group (30 subjects) underwent AP after listening to Mozart's Sonata for Two Pianos in D Major and the control group (30 subjects) underwent AP without previous exposure to the music.

Results.—The study group had significantly less fixation loss, false positive, and false negative rates compared to controls ($p < 0.05$).

Conclusion.—Listening to Mozart seems to improve AP performance in normal naive subjects.

▶ This novel study showed better first-time perimetry performance in normal subjects while listening to Mozart's Sonata for Two Pianos in D Major. The music group had fewer fixation losses, false positives, and false negatives.

Whether that would be true for patients with glaucoma, and whether it would be true for experienced testers is unknown. However, I applaud the idea of trying such a simple modification to improve a difficult test.

J. S. Myers, MD

Intravitreal Bevacizumab (Avastin®) in the Treatment of Neovascular Glaucoma
Iliev ME, Domig D, Wolf-Schnurrbursch U, et al (Univ of Bern, Switzerland)
Am J Ophthalmol 142:1054-1056, 2006   3–22

Purpose.—To describe a case series of neovascular glaucoma (NVG) caused by central retinal vein occlusion (CRVO) that was treated with intravitreal bevacizumab (IVB; Avastin®).

Design.—Retrospective interventional case series.

Methods.—Six consecutive patients with NVG and a refractory, symptomatic elevation of intraocular pressure (IOP) and pronounced anterior segment congestion received IVB (1.25 mg/0.05 ml). Diode laser cyclophotocoagulation was carried out only if pressure was controlled insufficiently by topical medication. Follow-up examinations occurred at four to 16 weeks.

Results.—IVB resulted in a marked regression of anterior segment neovascularization and relief of symptoms within 48 hours. IOP decreased substantially in three eyes; in the other three eyes, adjuvant cyclophotocoagulation was necessary. No side effects were observed. Panretinal photocoagulation (PRP) was performed as soon as feasible, five to 12 weeks after IVB treatment.

Conclusion.—IVB leads to a rapid regression of iris and angle neovascularization and should be investigated more thoroughly as an adjunct in the management of NVG.

▶ Bevacizumab, an antibody against vascular endothelial growth factor, has gained wide acceptance for posterior segment applications for neovascular conditions such as macular degeneration. Iliev et al detail the potential use of this agent to help regress anterior segment neovascularization, and which, in 3 of 6 NVG eyes, also reduced the IOP.

L. J. Katz, MD

Selective laser trabeculoplasty versus argon laser trabeculoplasty: results from a 1-year randomised clinical trial
Damji KF, Bovell AM, Hodge WG, et al (Univ of Ottawa Eye Inst, Ont, Canada)
Br J Ophthalmol 90:1490-1494, 2006   3–23

Aims.—To compare selective laser trabeculoplasty (SLT) and argon laser trabeculoplasty (ALT), in terms of intraocular pressure (IOP) lowering, in patients with open-angle glaucoma.

Methods.—176 eyes of 152 patients were enrolled in this study, 89 in the SLT and 87 in the ALT groups. Patients were randomised to receive either SLT or ALT treatment to 180° of the trabecular meshwork. Patients were followed up to 12 months after treatment. The main outcome measured was IOP lowering at 12 months after treatment, compared between the SLT and ALT groups.

Results.—No significant difference (p = 0.846) was found in mean decrease in IOP between the SLT (5.86 mm Hg) and ALT (6.04 mm Hg) groups at 1 year or at any other time points, nor were there any significant differences in the rate of early or late complications between the two groups.

Conclusions.—SLT is equivalent to ALT in terms of IOP lowering at 1 year, and is a safe and effective procedure for patients with open-angle glaucoma.

▶ In this good-sized, prospective, randomized study of 176 eyes of 152 patients, good results are seen with both SLT and ALT at 1 year after 180 degrees of treatment. There were no serious complications, and there were no significant differences between the 2 treatments. The success rate at 1 year was about 60% for both treatments.

Over the last half dozen years, there has been much speculation over whether the theoretic benefits of SLT over ALT, less energy and little or no tissue destruction, will translate into clinical benefits. One issue raised by Damji's earlier article[1] was whether SLT was superior to ALT in patients previously treated by ALT. This larger series, although limited in size does not show any evidence to suggest that SLT is superior to ALT with regard to pressure reduction, as shown in the tables. If one tried to "read into" the data that SLT was superior to ALT in patients with previous 360-degree ALT, then one would have to grant that ALT was superior to SLT in patients with previous 180-degree ALT and that SLT worked better in eyes with previous 360-degree ALT than in those without prior ALT. Given the numbers in these groups, the differences are likely chance, and overall, the conclusion has to be that ALT and SLT are fairly equal for all groups in this study.

Studies demonstrating that SLT can be repeated, with good success rates and a good duration of success, have so far not been reported in the peer-reviewed literature, although early reports have been presented at some recent meetings. SLT has clearly proven its equivalency to ALT, but more than 6 years into SLT use we continue to await clear evidence of superiority for repeat treatments.

J. S. Myers, MD

Reference

1. Damji KF, Shah KC, Rock WJ, et al: Selective laser trabeculoplasty v argon laser trabeculoplasty: A prospective randomised clinical trial.*Br J Ophthalmol* 83:718-722, 1999.

4 Cornea

Contact Lens Related Fusarium Keratitis

by Kristin M. Hammersmith, MD

Certainly one of the biggest ophthalmic-related new stories in 2006 was the outbreak of Fusarium keratitis in contact lens wearers. This outbreak, now known to be related the use of Renu with MoistureLoc (multipurpose disinfection solution) taught us several important lessons. First, is the importance of national and international communication. The initial reports of a problem with an increased rate of Fusarium occurred in Singapore in February 2006.[1] Physicians in Singapore noticed an unprecedented number of cases beginning in March of 2005 and alerted Singapore's Ministry of Health in February 2006, when 54 cases had been observed. Rapid data collection allowed investigators to determine that 93.9% of patients used Renu with MoistureLoc, while this product only occupied 30-40% of the market share. Unfortunately, although the solution was manufactured in the same center for distribution in Singapore, Hong Kong and the United States, sales were not suspended in the United States until mid-April of 2006.[2] The number of cases of Fusarium keratitis in the United States peaked in April. Perhaps many cases could have been prevented had the solution been withdrawn from the market earlier.

This outbreak also demonstrated the quick responsiveness of the Centers for Disease Control and Prevention (CDC). In one of the most important articles of the year by Chang et al, the CDC presents the results of the multistate outbreak in the United States.[3] This study presents 164 confirmed cases in the United States between June 1, 2005 and June 30, 2006. A case-control portion of the study analyzed the behaviors of 45 cases and 78 controls. This confirmed that cases were significantly more likely to have used Renu with MoistureLoc. Cases were also more likely to reuse their solutions than controls. Unfortunately, both patients and controls were noncompliant with recommended contact lens practices. As such, we continue to recommend daily disposable (single use) contact lenses in all patients in whom a fit with these lenses is possible. Events of early 2007, specifically the removal of Complete solution due to higher incidence of Acanthamoeba keratitis, support that currently available multipurpose solutions are often ineffective in preventing these infections.

On the clinical side, the recent increase in Fusarium keratitis has given us an opportunity to utilize a new antifungal therapy, voriconazole. We presented our initial case series of 9 patients in whom topical and oral voricon-azole were effective in management.[4] Since that series, we have treated many patients (some related to the MoistureLoc, some not) with this newer medication and had good results. Limitations of this new medicine remain that it is expensive and only available through compounding pharmacies. When taken orally, patients must have liver function tests and the knowledge that it may interact with other oral medications. Despite its limitations, this medication has resulted in medical cures in patients in whom standard antifungal therapy was ineffective.

References

1. Khor W-B, Aung A, Saw S-M, et al: An outbreak of fusarium keratitis associated with contact lens wear in Singapore. *JAMA* 29:2867-2873, 2006.
2. Cohen EJ: Fungal keratitis associated with contact lenses. *Arch Ophthalmol* 125:561-562, 2007.
3. Chang DC, Grant GB, O'Donnell K, et al: Multistate outbreak of Fusarium keratitis associated with use of a contact lens solution. *JAMA* 296:953-963, 2006.
4. Bunya VY, Hammersmith KM, Rapuano CJ, et al: Topical and oral voriconazole in the treatment of fungal keratitis. *Am J Ophthalmol* 143:151-153, 2007.

Long-term Graft Survival in Patients with Down Syndrome after Penetrating Keratoplasty

Wroblewski KJ, Mader TH, Torres MF, et al (Madigan Army Med Ctr, Tacoma, Wash)

Cornea 25:1026-1028, 2006   4–1

Purpose.—To determine graft survival and long-term visual outcome after penetrating keratoplasty (PK) for keratoconus in patients with Down syndrome.

Methods.—The records of all patients with Down syndrome who received PK by the same provider were reviewed. A retrospective analysis was performed to determine long-term graft survival, incidence of graft failure, and complication rate.

Results.—Twenty-one PKs were performed on 18 eyes of 13 patients with Down syndrome with keratoconus. Three repeat PKs were performed for secondary graft failure. All 18 eyes had clear grafts at the most recent examination. Follow-up ranged from 4 to 88 months, with a mean of 34.9 months. The average age of patients was 42 years, with a range of 20 to 63 years. Preoperative visual acuity ranged from 20/160 to count fingers. Postoperatively, visual acuity was objectively measurable in 12 eyes of 8 patients and ranged from 20/30 to 20/200, with a mean of 20/60. Broken sutures and difficulties with unsedated suture removal complicated postoperative care in some patients.

Conclusion.—Clear grafts and improvements in visual acuity can be obtained after PK in patients with Down syndrome, but consideration must be given to careful postoperative care by health care providers and home support personnel.

▶ This was a very good article on a subject that may not get as much attention as it should. That is, how do we best care for our patients with corneal problems and special needs? The challenges of caring for these individuals are familiar: the exam takes longer and is often less accurate, there may be issues of dangerous or self-destructive behaviors, the family or system support for them may be more complicated, etc. On the converse, these are individuals who have other physical challenges and in whom restoration of vision may be very important. When I see these patients, I try to honestly evaluate whether their quality of life is negatively impacted by their reduction in vision. This is accomplished through a discussion with the patient, when possible, and their care providers. When the visual problem, often keratoconus, as is the case in this article, seems to be impacting their ability to participate in a job or job workshops, to enjoy television or sports, or to ambulate, then the best intervention must be sought. I often ask for the assistance of pediatric ophthalmologists to do a cycloplegic refraction, as some patients will be much improved with glasses correction or contact lenses. But, some patients are best helped by keratoplasty.

This article, which evaluates the results of PK on 18 eyes of 13 patients with keratoconus and Down syndrome, gives encouraging results. The authors report a success rate of 83%, with a mean follow-up of just under 3 years. In those with failed grafts, neglected broken sutures were thought to be the culprit. The authors reinforce the importance of close follow-up, which may require additional trips to the operating room (but rarely did in this series), to help in the management. The future of corneal transplantation may involve more adhesives and fewer sutures, which may be especially beneficial in this group.

K. M. Hammersmith, MD

Epidemiological Characteristics of a Chicago-area *Acanthamoeba* Keratitis Outbreak

Joslin CE, Tu EY, McMahon TT, et al (Univ of Illinois at Chicago)
Am J Ophthalmol 142:212-217, 2006   4–2

Purpose.—To characterize *Acanthamoeba* keratitis (AK) cases and analyze the geographical distribution within the Chicago-Gary-Kenosha metropolitan area, Chicago, Illinois, USA.

Design.—Retrospective, population-based cohort study.

Methods.—All AK cases diagnosed at the University of Illinois at Chicago Cornea Service from June 1, 2003, to November 30, 2005, were included in analysis. Patients with keratitis were defined as cases through confocal microscopy, histology, and/or positive cultures. Exploratory analyses were performed to evaluate whether AK cases were unequally distributed geographically. County population data were extracted from US Census 2000 data, and rates were age-standardized to Cook County. Poisson regression analysis was used to estimate the age-standardized rate ratio (RR) between AK cases and county of residence. Current cases (June 1, 2003 to November 30, 2005) were compared with historical cases (June 1, 2000 to November 30,

2002) to determine if the current rate of AK diagnosis differed from historical rates.

Results.—Forty AK cases were diagnosed between June 1, 2003 and November 30, 2005. The average (±SD) age of patients with AK was 28.0 ± 15.0 years (range, 13 to 70 years), 52.5% were men, and 95.0% wore contact lenses. Estimated RR measures demonstrated increased rates for all counties relative to Cook, and were significant for both DuPage County (RR 3.59; 95% confidence interval [95% CI] 1.44, 8.39) and Will County (RR 3.66; 95% CI 1.18 to 9.56). Current AK diagnosis rates were significantly higher than historical rates (RR 6.67; 95% CI 3.05 to 17.52).

Conclusions.—AK cases are increasing in frequency. The increased rates are unevenly distributed in the study area. Further research is warranted to better understand the increase and unusual geographical distribution.

▶ This was a really interesting article, both in its description of the outbreak and in its hypothesis of the etiology. The authors report on 40 cases of AK diagnosed in 30 months in the Chicago area. In Philadelphia, we have seen a similar increase in cases of AK during the same period (2004 through present). This increase has been alarming, as nearly every patient who develops AK is greatly affected by this infection with significant pain and disruption of life. We have observed that all our patients with AK are soft contact lens wearers using multipurpose solutions. Data continue to accumulate that current multipurpose solutions are not effective against *Acanthamoeba*. Hiti et al[1] added more information to this body of literature in 2006 and tested most commercially available multipurpose solutions and found that cysts were still viable in all cases, even after 8 hours of soaking time. This is especially disconcerting given that the newer silicone hydrogel lenses may be even more "sticky" to *Acanthamoeba*.

What was truly unique in the study by Joslin et al was the discussion about the changing US Environmental Protection Agency standards for water disinfection that preceded the outbreak. The compliance deadlines for these changes, which reduced the allowable amount of carcinogenic disinfection byproducts, were January 2002 for large surface water systems and January 2004 for small surface water and group water systems. They found an uneven distribution of cases in their study area, suggesting that users further from treatment may be more likely to have microorganism-contaminated water and *Acanthamoeba*. More data on this will be very interesting and may help explain the increased rates of this troublesome infection.

K. M. Hammersmith, MD

Reference

1. Hiti K, Walochnik J, Haller-Schober EM, et al: Efficacy of contact lens storage solutions against different *Acanthamoeba* strains. *Cornea* 25:423-427, 2006.

Topical Cyclosporine A in Severe Steroid-Dependent Childhood Phlyctenular Keratoconjunctivitis

Doan S, Gabison E, Gatinel D, et al (Hôpital Bichat and Fondation A de Rothschild, Paris)

Am J Ophthalmol 141:62-66, 2006   4–3

Purpose.—To assess the efficacy of topical cyclosporine A (CsA) in children with phlyctenular keratoconjunctivitis associated with severe steroid-dependent corneal inflammation.

Design.—Prospective, noncomparative, interventional case series.

Methods.—PATIENTS: Children with phlyctenular keratoconjunctivitis associated with severe steroid-dependent corneal inflammation and not responding to oral antibiotics (cyclines or erythromycin). INTERVENTION: Topical CsA 2% four times daily, initially combined with topical dexamethasone for the first week. *Main Outcome Measures*: Efficacy was judged by the patients (symptoms and ocular redness) and by the ophthalmologist (ocular redness and corneal inflammation). The patients were monitored for adverse effects, and cyclosporinemia was determined every 3 months.

Results.—We studied 11 children (13 eyes) with a mean age of 9 years (range, 4 to 15 years). Inflammation was controlled in all the eyes within 14 days. Inflammation did not recur during CsA monotherapy, during a mean follow-up of 12 ± 8 months (range, 6 to 31 months). CsA therapy was stopped in eight patients (10 eyes) after a mean treatment duration of 13 ± 9 months (range, 6 to 31 months), and no recurrences occurred during 10 ± 3 months of follow-up (range, 6 to 12 months). Local tolerance of CsA was good. None of the patients had detectable CsA blood levels. CsA was withdrawn in one case after 6 months, because of generalized skin rash.

Conclusions.—Long-term topical CsA 2% therapy is safe and effective in children with phlyctenular keratoconjunctivitis associated with severe steroid-dependent corneal inflammation.

▶ We published data on a large series of children with blepharokeratoconjunctivitis in 2005. The patients in this study are similar to those that we have followed. It is interesting that the authors got such a fantastic response using CsA 2% in these patients. We have had a good response with oral erythromycin, lid hygiene, and interval low-potency steroids. We usually add CsA 0.05% in the management as well. It is unclear why the authors abandoned all other methods and used CsA as monotherapy, but it is impressive that they found control of the inflammation and no recurrences. The most interesting finding was that the patients tolerated the therapy so well. I have used CsA 2% after grafts in pediatric patients, and it is well tolerated, but I am surprised that it was so in these inflamed eyes. I will certainly think of using this in the future, and I look forward to larger randomized studies evaluating these different therapies.

K. M. Hammersmith, MD

Central Corneal Thickness and Corneal Hysteresis Associated With Glaucoma Damage

Congdon NG, Broman AT, Bandeen-Roche K, et al (Johns Hopkins Univ, Baltimore, Md; Johns Hopkins Bloomberg School of Public Health, Baltimore, Md)
Am J Ophthalmol 141:868-875, 2006   4–4

Purpose.—We sought to measure the impact of central corneal thickness (CCT), a possible risk factor for glaucoma damage, and corneal hysteresis, a proposed measure of corneal resistance to deformation, on various indicators of glaucoma damage.

Design.—Observational study.

Methods.—Adult patients of the Wilmer Glaucoma Service underwent measurement of hysteresis on the Reichert Ocular Response Analyzer and measurement of CCT by ultrasonic pachymetry. Two glaucoma specialists (H.A.Q., N.G.C.) reviewed the chart to determine highest known intraocular pressure (IOP), target IOP, diagnosis, years with glaucoma, cup-to-disk ratio (CDR), mean defect (MD), pattern standard deviation (PSD), glaucoma hemifield test (GHT), and presence or absence of visual field progression.

Results.—Among 230 subjects, the mean age was 65 ± 14 years, 127 (55%) were female, 161 (70%) were white, and 194 (85%) had a diagnosis of primary open-angle glaucoma (POAG) or suspected POAG. In multivariate generalized estimating equation models, lower corneal hysteresis value ($P = .03$), but not CCT, was associated with visual field progression. When axial length was included in the model, hysteresis was not a significant risk factor ($P = .09$). A thinner CCT ($P = .02$), but not hysteresis, was associated with a higher CDR at the most recent examination. Neither CCT nor hysteresis was associated with MD, PSD, or GHT "outside normal limits."

Conclusions.—Thinner CCT was associated with the state of glaucoma damage as indicated by CDR. Axial length and corneal hysteresis were associated with progressive field worsening.

▶ This is a thoughtful and well-executed study that seeks to measure the impact of CCT and corneal hysteresis on glaucoma damage. CCT became a standard discussion after the Ocular Hypertension Treatment Study, which found that CCT is an important and independent risk factor for glaucoma damage progression. But, what is this "hysteresis" thing all about? The corneal hysteresis is measured by the Ocular Response Analyzer, which measures the rapid motion of the cornea in response to a short-duration air impulse. The air causes inward corneal deformation (inward applanation), and the cornea then returns from concavity to its normal convex curvature (outward applanation). The difference in these 2 applanation pressures is determined by viscoelastic properties of the corneal shell. (The more stiff the eye, the greater the pressure difference, and the higher the hysteresis value. The more distensible the eye, the lower the pressure difference, and the lower the hysteresis value.) This study found that lower values for hysteresis were associated with visual field progression. How could this knowledge be useful for a cornea specialist? Patients with keratoconus have very low hysteresis. It is the observation of some in our group that patients with keratoconus quietly and quickly can develop visual field loss from glaucoma. This question will be addressed in a pilot study in the near future.

K. M. Hammersmith, MD

Comparative Study of Ocular Herpes Simplex Virus in Patients With and Without Self-Reported Atopy
Rezende RA, Hammersmith K, Bisol T, et al (Federal Univ of Sao Paulo, Brazil; Wills Eye Hosp, Philadelphia; Central Hosp of Brazilian Air-Force, Rio Comprido, Brazil; et al)
Am J Ophthalmol 141:1120-1125, 2006   4–5

Purpose.—To compare the characteristics of ocular herpes simplex virus (HSV) in patients with and without atopy.

Design.—Retrospective cohort comparative study.

Methods.—Patients who presented at the Cornea Service, Wills Eye Hospital, between March 2003 and March 2004 who had been previously diagnosed in the same institution as having ocular HSV diagnosis or were just diagnosed as having the disease were asked to complete a study questionnaire that enabled categorization into atopic and nonatopic. In April 2005, 223 patients who agreed to be in the study had their charts reviewed, and 125 patients were excluded according to exclusion criteria: immunosuppression, follow-up less than one year, previous history of penetrating keratoplasty (PK) out of the Cornea Service, and no active HSV episode during follow-up. MAIN OUTCOME MEASURES: Incidence of all types of HSV recurrences. SECONDARY OUTCOME MEASURES: Bilaterality, visual loss, need for PK, and secondary bacterial infection in both groups. HSV episodes were classified into infectious, inflammatory, and mixed for analysis.

Results.—Ninety eight patients (110 eyes) were included in the study. Atopic/nonatopic (P value): the mean follow-up was 11.6 ($\pm$ 10.6)/8.8 years ($\pm$8.4) ($P = .14$); the mean incidence of HSV episodes per year of follow-up was: total episodes 0.32 ($\pm$ 0.36)/0.28 ($\pm$ 0.33) ($P = .14$), infectious 0.16 ($\pm$ 0.22)/0.10 ($\pm$ 0.14) ($P < .01$), inflammatory 0.11 ($\pm$ 0.19)/0.11 ($\pm$ 0.19) ($P < .01$), and mixed 0.09 ($\pm$ 0.20)/0.07 ($\pm$ 0.16) ($P = .06$); bilateral HSV was present in 9/3 patients ($P = .22$); the mean loss of vision was four lines of Snellen in both groups; PK was performed in 14 of 16 eyes ($P = .45$); secondary bacterial infection was present in two of four eyes ($P = .26$).

Conclusions.—Atopic patients had considerably more infectious and fewer inflammatory episodes when compared with nonatopics.

▶ This is the first of several articles addressing ocular herpes simplex in patients with atopic disease. This article examines the number and types of recurrences of HSV in atopic versus nonatopic patients. It is commonly discussed that people with atopic disease have "worse" HSV. This study attempts to break down the phenotype of HSV outbreaks in these atopic patients versus patients without atopy. Defining atopic disease was our first challenge, as we discovered it was not absolute. We opted to enlist a dermatologist to help us define atopy in our patients. He independently reviewed the patients' questionnaires and was blinded to their ocular pathology. What was quite interesting is that we had more atopic than nonatopic patients. This may represent the tertiary referral practice that we have, but may also reflect the increasing rates of atopy in industrialized nations. What we found was interesting and made scientific sense: the patients with atopic disease had more infectious outbreaks of HSV and fewer immune outbreaks.

It should be noted that the study involved patients receiving no oral antiviral therapy. This helped in our standardization but is not our routine practice (many years of follow-up from these patients were before the HEDS [Herpetic Eye Disease Study], etc). A separate study analyzed the effectiveness of acyclovir in atopic patients versus those without atopic disease.[1] Prophylaxis decreased infectious episodes by 44% in nonatopic patients and by 76% in atopic patients, and decreased inflammatory manifestations by 69% in the nonatopic group and by 8% in the atopic group. We recommend oral antiviral prophylaxis in these patients.

K. M. Hammersmith, MD

Reference

1. Rezende RA, Bisol T, Hammersmith K, et al: Efficacy of oral antiviral prophylaxis in preventing ocular herpes simplex virus recurrences in patients with and without self-reported atopy. *Am J Ophthalmol* 142:563-567, 2006.

Herpes Zoster Ophthalmicus in Otherwise Healthy Children

De Freitas D, Martins EN, Adan C, et al (Federal Univ of São Paulo, Brazil; Massachusetts Eye and Ear Infirmary, Boston)
Am J Ophthalmol 142:393-399, 2006   4–6

Purpose.—To evaluate the complications of herpes zoster ophthalmicus (HZO) in children.

Design.—Prospective-observational case series.

Methods.—Ten healthy patients (five boys, five girls) with HZO were prospectively followed. Data regarding best-corrected visual acuity, biomicroscopy, intraocular pressure, corneal sensitivity, and funduscopy were collected. The median duration of follow-up was 19 months (range eight to 78 months).

Results.—The mean age at presentation was 8.7 years (range two to 14 years ±3.95). At last visit, two patients (20%) had decreased visual acuity and nine (90%) had some degree of abnormal corneal sensitivity and corneal opacity despite good final visual acuity.

Conclusion.—In general, HZO seems to have a good prognosis in healthy children; nonetheless, some cases can present severe eye complications causing visual loss.

▶ The question of when to do a workup for immunosuppression in a patient who presents with HZO is controversial. I was in medical school in the late 1990s when HIV rates were soaring. I was taught that an immunosuppressive workup, especially HIV testing, was indicated in all patients with shingles who were younger than 40 years. We recently had a discussion about this at a monthly cornea meeting, and I was surprised that my older partners did not have the same mindset. This series presents immunocompetent children with HZO. The authors note that many series have reported on healthy children with zoster. In fact, a local pediatrician reported to me that immune workups are not routinely done in kids with zoster. These children do need systemic antivirals at presentation, and a discussion with the child's pediatrician about the findings and medications still seems prudent.

The discussion section of the article has several additional interesting points, including the reminder that children who have varicella during the first year of life develop zoster at an increased incidence (4.1/1000 patient-years vs 0.45/1000 patient-years in those who have varicella after the first year of life). The authors also discuss that zoster appears to be less common in pediatric patients who have had the varicella vaccine than in pediatric patients who have not. It will be interesting to see how this vaccine, along with the new adult shingles vaccine, may greatly reduce the occurrence of this very frustrating disease.

K. M. Hammersmith, MD

Efficacy of Topical Cyclosporine 0.05% for Prevention of Cornea Transplant Rejection Episodes
Price MO, Price FW Jr (Cornea Research Found of America, Indianapolis, Ind; Price Vision Group, Indianapolis, Ind)
Ophthalmology 113:1785-1790, 2006   4–7

Purpose.—To assess the incidence of immunologic corneal graft rejection episodes in a prospective case series of patients treated 4 times a day with topical cyclosporine 0.05%.

Design.—Prospective, single-center, institutional review board–approved study.

Participants.—Fifty-two cornea transplant recipients considered low risk for graft rejection.

Methods.—Primary indications for transplantation were keratoconus, Fuchs' dystrophy, or nonherpetic, nonvascularized scars. Subjects completely tapered off prednisolone acetate 1% by 13 weeks after transplantation and used topical cyclosporine 0.05% 4 times a day, beginning either 1 or 10 weeks posttransplant, with use continued until 1 year posttransplant. One subgroup supplemented cyclosporine use with pulsed prednisolone acetate 1% dosing, 4 times a day for 4 days every 6 weeks. The incidence of immunologic corneal graft rejection episodes was compared with that in Fuchs' and keratoconus historical control subjects, who used topical steroids a median of 7 months after penetrating keratoplasty.

Main Outcome Measure.—Incidence of immunologic graft rejection episodes.

Results.—Graft rejection episodes occurred earlier and with higher incidence in subjects using cyclosporine 0.05% compared with historical control subjects who used steroids for a longer period of time ($P<0.0001$). Cyclosporine subjects who pulse-dosed prednisolone had a significantly higher incidence of graft rejection compared with those who did not pulse steroids ($P = 0.04$).

Conclusion.—The results suggest that 4 times daily dosing with topical cyclosporine 0.05% is not as effective as use of topical prednisolone acetate 1% for prevention of graft rejection episodes in low-risk corneal transplants, and that periodic pulsing with corticosteroids may increase the risk of rejection episodes.

▶ The concept of using topical cyclosporine as a steroid-sparing agent in young patients after corneal transplantation is an exciting one. Unfortunately, the study design presented in this article was very disappointing and does not allow for conclusions about the efficacy of adjunctive cyclosporine A 0.05% in treating posttransplant patients. Patients were treated with prednisone acetate 1% four times a day for 10 weeks, at which point the steroids were tapered off over a 1-month period and cyclosporine 0.05% (Restasis) was initiated. Group A then received cyclosporine alone (4 times a day), and group B received cyclosporine (4 times a day) and was pulsed with steroids every 6 weeks for 4 days at a time. Not surprisingly, patients had higher rates of rejection than in previous studies. Interestingly, the group that received the pulsed steroids had an even higher rate of rejection than the one receiving cyclosporine alone. The authors note that their patients historically use topical steroids for a median of 7 months, but they tapered the patients off at 14 weeks in this study. From this, we know that cyclosporine, even at 4 times a day, is not a replacement for prednisone acetate or the like, but most of us didn't think it was. A more useful question is, does adjunctive cyclosporine lower our rates of rejection when we treat patients with our standard tapering regimen?

K. M. Hammersmith, MD

Results from the Multicenter Boston Type 1 Keratoprosthesis Study
Belin MW, for the Boston Type 1 Keratoprosthesis Study Group (Albany Med College, NY)
Ophthalmology 113:1779-1784, 2006   4–8

Purpose.—To report indications, practices, complications, and outcomes from the first multicenter study on the Boston Type 1 keratoprosthesis.

Design.—Prospective, noncomparative, interventional case series.

Participants.—We analyzed 141 Boston Type 1 keratoprosthesis surgical procedures, from 17 surgical sites, done from January 2003 through September 2005 in 136 eyes of 133 patients.

Methods.—Forms reporting 70 preoperative, intraoperative, and postoperative parameters were collected and analyzed at a central data collection site (Cornea Consultants of Albany, Albany Medical College, Albany, New York).

Main Outcome Measures.—Visual acuity (VA) and keratoprosthesis survival.

Results.—Common preoperative diagnoses were graft rejection, in 73 eyes (54%) (average prior grafts, 2.24); chemical injury (20 eyes [15%]); bullous keratopathy (19 eyes [14%]); and herpes simplex virus keratitis (9 eyes [7%]). Additionally, 82 eyes (60%) had preoperative glaucoma. Preoperative best-corrected VA ranged from 20/100 to light perception, and was <20/200 in 96% of eyes. At an average follow-up of 8.5 months (range, 0.03-24; standard deviation, 6.1; median, 12), postoperative vision improved to ≥20/200 in 57%. Among eyes at least 1 year after the operation (62 eyes), vision was ≥20/200 in 56% of eyes and ≥20/40 in 23%. At an average follow-up of 8.5 months, graft retention was 95%. Severe visual loss or failure to improve from keratoprosthesis was usually secondary to comorbidities such as advanced glaucoma, macular degeneration, or retinal detachment.

Conclusions.—The Boston Type 1 keratoprosthesis seems, based on early follow-up, to be a viable option after multiple failed corneal grafts or in some situations of a poor prognosis for primary penetrating keratoplasty.

▶ This was a nice collection of data on patients over a period of more than 2 years from many sites performing the Boston keratoprosthesis. The visual rehabilitation in patients was impressive, with the percentage of patients with best-corrected VA of 20/200 or better increasing from 3.6% preoperatively to 57% postoperatively; almost 20% of patients reached best-corrected VA of 20/40 or better. It should be reinforced that the indication for surgery affects the success rate, with multiple graft failures having the best chance for great visual outcomes. Unfortunately, patients with ocular cicatricial pemphigoid and Stevens-Johnson syndrome did less well, although the numbers are quite small in this study. One shortcoming of this study is that more than 50% of those implanting the Boston keratoprosthesis did not respond to the inquiry for data collection. It is certainly possible that those with less than optimal outcomes did not share their data, leaving the impression of a more favorable outcome than truly observed. In our experience, the Boston keratoprosthesis is very exciting. Many of our patients have had excellent visual outcomes in a short recovery period. However, as our experience grows, we have seen a few more complications; 2 patients have developed endophthalmitis, and some have progressive thinning and inflammation, leaving the fate of the keratoprosthesis unclear. The database presented in this article is important, as collective experience will help us learn more about these implants.

K. M. Hammersmith, MD

Salzmann's Nodular Corneal Degeneration Clinical Characteristics and Surgical Outcomes

Farjo AA, Halperin GI, Syed N, et al (Davis Duehr Dean, Madison, Wis; Univ of Iowa, Iowa City; Uniformed Services Univ of the Health Sciences, Bethesda, Md; et al)
Cornea 25:11-15, 2006   4–9

Purpose.—To characterize the clinical characteristics and surgical outcomes for Salzmann's nodular corneal degeneration (SNCD).

Methods.—In this retrospective, noncomparative, observational case series, all patients coded with a diagnosis of SNCD between January 1, 1996, and April 30, 2002 were included. Cases whose clinical description did not match the classic description of this disorder were excluded. Clinical characteristics, surgical procedures, and qualitative outcomes were recorded.

Results.—Among 103 patients diagnosed with SNCD, 93 (152 eyes) met inclusion criteria. Eighty-three patients (89.2%) were women ($P < 0.00001$), and 59 patients (63.4%) had bilateral disease. A normal age distribution was noted, with a mean age of 54.3 years (median, 53 years; standard deviation = 16.9). Meibomian gland dysfunction was noted in 51 patients (54.8%), contact lens wear in 31 patients (33.3%), peripheral vascularization in 29 patients (31.2%), pterygium in 15 patients (16.1%), keratoconjunctivitis sicca in 9 patients (9.7%), and exposure keratitis in 4 patients (4.3%). Forty-nine eyes (32.2%) of 37 patients (39.8%) required a total of 62 surgical procedures. Impaired vision led to 53 (85.5%) of these procedures and resulted in improved vision in 42 (79.2%) of these cases. Seven eyes (4.6%) underwent surgical intervention for subjective discomfort or contact lens intolerance, and all had improved symptoms at last follow-up.

Conclusions.—SNCD appears to be a disorder that occurs predominantly in middle-aged women and may be associated with chronic ocular surface inflammation and/or irritation. It is important to diagnose properly because of the good prognosis with medical and surgical therapy.

▶ SNCD is not an uncommon condition for a cornea specialist; however, not much is written on the subject. This case series, which represents the largest one to date, reports on 103 patients with SNCD. As is commonly seen in our practice, the female preponderance is impressive. Further studies to assess the hormonal relationship to this hypertrophic growth may be interesting. The authors note significant posterior blepharitis in more than half of the patients. This is an important finding, as treatment of blepharitis often helps ease the discomfort noted by these patients. This medical therapy may prevent the need for a surgical intervention. Most of the patients who underwent surgical intervention did so because of visual concerns, not because of discomfort.

K. M. Hammersmith, MD

Histology of Dislocations in Endothelial Keratoplasty (DSEK and DLEK): A Laboratory-Based, Surgical Solution to Dislocation in 100 Consecutive DSEK Cases

Terry MA, Hoar KL, Wall J, et al (Devers Eye Inst, Portland, Ore; Lions Vision Research Lab of Oregon, Portland)
Cornea 25:926-932, 2006   4–10

Purpose.—Laboratory studies were performed to evaluate the histologic differences between the recipient bed after deep lamellar endothelial keratoplasty (DLEK) surgery and Descemet's-stripping endothelial keratoplasty (DSEK) surgery. Relevant new surgical strategies to prevent dislocation in DSEK surgery were initiated in our first 100 consecutive clinical cases.

Methods.—Ten pairs of cadaver eyes had a DLEK in 1 eye and a DSEK in the fellow eye, and the posterior stromal surface was analyzed by scanning electron microscopy at ×50 magnification. Based on the findings in these cadaver eyes, our DSEK procedure was modified to include surgical roughening in the peripheral recipient bed in 100 consecutive eyes. One hundred percent of these eyes were followed for at least 60 days after surgery to determine the rate of donor dislocation.

Results.—In all 10 pairs of cadaver eyes, the DSEK stromal interface showed a smoother surface than DLEK eyes, without the presence of cut stromal fibrils. The DLEK surface was less smooth than the DSEK eyes, but with the presence of uniformly cut fibrils over the entire surface. Subsequent surgical modifications to the DSEK procedure to include scraping and roughening of the recipient peripheral bed in humans resulted in only a 4% (4/100) dislocation rate of the donor tissue into the anterior chamber. One of these 4 dislocated donors was seen on the first postoperative day and was the only primary graft failure in the series. The other 3 cases were fully attached on the first postoperative day with no interface fluid, but they dislocated later on postoperative days 2, 3, and 4.

Conclusion.—The high rate of dislocation of the donor disc in DSEK may be caused by the absence of recipient stromal fibrils to initially bind to the donor stromal fibrils. Clinical success with a surgical technique of selectively scraping the peripheral recipient bed to promote donor edge adhesion (while leaving the central bed untouched for vision) may aid in the prevention of donor dislocation in DSEK surgery. Reduction of dislocation in DSEK surgery has also been associated with a reduced rate of iatrogenic primary graft failure (PGF) to 1%.

▶ Last year, I wrote about the excitement surrounding the innovations in lamellar keratoplasty, especially the innovative new surgery DSEK. This year DSEK continues to be a popular topic at national and international meetings, as well as in the literature. From personal observation and public discussion, 2 things seem clear about DSEK: It is great when it works, but it doesn't always work.

The adherence of the thin posterior lamellar graft to the posterior stroma is the "make it or break it" part of this surgery. This article addresses maneuvers that Mark Terry, who used to be the champion of DLEK and has now converted to DSEK, has undertaken to minimize dislocations. He recommends using a scraper to roughen the surface and promote adhesion. While this procedure is very exciting, the manipulation required to perform this surgery, and to reposition, if needed, may decrease the endothelial cell counts. In addition, reinflating the anterior chamber with air in the office, a nonsterile environment, may increase the risk of endophthalmitis. Long-term data are necessary to monitor the survival and infection rates of these grafts.

K. M. Hammersmith, MD

Descemet's Stripping with Endothelial Keratoplasty: Comparative Outcomes with Microkeratome-Dissected and Manually Dissected Donor Tissue
Price MO, Price FW Jr (Cornea Research Found of America, Indianapolis, Ind; Price Vision Group, Indianapolis, Ind)
Ophthalmology 113:1936-1942, 2006   4–11

Purpose.—To compare outcomes with 2 donor dissection methods for Descemet's stripping with endothelial keratoplasty (DSEK).

Design.—Retrospective, comparative, nonrandomized case series.

Participants.—Three hundred thirty consecutive transplants, 114 with manually dissected and 216 with microkeratome-dissected donor tissue.

Methods.—Donor posterior stroma/endothelium was transplanted, after stripping recipient Descemet's membrane/endothelium and dissecting the donor tissue by hand or with a microkeratome.

Main Outcome Measures.—Incidences of donor perforation and donor detachment were compared for all eyes. Visual and refractive outcomes were compared for the first 100 consecutive eyes in each group.

Results.—Visual recovery was faster with microkeratome-dissected donor tissue, as evidenced by statistically better best spectacle-corrected visual acuity (VA) in that group 1 month after surgery ($P = 0.015$). Best spectacle-corrected VA was statistically comparable for the 2 groups preoperatively and 3 and 6 months postoperatively. Best spectacle-corrected VA was not correlated significantly with postoperative central corneal thickness ($P = 0.25$). Corneal thickness was significantly higher in the microkeratome group (690 ± 77 μm, compared with 610 ± 62 μm after hand dissection; $P<0.0001$). Mean refractive astigmatism was 1.5 diopters (D) preoperatively and 6 months postoperatively in both groups. Spherical equivalent refraction did not change in the microkeratome group ($P = 0.64$) but increased by 0.66 D in the hand dissection group ($P = 0.0007$). Methods designed to remove fluid from the donor/recipient graft interface ultimately reduced the detachment rate to <1% (1 in the last 140 cases). No donor perforations occurred in 216 microkeratome dissections, compared with 5 in 114 hand dissections ($P = 0.002$).

Conclusions.—Microkeratome dissection reduced the risk of donor tissue perforation, provided faster visual recovery after DSEK, and did not alter the refractive outcome.

▶ This is another article from a busy DSEK surgeon. He reports excellent results with the microkeratome-dissected tissue when compared with manually dissected tissue. It should be reinforced that the technique evolved in many ways, and the surgeon became more experienced since the first cases, which were manual. Thus, the comparison between the two may not be totally fair since the detachment rate was higher in the manually dissected group. The authors report 2 new techniques that they believe helped reduce the detachment rate—massage with a Lindstrom LASIK roller and fenestration.

K. M. Hammersmith, MD

Top Hat Wound Configuration for Penetrating Keratoplasty Using the Femtosecond Laser: A Laboratory Model
Ignacio TS, Nguyen TB, Chuck RS, et al (Univ of California, Irvine; Johns Hopkins Hosp, Baltimore, Md)
Cornea 25:336-340, 2006   4–12

Purpose.—To evaluate the mechanical stability and induced astigmatism of a modified multiplanar "top hat" wound configuration for full-thickness penetrating keratoplasty (PK) using the femtosecond laser as compared with PK in a laboratory model.

Methods.—Eight human corneoscleral rims were mounted on an artificial anterior chamber. Four samples were assigned to the traditional PK group. Four samples underwent full-thickness keratoplasty with the femtosecond laser: a 9.0-mm cylindrical cut was made from the anterior chamber into the stroma, followed by a ring-shaped (outer diameter 9.0 mm, inner diameter 7.0 mm) horizontal lamellar resection at two-thirds corneal depth and a 7.0-mm cylindrical cut from the lamellae to the corneal surface. Mechanical stability was evaluated after placement of the cardinal sutures and the running sutures.

Results.—In the "top hat" PK group, wound leakage occurred at 19 ± 3.36 mm Hg after placement of the cardinal sutures and at 86.25 ± 9.74 mm Hg after placement of the running sutures. In the traditional PK group, leakage occurred at 0 ± 0 mm Hg and 76.25 ± 20.98 mm Hg after placement of the cardinal sutures and running sutures, respectively. Both techniques induced steepening of the corneal curvature postop. The modified wound group showed a mean change in average K of 3.43 ± 3.62 D, whereas the traditional PK group showed a mean change in average K of 3.21 ± 6.67 D.

Conclusion.—The femtosecond laser-produced "top hat" wound configuration for PK was found to be more mechanically stable than that produced by the traditional method.

▶ At this year's Cornea Society meeting, the use of the femtosecond laser in PK surpassed Descemet's-stripping endothelial keratoplasty (DSEK) in enthusiasm. While this study reports on a laboratory model, using the "top hat" configuration, many have reported on in vivo cases. Several configurations ("top hat," "mushroom," "zig-zag") have been described, each with a special niche given the host. These wounds may be more stable (as described in this article) and may lend more to a "cut and paste" corneal transplant. With overlapping shapes, better incision sealing with looser suture tension may be possible. The downsides to this technology remain the logistics and cost. With regard to the former, the recipient and donor corneas are cut with the femtosecond laser, which is typically housed in the refractive surgery area. The patient and donor are then taken to the operating room, where the recipient incision is manually completed and transplantation is performed.

K. M. Hammersmith, MD

Trends in Herpes Simplex Virus Type 1 and Type 2 Seroprevalence in the United States
Xu F, Sternberg MR, Kottiri BJ, et al (Ctrs for Disease Control and Prevention, Atlanta, Ga; Emory Univ, Atlanta, Ga)
JAMA 296:964-973, 2006   4–13

Context.—Herpes simplex virus type 1 (HSV-1) and type 2 are common infections worldwide. Herpes simplex virus type 2 (HSV-2) is the cause of most genital herpes and is almost always sexually transmitted. In contrast, HSV-1 is usually transmitted during childhood via nonsexual contacts. Preexisting HSV-1 antibodies can alleviate clinical manifestations of subsequently acquired HSV-2. Furthermore, HSV-1 has become an important cause of genital herpes in some developed countries.

Objective.—To examine trends in HSV-1 and HSV-2 seroprevalence in the United States in 1999-2004 compared with 1988-1994.

Design, Settings, and Participants.—Cross-sectional, nationally representative surveys (US National Health and Nutrition Examination Surveys [NHANES]), were used to compare national seroprevalence estimates from 1999-2004 with those from 1988-1994, and changes in HSV-1 and HSV-2 seroprevalence since 1976-1980 were reviewed. Persons aged 14 to 49 years were included in these analyses.

Main Outcome Measures.—Seroprevalence of HSV-1 and HSV-2 antibodies based on results from type-specific immunodot assays; diagnosis of genital herpes.

Results.—The overall age-adjusted HSV-2 seroprevalence was 17.0% (95% confidence interval [CI], 15.8%-18.3%) in 1999-2004 and 21.0% (95% CI, 19.1%-23.1%) in 1988-1994, a relative decrease of 19.0% between the 2 surveys (95% CI, −28.6% to −9.5%; *P*<.001). Decreases in HSV-2 seroprevalence were especially concentrated in persons aged 14 to 19 years between 1988 and 2004. In adolescents aged 17 to 19 years and young adults, the decreases in HSV-2 seroprevalence were significant even after adjusting for changes in sexual behaviors. Among those infected with HSV-2, the percentage who reported having been diagnosed with genital herpes was statistically different (14.3% in 1999-2004 and 9.9% in 1988-1994; *P*=.02). Seroprevalence of HSV-1 decreased from 62.0% (95% CI, 59.6%-64.6%) in 1988-1994 to 57.7% (95% CI, 55.9%-59.5%) in 1999-2004, a relative decrease of 6.9% between the 2 surveys (95% CI, −11.6% to −2.3%; *P*=.006). Among persons infected with HSV-1 but not with HSV-2, a higher percentage reported having been diagnosed with genital herpes in 1999-2004 compared with 1988-1994 (1.8% vs 0.4%, respectively; *P*<.001).

Conclusions.—These data show declines in HSV-2 seroprevalence, suggesting that the trajectory of increasing HSV-2 seroprevalence in the United States has been reversed. Seroprevalence of HSV-1 decreased but the incidence of genital herpes caused by HSV-1 may be increasing.

▶ This article is interesting for those of us who treat a lot of patients with HSV. While this article focuses on the decreasing rates of HSV-2, it is notable that HSV-1 seroprevalence is also on the decline. This was most impressive in US-born patients, in whom the HSV-1 seroprevalence decreased by 10% from 59.4% in 1988-1994 to 53.3% in 1999-2004. This decline is a continuation of dropping rates of seroprevalence, when compared with the original NHANES study in 1976-1980. In recent years, we have ordered more HSV titers in patients with stromal keratitis of unknown etiology. The results have been interesting and, when negative, are helpful in management. It was encouraging that the largest decline in HSV-2 seroprevalence was in persons aged 14 to 19 years.

K. M. Hammersmith, MD

Alcohol Delamination of the Corneal Epithelium: An Alternative in the Management of Recurrent Corneal Erosions

Dua HS, Lagnado R, Raj D, et al (Univ of Nottingham, England)
Ophthalmology 113:404-411, 2006   4–14

Purpose.—To investigate the efficacy of alcohol delamination in the management of recurrent corneal erosions (RCEs).

Design.—Prospective single-center consecutive descriptive case series.

Participants.—Twelve patients with RCEs who did not respond to conservative management were treated with alcohol delamination.

Methods.—A consecutive case series of 12 patients with RCEs who did not respond to conservative management were treated by alcohol delamination. A pain score was generated based on a visual analog scale of pain intensity. The duration of pain and frequency were also recorded. Patients were followed up at 1 week, 4 weeks, 3 months, 6 months, and 1 year and then at yearly intervals and monitored for recurrence of symptoms and corneal morphology. The removed epithelial sheet was examined by electron microscopy in 4 patients.

Intervention.—The affected area of epithelium was peeled off after an application of 20% alcohol for 40 seconds under topical anesthesia. Eyes of patients were treated with an antibiotic and preservative-free artificial tear medication, and a bandage contact lens was inserted until epithelial healing was complete.

Main Outcome Measures.—Frequency of recurrence of erosions and duration and intensity of symptoms after alcohol delamination were studied.

Results.—Eleven of the 12 eyes of patients had dramatic relief of symptoms over the follow-up period, ranging from 6 to 40 months. Eight patients were symptom free, and 1 patient had 2 mild symptom episodes in the first posttreatment month before becoming symptom free. The average follow-up period was 23.5 months. There were no residual effects from the application of alcohol noted in any patient. Electron microscopy of removed epithelium showed features of the underlying pathology. The separation of the epithelium occurred at the interface of the subepithelial abnormal deposit and the surface of Bowman's zone.

Conclusion.—Alcohol delamination appears to be a novel, simple, inexpensive treatment for RCEs. Unlike other methods, the removed epithelium is available as a sheet that may be subjected to further examination, though some of the changes observed may reflect the effect of alcohol on the epithelium.

▶ Recurrent erosion syndrome is one of the more maddening ophthalmic conditions, which interrupts patients' sleep and lifestyle. The surgical treatments available are pretty good, which make treating these patients very rewarding. This article presents a new alternative to anterior stromal puncture (ASP), diamond burr polishing, and phototherapeutic keratectomy (PTK). The authors report that the idea for this treatment came from the observation that retreatment cases of laser epithelial keratomileusis (LASEK) had very adherent epithelium. The major advantage of this procedure is the lack of anterior haze or scarring, as alcohol delamination leaves a very smooth surface. A disadvantage of this technique is the necessity to use an operating microscope, while the other procedures (except PTK) can be done at the slit lamp. This does not offer any advantage over the other procedures in terms of postoperative pain, which is the least attractive part of all the available therapies. Overall, the authors have provided an attractive alternative. Further studies that compare the available treatment options and provide longer follow-up are important to help us provide the best care to these very frustrated patients.

K. M. Hammersmith, MD

The RPS Adeno Detector for Diagnosing Adenoviral Conjunctivitis

Sambursky R, Tauber S, Schirra F, et al (Manatee Sarasota Eye Clinic & Laser Ctr, Bradenton, Fla; St Johns Ophthalmology Clinic, Springfield, Mo; Universitätsklinikum des Saarlandes, Homburg, Germany; et al)
Ophthalmology 113:1758-1764, 2006   4–15

Purpose.—To compare the sensitivity, specificity, and accuracy of the RPS Adeno Detector (Rapid Pathogen Screening Inc., South Williamsport, PA) against both viral cell culture with confirmatory immunofluorescence staining (CC-IFA) and the polymerase chain reaction (PCR) for diagnosing adenoviral conjunctivitis.

Design.—Prospective, nonrandomized, masked, multicenter clinical trial.

Participants.—One hundred eighty-six consecutive patients from 5 clinical centers seeking treatment within 1 week of developing a red eye and thought to have acute conjunctivitis.

Methods.—The RPS Adeno Detector is a 10-minute in-office lateral flow immunoassay. Patients were tested with the RPS Adeno Detector, CC-IFA, and PCR to detect the presence of adenovirus.

Main Outcome Measures.—The sensitivity, specificity, and accuracy of the RPS Adeno Detector were assessed for identifying cases of adenoviral conjunctivitis.

Results.—Compared with CC-IFA, the RPS Adeno Detector was 88% sensitive and 91% specific at detecting adenoviral conjunctivitis. Using PCR as a reference method, the sensitivity of the RPS Adeno Detector increased to 89% and the specificity increased to 94%. Compared with PCR, CC-IFA was found to be 91% as sensitive and 100% as specific.

Conclusions.—The RPS Adeno Detector demonstrated sufficient sensitivity and specificity to be used in the physician's office for the detection of adenoviral conjunctivitis.

▶ This article reports on an exciting new office-based diagnostic test for adenovirus. This test, which has impressive sensitivity and specificity, may be especially helpful in the primary care doctor's office. It will help decrease the administration of unnecessary antibiotics and provide documentation for school and work excuses. We were part of this study and have found the test very easy to use (much like a pregnancy test). The technology also has potential to diagnose other infections such as herpes simplex virus, varicella-zoster virus, and chlamydia, which may spread its worldwide usefulness.

K. M. Hammersmith, MD

5 Retina

Early Results for VEGF Inhibitors for ARMD

by James F. Vander, MD

Years ago, US Surgeon General, William Stewart, upon considering the development of antibiotics, boldly told the US Congress it was time to "close the books on infectious diseases."

Although perhaps not quite in the same league as pestilence and plague, age-related macular degeneration is undoubtedly a major public health issue in the United States in the 21st century. Until very recently our treatments for age-related macular degeneration (ARMD) were only marginally better than bloodletting. With the development of ranibizumab (Lucentis) and recognition of the utility of bevacizumab (Avastin) we now have therapeutic options that can provide genuine hope for physicians and patients alike, and especially for patients with wet ARMD. Of course, there is still nothing to offer the many patients with large areas of geographic atrophy or pre-existing disciform scars. Nevertheless, for those individuals with early exudative ARMD, there is finally reason to hope for, if not expect, stabilization or even meaningful improvement of vision.

As we review the retina literature for 2006, we see many articles concerning the growing experience with these vascular endothelial growth factor (VEGF) inhibitors in the treatment of ARMD. The range of papers is broad, as one would expect. There are multiple larger reports, some well controlled and prospective, including the primary projects which earned FDA approval for ranibizumab, finally making it into print. There are smaller retrospective pilot studies assessing various sub-groups and combination treatment strategies. The sub-group analysis reflects the diversity of ARMD, with lesion size and character among the principle variables to consider. The use of combination treatment strategies, however, reflects a recognition of the realities of anti-VEGF treatment for wet ARMD.

Most patients with wet ARMD will demonstrate a response to intravitreal bevacizumab or ranibizumab. In many cases this response is quite dramatic. The macular appearance a few weeks after the first or second injection will show substantial reduction in fluid and the reduction in activity is confirmed on OCT and fluorescein angiography. Patients will often report a significant reduction in metamorphopsia and improvement in overall vision. Although not invariable, this sequence of events is common.

The problem arises after the 3rd, 5th, or 10th injection. At some point the therapeutic response typically plateaus, sometimes with complete resolution of fluid, sometimes not. Sometimes the intraretinal fluid is gone but the sub-retina pigment epithelial (RPE) fluid is not. There is some evidence to suggest that patients who receive monthly injections, even if the macula is by all assessments dry, do a little better than those for whom the injections are halted. Whether this advantage is real and sufficiently large to offset the expense, inconvenience and risk of sustaining the injections remains controversial. Many experienced physicians will stop injecting after a period of time and watch, resuming treatment at the first sign of relapse.

The bigger question is, what happens after year 2 or 3? Will most patients remain free of exudation after a certain number of injections (whatever that number is), or will we be maintaining patients on periodic injections for life? This is where the notion of combination treatments comes in. As with the immediate enthusiasm of the 1940s when antibiotics first came in to popular use, the honeymoon period lasts a short while before reality sets in. Development of drug resistance to antibiotics has led to the use of combination drug strategies and forced the development of newer, stronger drugs. Similarly, our justifiable excitement over new anti-VEGF drugs is now moving to what happens after the honeymoon. Sadly, we are not yet ready to "close the book" on vision loss from macular degeneration.

Diabetes

Effect of Ruboxistaurin on Visual Loss in Patients with Diabetic Retinopathy
Aiello LP, for the PKC-DRS2 Group (Harvard Med School, Boston; et al)
Ophthalmology 113:2221-2230, 2006   5–1

Objective.—To evaluate the effect of ruboxistaurin, an orally administered protein kinase C β (PKC β) isozyme-selective inhibitor, on vision loss in patients with diabetes.

Design.—Thirty-six-month, randomized, double-masked, placebo-controlled, parallel, multicenter trial.

Participants.—Six hundred eighty-five patients randomized at 70 clinical sites.

Methods.—Ophthalmologic examination was performed at screening and at each 3-month visit. Retinopathy status was assessed every 6 months with Early Treatment Diabetic Retinopathy Study (ETDRS) standard 7-field 30° color stereoscopic fundus photography. Levels of diabetic retinopathy and diabetic macular edema were determined by 2 independent graders masked to site and treatment assignment, with additional independent adjudication as required. Eligible patients had a best-corrected visual acuity (VA) score of ≥ 45 letters, retinopathy level ≥ 47A and ≤ 53E, and no prior panretinal photocoagulation in at least one eye.

Main Outcome Measure.—Effect of oral ruboxistaurin (32 mg/day) on reduction of sustained moderate visual loss (≥15-letter decrease in ETDRS VA score maintained ≥6 months) in patients with moderately severe to very severe nonproliferative diabetic retinopathy.

Results.—Sustained moderate visual loss occurred in 9.1% of placebo-treated patients versus 5.5% of ruboxistaurin-treated patients (40% risk reduction, $P = 0.034$). Mean VA was better in the ruboxistaurin-treated patients after 12 months. Baseline–to–end point visual improvement of ≥ 15 letters was more frequent (4.9% vs. 2.4%) and ≥ 15-letter worsening was less frequent (6.7% vs. 9.9%) in ruboxistaurin-treated patients relative to placebo ($P = 0.005$). When clinically significant macular edema was >100 µm from the center of the macula at baseline, ruboxistaurin treatment was associated with less frequent progression of edema to within 100 µm (68% vs. 50%, $P = 0.003$). Initial laser treatment for macular edema was 26% less frequent in eyes of ruboxistaurin-treated patients ($P = 0.008$).

Conclusion.—Oral ruboxistaurin treatment reduced vision loss, need for laser treatment, and macular edema progression, while increasing occurrence of visual improvement in patients with nonproliferative retinopathy.

▶ This is the latest report regarding this promising drug being developed for the treatment of complications of diabetes, particularly diabetic retinopathy. It is a multicenter, double-blinded, randomized, phase III clinical trial of 685 patients who received either this PKC β inhibitor or placebo over the course of 3 years. Eligible patients had moderate nonproliferative retinopathy. The drug is well tolerated and does have a measurable effect on maculopathy. Patients had a reduction in progression of macular edema, were less likely to need focal laser, and had a reduction in the rate of vision loss due to macular edema. The rate of vision loss in the treated group was 5.5% versus 9.1% in the control group. It is important to realize that the event rate in the control group is fairly low. Therefore, a large number of patients must be treated to demonstrate a therapeutic benefit for a relatively small number of patients, at least over a 3-year time frame. Given the huge issues of cost of treatment and compliance in the management of diabetes, it is not clear yet where this drug, once approved, will fit into the regimen for managing diabetic patients. While longer-term data may show a more substantial benefit with widespread usage among diabetics, at this stage treatment may be more appropriate just for those with existing retinopathy of a moderate degree.

J. F. Vander, MD

Diabetic macular edema associated with glitazone use

Ryan EH Jr, Han DP, Ramsay RC, et al (VitreoRetinal Surgery, PA, Minneapolis, Minn)
Retina 26:562-570, 2006   5–2

Purpose.—To describe diabetic macular edema (DME) in patients who developed fluid retention as a consequence of glitazone use.

Methods.—A chart review identified 30 patients who used pioglitazone or rosiglitazone and had both lower extremity edema and macular edema. Clinical reports, photographs, and fluorescein angiograms were reviewed. Patients followed for >3 months were analyzed separately.

Results.—Seventeen patients took oral pioglitazone, 11 took rosiglitazone, and 2 took both drugs at different times. Eleven patients were observed for >3 months after cessation of glitazones. Mean weight gain during drug administration in this group was 30 lb, and mean weight loss after drug discontinuation was 19 lb. Rapid reduction in macular edema off drug occurred in only 4 of 11 patients, but 8 of 11 had reduced edema over 2 years. Mean visual acuity in this group at the initial visit was 20/60, and at the final visit, it was 20/85. Four eyes of three patients had resolution of diffuse macular edema with improved vision after cessation of glitazones without laser treatment.

Conclusions.—Fluid retention occurs in 5% to 15% of patients taking glitazones. In some of these patients, glitazone use appears to be a cause of macular edema, and drug cessation appears to result in rapid resolution of both peripheral and macular edema. Fluid retention associated with glitazone use should be considered when assessing treatment options for patients with DME, especially those with concomitant peripheral edema.

▶ Glitazones are widely used drugs prescribed for glycemic control either as monotherapy or in combination with oral agents or insulin. Two drugs, rosiglitazone (Avandia) and pioglitazone (Actos), are commonly used in the United States. This study is a retrospective chart review of patients with a combination of macular edema and lower extremity edema associated with the use of a glitazone. The most important aspect of the report is the effect of drug withdrawal on patients with macular edema. There are only 11 patients with follow-up ≥3 months off drug, so it is difficult to draw precise conclusions. Nevertheless, some interesting results were reported. Four of 11 patients had rapid reduction in macular edema on drug cessation with no other intervention. Eight of 11 had reduction in edema over 2 years. Although factors such as renal failure or cardiac failure must also be considered, one should consider stopping glitazone usage for patients with macular edema, especially if associated with lower extremity edema or if not responsive to focal laser.

J. F. Vander, MD

Intravitreal Triamcinolone for Refractory Diabetic Macular Edema: Two-Year Results of a Double-Masked, Placebo-Controlled, Randomized Clinical Trial
Gillies MC, Sutter FKP, Simpson JM, et al (Univ of Sydney, Australia)
Ophthalmology 113:1533-1538, 2006   5–3

Objective.—To report 2-year safety and efficacy outcomes from a trial of intravitreal triamcinolone acetonide (TA) injections (4 mg) in eyes with diabetic macular edema and impaired vision that persisted or recurred after laser treatment.

Design.—Prospective, double-masked, placebo-controlled, randomized clinical trial.

Participants and Controls.—Sixty-nine eyes of 43 patients were entered into the study, with 34 eyes randomized to receive active treatment and 35 placebo. Two-year data were available for 60 of 69 (87%) eyes of 35 of 41 (85%) patients; 9 eyes of 6 patients were lost to follow-up, of which 6 received a placebo and 3 received intravitreal TA.

Intervention.—Triamcinolone acetonide (0.1 ml) was injected through the pars plana using a 27-gauge needle. Eyes randomized to placebo received a subconjunctival injection of saline.

Main Outcome Measures.—Improvement of best-corrected logarithm of the minimum angle of resolution visual acuity (VA) by ≥ 5 letters after 2 years and incidence of moderate or severe adverse events.

Results.—Improvement of ≥ 5 letters' best-corrected VA was found in 19 of 34 (56%) eyes treated with intravitreal TA, compared with 9 of 35 (26%) eyes treated with the placebo ($z_{generalized\ estimating\ equation} = 2.73$, $P = 0.006$). The mean improvement in VA was 5.7 letters (95% confidence interval, 1.4–9.9) more in the intravitreal TA–treated eyes than in those treated with the placebo. An increase of intraocular pressure (IOP) of ≥ 5 mmHg was observed in 23 of 34 (68%) treated versus 3 of 30 (10%) untreated eyes ($P<0.0001$). Glaucoma medication was required in 15 of 34 (44%) treated versus 1 of 30 (3%) untreated eyes ($P = 0.0002$). Cataract surgery was performed in 15 of 28 (54%) treated versus 0 of 21 (0%) untreated eyes ($P<0.0001$). Two eyes in the intravitreal TA–treated group required trabeculectomy. There was one case of infectious endophthalmitis in the treatment group.

Conclusion.—Intravitreal TA improves vision and reduces macular thickness in eyes with refractory diabetic macular edema. This beneficial effect persists for up to 2 years with repeated treatment. Progression of cataract and elevation of IOP commonly occur but appear manageable. Spontaneous improvement over years can still occur in eyes that are apparently severely affected by diabetic macular edema.

▶ It has now been several years since the first reported use of intravitreal steroid injection for the treatment of diabetic macular edema. Nearly all the prior reports were case reports, small series, or retrospective reviews, and most had limited follow-up. This report describes a fairly large number of patients studied in a prospective, randomized clinical trial of TA injections, thereby providing a higher quality of data. It turns out, however, that the conclusions are, for the most part, confirmatory rather than transformative. A majority of patients will demonstrate a reduction in macular edema, which is usually temporary. Repeat injections are needed for sustained effect. Progression of cataract is likely, especially with repeated injections. A sizable minority (44% in this report) develop a significant IOP increase, usually manageable with topical medications. Serious reactions such as severe glaucoma or endophthalmitis are uncommon.

J. F. Vander, MD

Macular grid photocoagulation after intravitreal triamcinolone acetonide for diffuse diabetic macular edema

Kang SW, Sa HS, Cho HY, et al (Sungkyunkwan Univ, Seoul, Korea)
Arch Ophthalmol 124:653-658, 2006   5–4

Objective.—To evaluate the clinical outcomes of macular laser photocoagulation after the intravitreal injection of 4 mg of triamcinolone acetonide (IVTA) for diffuse diabetic macular edema (DME).

Methods.—Eighty-six eyes of 74 patients with diffuse DME were randomized into 2 groups. The laser group eyes (n = 48) were subjected to a macular grid laser photocoagulation 3 weeks after IVTA. The control group eyes (n = 38) underwent only IVTA. Both groups were compared with regard to the changes in visual acuity and central macular thickness at 3 weeks, 3 months, and 6 months after IVTA.

Results.—The mean central macular thickness before, 3 weeks after, and 3 and 6 months after IVTA were 538, 250, 295, and 301 μm in the laser group vs 510, 227, 302, and 437 μm in the control group, respectively. The logMAR visual acuities were not significantly different between the 2 groups at baseline and at 3 weeks after IVTA but were significantly better in the laser group at 3 ($P = .02$) and 6 months ($P<.001$) after IVTA.

Conclusions.—Macular laser coagulation effectively maintains improved visual acuity after IVTA for diffuse DME and is believed to reduce recurrent DME after IVTA.

▶ Given the high recurrence rate of macular edema after intravitreal steroid injection (see Abstract 5–3) recent efforts have been directed toward reducing the need for repeated injections by combining therapeutic approaches. In this report, a prospective randomized trial, all patients received steroid injections. The treatment group also received typical focal laser about 2 weeks after the injection. The initial responses were, not surprisingly, similar in the 2 groups. By 6 months, however, the steroid-only group showed a strong tendency for recurrence of edema, whereas the combination treatment patients retained most of the initial therapeutic response. Similarly, visual acuities were better in the combination group at 6 months. What is missing here is longer follow-up, which will be necessary to confirm this report. Nevertheless, a combination of steroid injection, followed shortly thereafter by focal laser may well prove to be the preferred strategy for managing DME if laser alone is not adequate.

J. F. Vander, MD

Intravitreal Injection of Bevacizumab (Avastin) as Adjunctive Treatment of Proliferative Diabetic Retinopathy

Mason JO III, Nixon PA, White MF (Retina Consultants of Alabama, Birmingham; Univ of Alabama at Birmingham School of Medicine)
Am J Ophthalmol 142:685-688, 2006   5–5

Purpose.—To report the use of intravitreal bevacizumab (Avastin) as an adjunctive treatment for proliferative diabetic retinopathy (PDR).

Design.—Retrospective case review.

Methods.—Institutional review board approval to review patient data was obtained for this retrospective study. Three patients underwent intravitreal injection of bevacizumab as part of their treatment for PDR after informed consent was signed. Each patient also underwent fundus photographs before the bevacizumab injection and then one to three weeks after.

Results.—All three patients showed complete regression of their neovascularization elsewhere (NVE) and neovascularization of the disk (NVD) between one and three weeks after injection.

Conclusions.—The speed and degree of neovascular regression after the injection of intravitreal bevacizumab may make this procedure an important adjunctive treatment in the management of selected cases with severe PDR.

Intravitreal Bevacizumab (Avastin) in the Treatment of Proliferative Diabetic Retinopathy

Avery RL, Pearlman J, Pieramici DJ, et al (California Retina Consultants, Santa Barbara; Retina Consultants, Sacramento, Calif)
Ophthalmology 113:1695-1705, 2006   5–6

Purpose.—To report the biologic effect of intravitreal bevacizumab in patients with retinal and iris neovascularization secondary to diabetes mellitus.

Design.—Interventional, consecutive, retrospective, case series.

Participants.—Forty-five eyes of 32 patients with retinal and/or iris neovascularization secondary to diabetes mellitus.

Methods.—Patients received intravitreal bevacizumab (6.2 µg–1.25 mg). Ophthalmic evaluations included nonstandardized Snellen visual acuity (VA), complete ophthalmic examination, fluorescein angiography, and optical coherence tomography.

Main Outcome Measures.—Change in fluorescein angiographic leakage of the proliferative diabetic retinopathy (PDR). Secondary outcomes included changes in Snellen VA.

Results.—No significant ocular or systemic adverse events were observed. All patients with neovascularization demonstrated by fluorescein angiography (44/44 eyes) had complete (or at least partial) reduction in leakage of the neovascularization within 1 week after the injection. Complete resolution of angiographic leakage of neovascularization of the disc was noted in 19 of 26 (73%) eyes, and leakage of iris neovascularization completely resolved in 9 of 11 (82%) eyes. The leakage was noted to diminish as early as 24 hours after injection. In addition to the reduction in angiographic leakage, the neovascularization clinically appeared to involute in many patients with a reduction in the caliber or presence of perfused blood vessels. In 2 cases, a subtle decrease in leakage of retinal or iris neovascularization in the fellow uninjected eye was noted, raising the possibility that therapeutic systemic levels were achieved after intravitreal injection. Recurrence of fluorescein leakage varied. Recurrent leakage was seen as early as 2 weeks in one case, whereas in other cases, no recurrent leakage was noted at last follow-up of 11 weeks.

Conclusions.—Short-term results suggest that intravitreal bevacizumab is well tolerated and associated with a rapid regression of retinal and iris neovascularization secondary to PDR. A consistent biologic effect was noted, even with the lowest dose (6.2 µg) tested, supporting proof of concept. The observation of a possible therapeutic effect in the fellow eye raises concern that systemic side effects are possible in patients undergoing treatment with intravitreal bevacizumab (1.25 mg), and lower doses may achieve a therapeutic result with less risk of systemic side effects. Further study is indicated.

▶ These reports (Abstracts 5–5 and 5–6) are just 2 of the numerous articles that appeared this year regarding the use of bevacizumab (Avastin) for the treatment of disc, retinal, and iris neovascularization in proliferative retinopathy, particularly diabetes. The drug is a potent vascular endothelial growth factor (VEGF) inhibitor, which is approved by the Food and Drug Administration (FDA) for the treatment of colorectal carcinoma. Its off-label use in the eye was first described in age-related macular degeneration but, given the important role of VEGF in the progression of proliferative retinopathy, it also has application in diabetic patients.

The first article by Mason et al (Abstract 5–5) presents 3 patients with an impressive resolution of NVD and NVE between 1 and 3 weeks after injection.

The report by Avery et al (Abstract 5–6) presents a sizable series, 45 eyes in 32 patients, and in every case, there was at least a partial reduction in neovascular activity by 1 week. This response included retinal and iris neovascularization. Not all cases showed complete resolution of neovascularization and in those patients with preexisting fibrosis, only the vascular part of the proliferation regressed. Furthermore, the follow-up is very limited, with less than 3 months reported, so the long-term efficacy and the need for reinjection remain uncertain.

J. F. Vander, MD

A Pilot Study of Multiple Intravitreal Injections of Ranibizumab in Patients with Center-Involving Clinically Significant Diabetic Macular Edema

Chun DW, Heier JS, Topping TM, et al (Ophthalmic Consultants of Boston; Tufts–New England Med Ctr, Boston)
Ophthalmology 113:1706-1712, 2006   5–7

Objective.—To evaluate the biologic activity of multiple intravitreal injections of ranibizumab in patients with center-involving clinically significant diabetic macular edema (DME) and to report any associated adverse events.

Design.—Single-center, open-label, dose-escalating pilot study.

Participants.—A total of 10 eyes of 10 patients (mean age, 69.3 years [range, 59–81]) with DME involving the center of the macula and best-corrected visual acuity (BCVA) in the study eye between 20/63 and 20/400.

Intervention.—Three intravitreal injections of ranibizumab (0.3 mg or 0.5 mg each injection) administered on day 0, month 1, and month 2, and observation until month 24.

Main Outcome Measures.—Primary end points were the frequency and severity of ocular and systemic adverse events. Secondary end points were BCVA and measurement of retinal thickness by optical coherence tomography.

Results.—Of the 10 patients enrolled, 5 received 0.3-mg and 5 received 0.5-mg ranibizumab. Intravitreal injections of ranibizumab were well tolerated. No systemic adverse events were reported. Five occurrences of mild to moderate ocular inflammation were reported. At month 3, 4 of 10 patients gained $\geq$15 letters, 5 of 10 gained $\geq$10 letters, and 8 of 10 gained $\geq$1 letters. At month 3, the mean decrease in retinal thickness of the center point of the central subfield was 45.3±196.3 µm for the low-dose group and 197.8±85.9 µm for the high-dose group.

Conclusions.—Ranibizumab appears to be a well-tolerated therapy for patients with DME. This pilot study demonstrates that ranibizumab therapy has the potential to maintain or improve BCVA and reduce retinal thickness in patients with center-involved clinically significant DME.

▶ Vascular endothelial growth factor (VEGF) activity is not only important in the development of proliferative retinopathy, but it also has a role in the progression of exudative retinal vascular disease. In this open-label pilot study, 10 patients received intravitreal injections of ranibizumab (Lucentis)—3 injections were given over 3 months—for the primary treatment of DME. Most patients showed a good reduction in macular edema with only mild side effects, uveitis, developing in some. No conclusions can be drawn about long-term effects, need for reinjection, and how this approach fits into the management of DME at this time. Injection of a VEGF inhibitor, possibly combined with focal laser, will undoubtedly be the subject of many reports in the coming year.

J. F. Vander, MD

Macular Degeneration

Dietary fatty acids and the 5-year incidence of age-related maculopathy
Chua B, Flood V, Rochtchina E, et al (Univ of Sydney Eye Clinic, Westmead, NSW, Australia)
Arch Ophthalmol 124:981-986, 2006   5–8

Objective.—To assess longitudinal associations between dietary fat and incident age-related maculopathy (ARM) in an older, population-based, historical cohort.

Methods.—A total of 3654 persons, 49 years or older, participated in the Blue Mountains Eye Study (1992-1994); 2335 (75.1% of survivors) were reexamined after 5 years (1997-1999). Dietary data were collected from 2895 people (79%) at baseline by means of a semiquantitative food frequency questionnaire to calculate dietary fat intakes. Presence of ARM was graded from retinal photographs (Wisconsin ARM Grading System). Logistic regression adjusted for age, sex, vitamin C intake, and smoking.

Results.—Participants with the highest vs lowest quintiles of n-3 polyunsaturated fat intake had lower risk of incident early ARM (odds ratio [95% confidence interval], 0.41 [0.22-0.75). A 40% reduction of incident early ARM was associated with fish consumption at least once a week (odds ratio [95% confidence interval], 0.58 [0.37-0.90]), whereas fish consumption at least 3 times per week could reduce the incidence of late ARM (odds ratio [95% confidence interval], 0.25 [0.06-1.00]). We found no association between incident ARM and butter, margarine, or nut consumption.

Conclusions.—A regular diet high in n-3 polyunsaturated fat, especially from fish, suggests protection against early and late ARM in this older Australian cohort. Our study could not confirm deleterious effects of higher polyunsaturated fat intakes reported by other clinic-based studies.

Cigarette smoking, fish consumption, omega-3 fatty acid intake, and associations with age-related macular degeneration: the US Twin Study of Age-Related Macular Degeneration
Seddon JM, George S, Rosner B (Harvard Med School, Boston)
Arch Ophthalmol 124:995-1001, 2006   5–9

Objective.—To evaluate modifiable risk and protective factors for age-related macular degeneration (AMD) among elderly twins.

Methods.—The US Twin Study of Age-Related Macular Degeneration comprises elderly male twins from the National Academy of Sciences-National Research Council World War II Veteran Twin Registry. To determine genetic and environmental risk factors for AMD, twins were surveyed for a prior diagnosis of AMD and underwent an eye examination, fundus photography, and food frequency and risk factor questionnaires. This environmental component of the study includes 681 twins: 222 twins with AMD (intermediate or late stages) and 459 twins with no maculopathy or early signs. Risk for AMD according to cigarette smoking and dietary fat intake was estimated using logistic regression analyses.

Results.—Current smokers had a 1.9-fold increased risk (95% confidence interval, 0.99-3.68, P = .06) of AMD while past smokers had about a 1.7-fold increased risk (95% confidence interval, 1.2-2.6, P = .009). Increased intake of fish reduced risk of AMD, particularly for 2 or more servings per week (P trend = .04). Dietary omega-3 fatty intake was inversely associated with AMD (odds ratio, 0.55; 95% confidence interval, 0.32-0.95) comparing the highest vs lowest quartile. Reduction in risk of AMD with higher intake of omega-3 fatty acids was seen primarily among subjects with low levels (below median) of linoleic acid intake, an omega-6 fatty acid (P trend <.001). The attributable risk percentage was 32% for smoking and the preventive fraction was 22% for higher omega-3 intake.

Conclusions.—This study of twins provides further evidence that cigarette smoking increases risk while fish consumption and omega-3 fatty acid intake reduce risk of AMD.

▶ These 2 reports (Abstracts 5–8 and 5–9) are large studies using somewhat different methodologies to come to similar conclusions about the role of diet in the avoidance of progressive AMD in older individuals. The first trial by Chua et al (Abstract 5–8) is part of the Australian Blue Mountains Eye Study looking at 3654 patients over a 5-year period. Baseline characteristics were assessed and then reassessed at a 5-year follow-up visit. Dietary data were obtained by questionnaire. Fish consumption of at least once weekly was associated with a lower rate of early AMD, and fish consumption 3 times per week was associated with a lower rate of advanced ARMD.

The second study by Seddon et al (Abstract 5–9) is not longitudinal but simply a one-time survey of over 1200 twins looking for risk factors associated with AMD. In this particular study, attention was limited to 681 twins, and the data show an apparent protective effect with fish intake, especially if 2 or more servings per week are consumed. Omega-3 fatty intake is inversely proportional to the risk of developing AMD, and as has been shown previously, cigarette smoking is a significant risk factor for developing AMD.

Taken together, these 2 studies lend considerable support to the recommendation that regular consumption of fish, especially those high in omega-3 fatty acids, may help to reduce the development or the progression of AMD.

J. F. Vander, MD

Complement Factor H Increases Risk for Atrophic Age-Related Macular Degeneration

Postel EA, Agarwal A, Caldwell J, et al (Duke Univ Eye Ctr, Durham, NC; Vanderbilt Eye Inst, Nashville, Tenn; Duke Univ Ctr for Human Genetics, Durham, NC; et al)

Ophthalmology 113:1504-1507, 2006   5–10

Objective.—To determine if the complement factor H gene (*CFH*) determines risk for development of geographic atrophy (GA).

Design.—Retrospective case-control study.

Participants and Controls.—The independent case-control data set contained 647 age-related macular degeneration (AMD) cases (grades 3, 4, or 5) and 163 controls (grades 1 or 2).

Methods.—To determine if *CFH* had any effect on determining risk for development of GA in an independent case-control data set of 647 AMD cases and 163 controls, the rs1061170 single-nucleotide polymorphism was tested for association, separating grades and analyzing them independently against the controls. Odds ratios were calculated using standard logistic regression models.

Main Outcome Measures.—The outcome variable was AMD affection status, and genotypes were coded according to a log-additive model.

Results.—There were 407 grade 5, 107 grade 4, 133 grade 3, 35 grade 2, and 128 grade 1 individuals. There was significant association with AMD when comparing grades 3, 4, and 5 versus the controls. The highest odds ratio was obtained when analyzing the grade-4 cases versus the grade-1 controls (OR = 3.217, $P<0.0001$).

Conclusions.—Our results indicate that *CFH* increases the risk of developing GA (grade 4) as well as neovascular (grade 5) and milder (grade 3) disease. Although neovascular disease is responsible for the majority of severe vision loss with AMD, GA is also a significant cause of vision loss, and without effective treatment. Therefore, an attempt to clarify its pathogenesis is of the utmost importance.

Complement Factor H and Macular Degeneration: The Genome Yields an Important Clue

Wiggs JL (Harvard Med School)

Arch Ophthalmol 124:577, 2006   5–11

Background.—The Human Genome Project has provided important tools for understanding the molecular events that predispose to human disease. Information obtained by the Project has played a critical role in 5 recent investigations that have identified complement factor H as an important susceptibility gene for age-related macular degeneration (AMD). A perspective is provided regarding the potential role of complement factor H in the development of AMD.

Overview.—More than 10 million Americans are affected by AMD, which is the leading cause of blindness among elderly persons. This form of macular degeneration is a complex disease that results from interactions between genetic and environmental factors. The risk of macular degeneration is increased with older age, smoking, and excess dietary lipids. The identification of genes that contribute to a common age-related disorder is difficult. The successful identification of complement factor H as a susceptibility factor for AMD was the result of studies that used a newly characterized set of human single-nucleotide polymorphisms (SNPs) that are single-letter variations in a DNA base sequence. Complement factor H is an important regulator of complement activation, which is a major part of the immune reaction against microbial infection. Findings from recent studies have suggested that activation of complement contributes to the development of macular degeneration. Older age and smoking, environmental factors related to AMD, have been shown to increase levels of complement factor H. The relationship between complement factor H and macular degeneration is suggestive of complement activation and inflammation in general as important contributing factors to the disease. However, from a diagnostic perspective, it is not known whether complement factor H is associated with drusen or with neovascularization or both. This is an important distinction because drusen alone do not typically cause severe visual disability, although neovascularization does.

Conclusions.—The discovery of an association between the complement factor H histidine 402 allele and macular degeneration is an important first step toward understanding the underlying molecular pathophysiologic nature of this disease.

▶ The first report (Abstract 5–10) in this pair of articles looks at more than 600 patients with AMD in a case-control method to determine if the presence of the complement factor H gene (CFH) is associated with a higher rate of advanced AMD. The highest association proved to be between the presence of the genotype and grade 4 findings, which were cases of geographic atrophy. It is not clear how the presence of this inflammatory marker might be connected with the development of advanced AMD, but this is an interesting avenue for future research.

The second article (Abstract 5–11) is an editorial prompted by several additional reports on this subject that have appeared recently in general scientific literature. Although the details vary, the basic conclusions of these studies are similar. All seem to suggest an association between this particular genetic locus and development of AMD. The overview in this editorial helps to put this work in perspective.

J. F. Vander, MD

Prophylactic Treatment of Age-Related Macular Degeneration Report Number 1: 810-Nanometer Laser to Eyes with Drusen. Unilaterally Eligible Patients

Friberg TR, and the PTAMD Study Group (Univ of Pittsburgh, Pa; et al)
Ophthalmology 113:612-622, 2006   5–12

Objective.—To determine the effects of subthreshold 810-nm-diode laser treatment on the rate of development of choroidal neovascularization (primary end point) and the effect on visual acuity (VA) in participants with multiple large drusen in one eye and a preexisting neovascular age-related macular degeneration (AMD) lesion in the other.

Design.—Multicenter, prospective, randomized controlled trial.

Participants.—Two hundred forty-four patients $\geq$50 years of age and with a neovascular or advanced AMD lesion in one eye and, in the fellow "study" eye, (1) at least 5 drusen $\geq$63 μm in diameter, (2) Early Treatment Diabetic Retinopathy Study best-corrected VA (BCVA) of 20/63 or better, and (3) no evidence of neovascularization at baseline.

Methods.—Patients were randomized to treatment or observation of their study eye at each of 22 centers. At each visit, the protocol specified that BCVA, a complete retinal examination, and fluorescein angiography be documented. Treated eyes had a grid of 48 extrafoveal, subthreshold diode (810 nm) laser spots, 125 μm in diameter, placed in an annulus outside of the foveola. Patients were seen at baseline and at 3, 6, 12, 18, 24, 30, and 36 months after randomization. No retreatments were allowed.

Main Outcome Measures.—Development of choroidal neovascularization (as confirmed by fluorescein angiography) and change in BCVA.

Results.—Throughout follow-up, the rate of choroidal neovascularization events in treated eyes consistently exceeded that in observed eyes. At 1 year, the difference was 15.8% versus 1.4% ($P = 0.05$). Most of the intergroup differences in choroidal neovascularization events occurred during the first 2 years of follow-up. Treated eyes showed a higher rate of VA loss ($\geq$3 lines) at 3- and 6-month follow-ups relative to observed eyes (8.3% vs. 1% and 11.4% vs. 4%, respectively; $Ps = 0.02, 0.07$). After 6 months, no significant differences were observed in VA loss between groups.

Conclusion.—Prophylactic subthreshold 810-nm-diode laser treatment to an eye with multiple large drusen in a patient whose fellow eye has already suffered a neovascular event places the treated eye at higher risk of developing choroidal neovascularization. We advise against using prophylactic subthreshold diode laser treatment in these eyes.

Laser Treatment in Patients with Bilateral Large Drusen: The Complications of Age-Related Macular Degeneration Prevention Trial

Complications of Age-Related Macular Degeneration Prevention Trial Research Group (Univ of Pennsylvania, Philadelphia; et al)
Ophthalmology 113:1974-1986, 2006   5–13

Objective.—To evaluate the efficacy and safety of low-intensity laser treatment in the prevention of visual acuity (VA) loss among participants with bilateral large drusen.

Design.—Multicenter randomized clinical trial. One eye of each participant was assigned to treatment, and the contralateral eye was assigned to observation.

Participants.—A total of 1052 participants who had ≥10 large (>125 µm) drusen and VA ≥20/40 in each eye enrolled through 22 clinical centers.

Intervention.—The initial laser treatment protocol specified 60 barely visible burns applied in a grid pattern within an annulus between 1500 and 2500 µm from the foveal center. At 12 months, eyes assigned to treatment that had sufficient drusen remaining were retreated with 30 burns by targeting drusen within an annulus between 1000 and 2000 µm from the foveal center.

Main Outcome Measure.—Proportion of eyes at 5 years with loss of ≥3 lines of VA from baseline. Secondary outcome measures included the development of choroidal neovascularization or geographic atrophy (GA), change in contrast threshold, change in critical print size, and incidence of ocular adverse events.

Results.—At 5 years, 188 (20.5%) treated eyes and 188 (20.5%) observed eyes had VA scores ≥3 lines worse than at the initial visit ($P = 1.00$). Cumulative 5-year incidence rates for treated and observed eyes were 13.3% and 13.3% ($P = 0.95$) for choroidal neovascularization and 7.4% and 7.8% ($P = 0.64$) for GA, respectively. The contrast threshold doubled in 23.9% of treated eyes and in 20.5% of observed eyes ($P = 0.40$). The critical print size doubled in 29.6% of treated eyes and in 28.4% of observed eyes ($P = 0.70$). Seven treated eyes and 14 observed eyes had an adverse event of a ≥6-line loss in VA in the absence of late age-related macular degeneration or cataract.

Conclusion.—As applied in the Complications of Age-Related Macular Degeneration Prevention Trial, low-intensity laser treatment did not demonstrate a clinically significant benefit for vision in eyes of people with bilateral large drusen.

Prophylactic Laser Treatment Hastens Choroidal Neovascularization in Unilateral Age-Related Maculopathy: Final Results of the Drusen Laser Study

Owens SL, and the Drusen Laser Study Group (Moorfields Eye Hosp, London; et al)

Am J Ophthalmol 141:276-281, 2006   5–14

Purpose.—The Drusen Laser Study evaluated macular laser to prevent choroidal neovascularization (CNV) and vision loss in high-risk age-related maculopathy (ARM).

Design.—Prospective, interventional, randomized, controlled clinical trial in five hospital centers.

Methods.—Patients in the unilateral group had neovascular ARM and drusen in the study eye. Study eyes were randomized to laser-treated or no-laser groups. For patients in the bilateral drusen group, eyes were randomized to right eye, laser or no laser; and left eye, alternative. Laser treatment comprised 12 argon spots. Outcome was best-corrected visual acuity and CNV signs, which were monitored for 3 years.

Results.—In the unilateral group, vision loss occurred in 21 (28.8%) of 73 patients in laser vs 13 (19.7%) of 66 no-laser patients ($P = .214$). Incidence of CNV was 27 (29.7%) of 91 in laser vs 15 (17.65%) of 85 no-laser patients ($P = .061$). CNV onset was approximately 6 months earlier in laser-treated compared with no-laser patients ($P = .05$). In the bilateral group, vision loss occurred in six (8.3%) of 72 laser-treated vs 10 (13.9%) of 72 fellow eyes ($P = .3877$). CNV incidence was 12 (11.6%) of 103 in laser-treated vs seven (6.8%) of 103 fellow eyes ($P = .225$). There was no difference in onset of CNV.

Conclusions.—Results do not support prophylactic laser of the fellow eye of patients with neovascular ARM. Its role in patients with bilateral drusen remains unclear.

▶ Several years ago, there was great enthusiasm for the potential use of laser treatment as prophylaxis for patients with age-related macular degeneration (ARMD). Application of a light grid treatment has been shown to induce resolution of drusen and, in some cases, modest improvement in vision. Concerns were raised about the risk of developing choroidal neovascularization (CNV), as well as the long-term visual results. These led to the initiation of several clinical trials to assess this method of treatment. Some studies looked at the fellow eye of patients with exudative ARMD, others looked at patients with bilateral high-risk dry disease, and others looked at both.

The first report by Friberg and the PTAMD Study Group (Abstract 5–12) described the arm of this prospective, randomized trial looking at the fellow eye of patients with wet ARMD treated with a grid of light laser. Prophylactic treatment in this group with this technique increases the risk of developing CNV and is not recommended.

The second report by the Complications of Age-Related Macular Degeneration Prevention Trial Research Group (Abstract 5–13) looks at patients with bilateral high-risk dry disease, also using a prospective, randomized structure, and found no difference between treated and control eyes at 5 years.

The third report by Owens and the Drusen Laser Study Group (Abstract 5–14) looked at both types of patients, again using a prospective, randomized format. The unilateral cases with wet disease in the fellow eye also had an increased risk of developing CNV in the treated eye. The bilateral dry cases showed no difference between treated and control groups.

To summarize, these 3 reports collectively indicate that prophylactic treatment of drusen for fellow eyes of patients with wet ARMD is definitely contraindicated. Prophylactic treatment for bilateral dry high-risk eyes has not been shown to be helpful at 5 years' follow-up and is probably not indicated, although conclusive results are not available.

J. F. Vander, MD

Verteporfin Therapy Combined with Intravitreal Triamcinolone in All Types of Choroidal Neovascularization due to Age-Related Macular Degeneration
Augustin AJ, Schmidt-Erfurth U (Klinikum Karlsruhe, Germany; Med Univ of Vienna)
Ophthalmology 113:14-22, 2006   5–15

Objective.—To evaluate the efficacy and safety of photodynamic therapy with verteporfin combined with intravitreal triamcinolone in choroidal neovascularization secondary to age-related macular degeneration (AMD).

Design.—Prospective, noncomparative, interventional case series.

Participants.—One hundred eighty-four patients undergoing treatment for neovascular AMD at one retinal referral center.

Methods.—One hundred eighty-four eyes of 184 consecutive patients (63.6% female, 36.4% male) with a mean age of 76.5 years and a follow-up of a median of 38.8 weeks (range, 12–103) were included in a case series. One hundred forty-eight (80.4%) patients had subfoveal choroidal neovascularization, 19 patients (10.3%) had juxtafoveal choroidal neovascularization, and 17 patients (9.2%) had extrafoveal choroidal neovascularization. Verteporfin photodynamic therapy was performed using the recommended standard procedure. A solution containing 25 mg of triamcinolone was injected intravitreally 16 hours after photodynamic therapy in 184 patients. The combined therapy procedure was repeated at the 3-month follow-up visits whenever persistent choroidal neovascularization leakage was documented angiographically.

Main Outcome Measures.—Mean change in best-refracted visual acuity (VA) between baseline and the last visit, and number of treatments necessary to achieve absence of leakage.

Results.—Visual acuity improved in the majority of patients (baseline VA, mean 20/125) by a mean increase of 1.22 Snellen lines and 1.43 lines using laser interferometry ($P<0.01$). The mean number of required treatments was 1.21. Twenty-three eyes (12.5%) required 2 treatments, 6 eyes (3.26%) required 3 treatments, and 1 eye (0.5%) required 4 treatments. The combination treatment including laser and intravitreal steroid administration was well tolerated. Forty-six patients (25%) required glaucoma therapy due to a transient steroid-induced intraocular pressure (IOP) increase. Twelve patients (6.5%) were on topical medication for preexisting glaucoma. Two patients (1%) whose IOP increase could not be controlled with topical therapy required surgery.

Conclusions.—Verteporfin photodynamic therapy combined with intravitreal triamcinolone may improve the outcome of standard verteporfin photodynamic therapy in the treatment of choroidal neovascularization secondary to AMD. A significant improvement in VA was observed in a majority of treated patients and was maintained during the maximum follow-up. In addition, retreatment rates were lower than anticipated.

Photodynamic Therapy with Intravitreal Triamcinolone in Predominantly Classic Choroidal Neovascularization: One-Year Results of a Randomized Study
Arias L, Garcia-Arumi J, Ramon JM, et al (Bellvitge Univ Hosp, Barcelona; Universitat Autonoma de Barcelona; Institut de Microcirurgia Ocular, Barcelona)
Ophthalmology 113:2243-2250, 2006   5–16

Purpose.—To determine whether intravitreal triamcinolone acetonide (IVTA) improves the efficacy of photodynamic therapy (PDT) with verteporfin in predominantly classic subfoveal choroidal neovascularization (CNV) secondary to age-related macular degeneration (AMD).

Design.—Prospective randomized study.

Participants.—Sixty-one patients with predominantly classic subfoveal CNV secondary to AMD.

Methods.—Patients were randomized to receive PDT (n = 30) or PDT followed by approximately 11 mg IVTA (n = 31), with retreatment every 3 months when leakage was documented by fluorescein angiography. At baseline and each follow-up visit, best-corrected visual acuity (VA) was measured with Early Treatment Diabetic Retinopathy Study charts by a certified examiner masked to the patient's treatment, lesion size on fluorescein angiography, and foveal thickness on optical coherence tomography.

Main Outcome Measures.—Mean change in VA (logarithm of the minimum angle of resolution [logMAR]) from baseline, percentage of patients losing fewer than 15 letters (3 lines) of VA, mean change in lesion size, mean change in foveal thickness, and retreatment rate.

Results.—At the 12-month follow-up, VA (mean logMAR change from baseline) was significantly better ($P = 0.001$) in the group of patients who received combined therapy. Seventy-four percent of patients treated with combined therapy compared with 61% treated with verteporfin alone lost fewer than 15 letters of VA ($P = 0.78$). Reduction in lesion size ($P = 0.001$) and in foveal thickness ($P = 0.03$) was significantly greater with combined therapy than with verteporfin. Retreatment rate was significantly lower ($P = 0.04$) in the combined therapy group. Triamcinolone-related adverse events included glaucoma (25.8%) and cataract progression (32%).

Conclusions.—Combined PDT and IVTA therapy seemed to be more effective than PDT alone for managing predominantly classic subfoveal lesions secondary to AMD. The triamcinolone-related adverse events included glaucoma and cataract progression.

▶ The availability of intravitreal vascular endothelial growth factor (VEGF) inhibitors has greatly reduced the use of PDT in the United States for treatment of CNV in AMD. PDT as monotherapy is typically associated with a progressive reduction in vision, and multiple treatments are needed over years to resolve the exudation. The introduction of combination therapy, using intravitreal steroids along with PDT, was met with great excitement that only waned when the newer intravitreal agents came along. In the first report by Augustin et al (Abstract 5–15), a prospective, nonrandomized study, we see that this form of combination therapy is not without merit, even when held up against intravitreal VEGF inhibitor treatment. Mean VA improved, and the number of treatments was only slightly above 1 per eye. Serious complications were infrequent. The main deficiency is a relatively short follow-up, with the mean only 38 weeks.

In the second article by Arias et al (Abstract 5–16) comparing PDT monotherapy versus combination PDT with steroid injection, we see similar data. There is a very slight reduction in mean VA over 1 year in the combination group, and almost 90% of patients needed only 1 or 2 treatments. While these VA data are not quite as encouraging as the data from the ranibizumab trials of intravitreal injection, they are better than those obtained from PDT as monotherapy. While this may not be the first choice of therapy for most wet AMD patients, there may yet be a role for this method in selected cases.

J. F. Vander, MD

Ranibizumab for Neovascular Age-Related Macular Degeneration
Rosenfeld PJ, for the MARINA Study Group (Univ of Miami, Fla; et al)
N Engl J Med 355:1419-1431, 2006   5–17

Background.—Ranibizumab—a recombinant, humanized, monoclonal antibody Fab that neutralizes all active forms of vascular endothelial growth factor A—has been evaluated for the treatment of neovascular age-related macular degeneration.

Methods.—In this multicenter, 2-year, double-blind, sham-controlled study, we randomly assigned patients with age-related macular degeneration with either minimally classic or occult (with no classic lesions) choroidal neovascularization to receive 24 monthly intravitreal injections of ranibizumab (either 0.3 mg or 0.5 mg) or sham injections. The primary end point was the proportion of patients losing fewer than 15 letters from baseline visual acuity at 12 months.

Results.—We enrolled 716 patients in the study. At 12 months, 94.5% of the group given 0.3 mg of ranibizumab and 94.6% of those given 0.5 mg lost fewer than 15 letters, as compared with 62.2% of patients receiving sham injections (P<0.001 for both comparisons). Visual acuity improved by 15 or more letters in 24.8% of the 0.3-mg group and 33.8% of the 0.5-mg group, as compared with 5.0% of the sham-injection group (P<0.001 for both doses). Mean increases in visual acuity were 6.5 letters in the 0.3-mg group and 7.2 letters in the 0.5-mg group, as compared with a decrease of 10.4 letters in the sham-injection group (P<0.001 for both comparisons). The benefit in visual acuity was maintained at 24 months. During 24 months, presumed endophthalmitis was identified in five patients (1.0%) and serious uveitis in six patients (1.3%) given ranibizumab.

Conclusions.—Intravitreal administration of ranibizumab for 2 years prevented vision loss and improved mean visual acuity, with low rates of serious adverse events, in patients with minimally classic or occult (with no classic lesions) choroidal neovascularization secondary to age-related macular degeneration. (ClinicalTrials.gov number, NCT00056836 [ClinicalTrials.gov].)

▶ This is one of the pivotal trials, the Minimally Classic/Occult Trial of the Anti-VEGF Antibody Ranibizumab in the Treatment of Neovascular Age-Related Macular Degeneration (MARINA), demonstrating the role of intravitreal vascular endothelial growth factor inhibitor injection in the treatment of wet age-related macular degeneration. In this randomized prospective trial, 716 patients with either minimally classic or pure occult lesions were randomly assigned to receive either 0.3 mg of ranibizumab (Lucentis) injections monthly, 0.5-mg dosing, or sham injections. About 95% of patients maintained stable vision over 2 years. Between one fourth and one third showed improvement of vision. These numbers are a marked improvement over any previously described method of treating these types of lesions. Furthermore, the quality of the data and duration of follow-up are excellent. Although many questions remain unanswered, such as the duration and frequency of injections that are needed, this is a landmark study reporting a breakthrough in care for a common and vexing problem.

J. F. Vander, MD

Ranibizumab versus Verteporfin for Neovascular Age-Related Macular Degeneration
Brown DM, for the ANCHOR Study Group (Methodist Hosp, Houston; et al)
N Engl J Med 355:1432-1444, 2006   5–18

Background.—We compared ranibizumab—a recombinant, humanized, monoclonal antibody Fab that neutralizes all active forms of vascular endothelial growth factor A—with photodynamic therapy with verteporfin in the treatment of predominantly classic neovascular age-related macular degeneration.

Methods.—During the first year of this 2-year, multicenter, double-blind study, we randomly assigned patients in a 1:1:1 ratio to receive monthly intravitreal injections of ranibizumab (0.3 mg or 0.5 mg) plus sham verteporfin therapy or monthly sham injections plus active verteporfin therapy. The primary end point was the proportion of patients losing fewer than 15 letters from baseline visual acuity at 12 months.

Results.—Of the 423 patients enrolled, 94.3% of those given 0.3 mg of ranibizumab and 96.4% of those given 0.5 mg lost fewer than 15 letters, as compared with 64.3% of those in the verteporfin group ($P<0.001$ for each comparison). Visual acuity improved by 15 letters or more in 35.7% of the 0.3-mg group and 40.3% of the 0.5-mg group, as compared with 5.6% of the verteporfin group ($P<0.001$ for each comparison). Mean visual acuity increased by 8.5 letters in the 0.3-mg group and 11.3 letters in the 0.5-mg group, as compared with a decrease of 9.5 letters in the verteporfin group ($P<0.001$ for each comparison). Among 140 patients treated with 0.5 mg of ranibizumab, presumed endophthalmitis occurred in 2 patients (1.4%) and serious uveitis in 1 (0.7%).

Conclusions.—Ranibizumab was superior to verteporfin as intravitreal treatment of predominantly classic neovascular age-related macular degeneration, with low rates of serious ocular adverse events. Treatment improved visual acuity on average at 1 year. (ClinicalTrials.gov number, NCT00061594 [ClinicalTrials.gov].)

▶ This study describes a head-to-head comparison of ranibizumab versus photodynamic therapy as primary treatment for classic subfoveal choroidal neovascularization in age-related macualar degeneration. This is a large, well-designed trial (the Anti-VEGF Antibody for the Treatment of Predominantly Classic Choroidal Neovascularization in Age-Related Macular Degeneration [ANCHOR] trial), and the clear winner is ranibizumab. The response to intravitreal injections was similar to that reported in other ranibizumab trials, with a roughly 95% stabilization rate and a significant minority showing improved vision. Verteporfin photodynamic therapy as monotherapy is clearly not as effective and should not be considered as primary therapy in age-related macualar degeneration for these lesions. Considering that classic lesions respond better to photodynamic therapy as opposed to minimally classic or occult lesions, the relative superiority of ranibizumab injections for these lesions would likely be even greater, although not assessed in this report.

J. F. Vander, MD

Systemic Bevacizumab (Avastin) Therapy for Neovascular Age-Related Macular Degeneration: Twenty-Four–Week Results of an Uncontrolled Open-Label Clinical Study

Moshfeghi AA, Rosenfeld PJ, Puliafito CA, et al (Univ of Miami, Fla; Univ Eye Hosp Vienna)

Ophthalmology 113:2002-2011, 2006   5–19

Purpose.—To evaluate the safety, efficacy, and durability of bevacizumab for the treatment of subfoveal choroidal neovascularization (CNV) in patients with neovascular age-related macular degeneration (AMD).

Design.—Open-label, single-center, uncontrolled clinical study.

Participants.—Age-related macular degeneration patients with subfoveal CNV (n = 18) and best-corrected visual acuity (VA) letter scores of 70 to 20 (approximate Snellen equivalent, 20/40–20/400).

Methods.—Patients were treated at baseline with an intravenous infusion of bevacizumab (5 mg/kg) followed by 1 or 2 additional doses given at 2-week intervals. Safety assessments were performed at all visits. Ophthalmologic evaluations included protocol VA measurements, ocular examinations, and optical coherence tomography (OCT) imaging at each visit. Retreatment with bevacizumab was performed if there was evidence of recurrent CNV.

Main Outcome Measures.—Assessments of safety and changes from baseline in VA scores and OCT measurements were performed through 24 weeks.

Results.—No serious ocular or systemic adverse events were identified through 24 weeks. The only adverse event identified was a mild elevation of mean systolic and diastolic blood pressure measurements ($+11$ mm Hg, $P = 0.004$; $+8$ mm Hg, $P < 0.001$) evident by 3 weeks and easily controlled with antihypertensive medications. By 24 weeks, the systolic and diastolic mean blood pressures were at or below baseline measurements. Visual acuity in the study eyes improved within the first 2 weeks, and by 24 weeks, the mean VA letter score increased by 14 letters in the study eyes ($P < 0.001$), and the mean OCT central retinal thickness measurement decreased by 112 μm ($P < 0.001$). By 24 weeks, retreatment was needed for only 6 of the 18 study eyes, and after retreatment, the recurrent leakage was eliminated, with restoration of any lost VA.

Conclusions.—Systemic bevacizumab therapy for neovascular AMD was well tolerated and effective for all 18 patients through 24 weeks. By 6 months, most patients did not require any additional treatment beyond the initial 2 or 3 infusions. Despite these impressive results, it is unlikely that systemic bevacizumab will be studied in a large clinical trial because of the potential risks associated with systemic anti-VEGF therapy and the perception that intravitreal therapy is safer.

▶ The use of bevacizumab for the management of CNV in AMD was inspired by its similarity to ranibizumab, which, while promising, was still in the Food and Drug Administration approval process and therefore not available.

Bevacizumab is approved by the Food and Drug Administration for treating colorectal carcinoma and is administered IV. This pilot study demonstrated a strong therapeutic effect and a reasonable safety profile for patients with wet AMD. Despite these very promising initial findings, there was great reservation about moving ahead with larger trials because of concerns about potential systemic side effects, primarily thromboembolic, given the effects reported in the cancer population. Since patients with AMD are likely to be at risk for stroke and coronary artery disease, this concern is valid. Out of consideration for these concerns and the demonstrated therapeutic effect of the systemic drug, intravitreal bevacizumab injections were a logical subsequent approach.

J. F. Vander, MD

Intravitreal Bevacizumab (Avastin) for Neovascular Age-Related Macular Degeneration
Avery RL, Pieramici DJ, Rabena MD, et al (California Retina Consultants, Santa Barbara)
Ophthalmology 113:363-372, 2006   5–20

Purpose.—To report the short-term safety, biologic effect, and a possible mechanism of action of intravitreal bevacizumab in patients with neovascular age-related macular degeneration (AMD).

Design.—Interventional, consecutive, retrospective case series.

Participants.—Eighty-one eyes of 79 patients with subfoveal neovascular AMD.

Methods.—Patients received intravitreal bevacizumab (1.25 mg) on a monthly basis until macular edema, subretinal fluid (SRF), and/or pigment epithelial detachment (PED) resolved. Ophthalmic evaluations included nonstandardized Snellen visual acuity (VA), complete ophthalmic examination, fluorescein angiography, and optical coherence tomography (OCT).

Main Outcome Measures.—Assessments of safety, changes in Snellen VA, OCT retinal thickness, and angiographic lesion characteristics were performed.

Results.—No significant ocular or systemic side effects were observed. Most patients (55%) had a reduction of >10% of baseline retinal thickness at 1 week after the injection. At 4 weeks after injection, 30 of 81 eyes demonstrated complete resolution of retinal edema, SRF, and PEDs. Of the 51 eyes with 8 weeks' follow-up, 25 had complete resolution of retinal thickening, SRF, and PEDs. At 1, 4, 8, and 12 weeks, the mean retinal thickness of the central 1 mm was decreased by 61, 92, 89, and 67 μm, respectively ($P<0.0001$ for 1, 4, and 8 weeks and $P<0.01$ for 12 weeks). At 4 and 8 weeks, mean VA improved from 20/200 to 20/125 ($P<0.0001$). Median vision improved from 20/200 to 20/80⁻ at 4 weeks and from 20/200 to 20/80 at 8 weeks.

Conclusions.—Short-term results suggest that intravitreal bevacizumab (1.25 mg) is well tolerated and associated with improvement in VA, decreased retinal thickness by OCT, and reduction in angiographic leakage in most patients, the majority of whom had previous treatment with photo-dynamic therapy and/or pegaptanib. Further evaluation of intravitreal bevacizumab for the treatment of choroidal neovascularization is warranted.

▶ One of many reports published recently regarding the use of this medication in an off-label, intraocular fashion. The data in this, as in all the reports so far, are short-term and uncontrolled. The response to injection of this drug is rapid and substantial, with reduction or elimination of fluid and improvement of vision seen in many patients. Most of the patients had previous treatment with photodynamic therapy or pegaptanib (Macugen), which makes the very dramatic responses described even more impressive. It is impossible to compare these data with those from the ranibizumab trials given the differences in study design and follow-up. We await a head-to-head trial to judge the relative effectiveness of the 2 drugs.

J. F. Vander, MD

Ranibizumab combined with verteporfin photodynamic therapy in neovascular age-related macular degeneration: year 1 results of the FOCUS Study

Heier JS, and the FOCUS Study Group (Ophthalmic Consultants of Boston)

Arch Ophthalmol 124:1532-1542, 2006   5–21

Objective.—To investigate the safety and efficacy of intravitreal ranibizumab treatment combined with verteporfin photodynamic therapy (PDT) in patients with predominantly classic choroidal neovascularization secondary to age-related macular degeneration.

Methods.—In this 2-year, phase I/II, multicenter, randomized, single-masked, controlled study, patients received monthly ranibizumab (0.5 mg) (n = 106) or sham (n = 56) injections. The PDT was performed 7 days before initial ranibizumab or sham treatment and then quarterly as needed.

Main Outcomes Measures.—Proportion of patients losing fewer than 15 letters from baseline visual acuity at 12 months (primary efficacy outcome) and the incidence and severity of adverse events.

Results.—At 12 months, 90.5% of the ranibizumab-treated patients and 67.9% of the control patients had lost fewer than 15 letters (P<.001). The most frequent ranibizumab-associated serious ocular adverse events were intraocular inflammation (11.4%) and endophthalmitis (1.9%; 4.8% if including presumed cases). On average, patients with serious inflammation had better visual acuity outcomes at 12 months than did controls. Key serious nonocular adverse events included myocardial infarctions in the PDT-alone group (3.6%) and cerebrovascular accidents in the ranibizumab-treated group (3.8%).

Conclusion/Application to Clinical Practice.—Ranibizumab + PDT was more efficacious than PDT alone for treating neovascular age-related macular degeneration. Although ranibizumab treatment increased the risk of serious intraocular inflammation, affected patients, on average, still experienced visual acuity benefit.

▶ This is a multicenter randomized trial comparing combined treatment using PDT plus ranibizumab versus PDT alone. Because it is a phase I/II study, we do not have enough data to make definitive judgments regarding efficacy, but there is a very strong suggestion that combination treatment is superior to PDT alone, and it is well tolerated. Given the results of another clinical trial showing that ranibizumab is superior to PDT as monotherapy (the ANCHOR trial, Abstract 5–18), this result is expected. This trial did not address the question as to whether ranibizumab combined with PDT is better than ranibizumab alone. Given the large number of injections needed with ranibizumab alone, combination treatment has some appealing possibilities, but we don't know the answer yet.

J. F. Vander, MD

Combined photodynamic therapy with verteporfin and intravitreal bevacizumab for choroidal neovascularization in age-related macular degeneration

Dhalla MS, Shah GK, Blinder KJ, et al (Barnes Retina Inst, St Louis)
Retina 26:988-993, 2006   5–22

Purpose.—To examine the 7-month results for patients treated with combined photodynamic therapy (PDT) with verteporfin and intravitreal bevacizumab for choroidal neovascularization (CNV) secondary to age-related macular degeneration (AMD).

Methods.—This is a retrospective series of 24 eyes with juxtafoveal or subfoveal CNV secondary to AMD. Patients were treated with PDT with verteporfin and 1.25 mg of intravitreal bevacizumab. All patients were naive to treatment and had either treatment within a 14-day interval. Main outcome measures were visual acuity stabilization (defined as no change or a gain in visual acuity) and retreatment rate.

Results.—At the 7-month follow-up, 20 (83%) of 24 patients had stabilization of visual acuity. Sixteen eyes (67%) had improvement in visual acuity. Mean improvement in visual acuity (n = 24) was 2.04 Snellen lines. Fifteen eyes (63%) required only a single combined treatment for CNV resolution. There were no complications, including endophthalmitis, uveitis, and ocular hypertension.

Conclusion.—The results of this study suggest that combined treatment of PDT with verteporfin and intravitreal bevacizumab may be useful in treating neovascular AMD by reducing retreatment rates and improving visual acuity. Further investigation with large, controlled trials is warranted to outline the appropriate treatment paradigm for combination therapy.

▶ This small retrospective series is the first step toward addressing the possible virtues of combination treatment for wet AMD using an intravitreal vascular endothelial growth factor inhibitor injection and PDT. In this case the drug is bevacizumab, and the short-term results are promising. Of particular note, almost two thirds of patients needed only a single combination treatment to induce resolution of neovascular activity. Unfortunately, there is only 7 months of follow-up, and we will need better data to resolve this question. Additional issues include the timing for each step of the 2-step treatment and whether the settings for the PDT laser should be adjusted to minimize the risk of early vision loss, which can be seen with PDT alone.

J. F. Vander, MD

Intraocular Infection

Vitreous and aqueous penetration of orally administered moxifloxacin in humans
Hariprasad SM, Shah GK, Mieler WF, et al (Univ of Chicago)
Arch Ophthalmol 124:178-182, 2006   5–23

Objective.—To investigate intraocular penetration of moxifloxacin hydrochloride after oral administration.

Methods.—Prospective study of 15 patients scheduled for vitrectomy between September and November 2004 at the Barnes Retina Institute, St Louis, MO. Aqueous, vitreous, and serum samples were analyzed from 15 patients after oral administration of 2 tablets containing 400 mg of moxifloxacin. Assays were performed using high-performance liquid chromatography.

Results.—The mean ± SD moxifloxacin concentrations in plasma (n = 15), vitreous (n = 13), and aqueous (n = 13) samples were 3.56 ± 1.31 microg/mL, 1.34 ± 0.66 microg/mL, and 1.58 ± 0.80 microg/mL, respectively. Mean ± SD sampling times after oral administration of the second moxifloxacin tablet for plasma, vitreous, and aqueous were 2.94 ± 0.81 hours, 3.77 ± 0.92 hours, and 3.71 ± 0.89 hours, respectively. The percentages of plasma moxifloxacin concentration in the vitreous and aqueous were 37.6% and 44.3%, respectively. Minimal inhibitory concentrations against 90% levels were exceeded against a wide spectrum of gram-positive and gram-negative pathogens in the vitreous and aqueous.

Conclusions.—Moxifloxacin has a spectrum of coverage that encompasses the most common organisms in endophthalmitis. The pharmacokinetic findings of this investigation reveal that orally administered moxifloxacin achieves therapeutic levels in the noninflamed eye. Because of their broad spectrum of coverage, low minimal inhibitory concentration against 90% levels, good tolerability, and excellent oral bioavailability, fourth-generation fluoroquinolones may represent a major advance for managing posterior segment infections.

▶ In an era when ophthalmologists spend very little time in an inpatient hospital setting, the need for IV antibiotics may provide a rare occasion for hospitalization in cases of foreign body, ruptured globe, or intraocular infection. The standard of care requiring IV antibiotics is based on dated practices from a period when oral antibiotics were ineffectual at penetrating the eye and IV drugs were only marginally better. This study looks at a modest number of noninflamed eyes and demonstrates excellent penetration with oral administration. Furthermore, the spectrum of coverage is as good or better than those protocols utilizing older IV drugs with notoriously limited penetration. While this method of delivery will not likely supplant intravitreal administration for actively infected eyes, by any objective assessment, it should become the standard of care for prophylaxis, and a supplement to injections for cases of active infection.

J. F. Vander, MD

In vitro fluoroquinolone resistance in staphylococcal endophthalmitis isolates

Miller D, Flynn PM, Scott IU, et al (Univ of Miami, Fla)
Arch Ophthalmol 124:479-483, 2006   5–24

Objective.—To evaluate the in vitro susceptibility and cross-resistance of gatifloxacin and moxifloxacin vs older fluoroquinolones among coagulase-negative staphylococci recovered from patients with clinical endophthalmitis.

Methods.—A combination of E tests and disk diffusion methods was used to determine in vitro susceptibility and cross-resistance for 111 coagulase-negative staphylococci isolates recovered during a 15-year period (January 1, 1990, to December 31, 2004) against 5 fluoroquinolones.

Results.—In vitro susceptibilities (percentage sensitive) in descending order were as follows: gatifloxacin, 74.5%; moxifloxacin, 72.1%; levofloxacin, 69.3%; ciprofloxacin, 65.6%, and ofloxacin, 60.4%. More than 65% of the coagulase-negative staphylococci resistant to ciprofloxacin (n = 38) demonstrated in vitro cross-resistance to gatifloxacin (25 [65.8%] of 38) and moxifloxacin (27 [71.1%] of 38). During the initial 5 years (January 1, 1990, to December 31, 1994), 96.6% of the coagulase-negative staphylococci were sensitive to gatifloxacin and moxifloxacin, with minimal inhibitory concentration required to inhibit or kill 90% of the isolates of 0.19 microg/mL and 0.12 microg/mL, respectively. During the last 5-year period (January 1, 2000, to December 31, 2004), the percentage of sensitive coagulase-negative staphylococci declined to 65.4% for gatifloxacin and moxifloxacin (P=.02). Minimal inhibitory concentration required to inhibit or kill 90% of the isolates was 32 microg/mL or greater for both drugs.

Conclusions.—Gatifloxacin and moxifloxacin demonstrated an in vitro efficacy of less than 80% for coagulase-negative staphylococci endophthalmitis in the present study. Ciprofloxacin resistance may serve as a surrogate for concurrent in vitro resistance for gatifloxacin and moxifloxacin. Resistance increased significantly during the last 5 years. Declining in vitro susceptibility to gatifloxacin and moxifloxacin may have important implications for the prevention and treatment of postoperative endophthalmitis.

▶ The development of resistance to antibiotics has been a source of repeated frustration for infectious disease experts and pharmacologic researchers for decades. Each generation of new antibiotics has been heralded with great expectations of resistance to the development of resistance. This is particularly true of the newest generation of fluoroquinolones, gatifloxacin and moxifloxacin, which were developed with modifications specifically engineered to prevent development of resistance. This study reveals an efficacy of less than 80% for these drugs against the most common organism to cause postoperative endophthalmitis, *Staphylococcus epidermidis*. It is fortunate that this particular organism tends to cause a less virulent form of endophthalmitis and, with luck, other more aggressive organisms may be more sensitive to these drugs. Nevertheless, we are reminded that we still do not have, and will likely never have, the long-lasting silver bullet to prevent or treat intraocular infections.

J. F. Vander, MD

Acute Endophthalmitis in Eyes Treated Prophylactically with Gatifloxacin and Moxifloxacin

Deramo VA, Lai JC, Fastenberg DM, et al (Albert Einstein College of Medicine, New Hyde Park, NY; Long Island Vitreoretinal Consultants, Great Neck, NY)
Am J Ophthalmol 142:721-725, 2006   5–25

Purpose.—To study the use of prophylactic fourth-generation fluoroquinolone antibiotics, gatifloxacin and moxifloxacin, and bacterial sensitivity in cases of acute postoperative endophthalmitis following cataract surgery.

Design.—Retrospective, consecutive, observational case series.

Methods.—Forty-two eyes of 42 patients with acute endophthalmitis occurring within six weeks after cataract surgery were identified. All patients were seen in a referral vitreoretinal practice over a two-year time interval. The number of patients using prophylactic gatifloxacin or moxifloxacin and results of bacterial culture and sensitivity to all fluoroquinolone antibiotics were recorded.

Results.—Thirty-one of 42 eyes (74%) were treated with perioperative gatifloxacin or moxifloxacin and 24 eyes (57%) were continuously taking one of these antibiotics at the time of diagnosis. Nineteen eyes (45%) had a positive bacterial culture. The most frequent organism isolated was coagulase-negative *Staphylococcus*. Sensitivities were performed for 14 gram-positive organisms, and sensitivities to ciprofloxacin (50%), ofloxacin (44%), levofloxacin (46%), gatifloxacin (38%), and moxifloxacin (38%) were noted. Five organisms were resistant to gatifloxacin and moxifloxacin with a minimum inhibitory concentration of 8 µg/ml. All gram-positive organisms were sensitive to vancomycin. Median visual acuity improved from hand motions to 20/40 at last follow-up.

Conclusion.—Acute endophthalmitis can develop after cataract surgery despite the prophylactic use of fourth-generation fluoroquinolone antibiotics. Gram-positive organisms causing acute endophthalmitis are frequently resistant to all fluoroquinolones, including a significant number of cases resistant to gatifloxacin and moxifloxacin.

▶ This study reflects the clinical consequences of the in vitro characteristics described in the previous report (Abstract 5–24) A retrospective analysis of 42 cases of postoperative endophthalmitis from a busy retina practice reveals that *Staphylococcus epidermidis* remains the most common isolate from these infected eyes and that infections develop even in cases where the most current prophylactic topical antibiotic agents are being used. Most patients did well after appropriate treatment for endophthalmitis. Although no clear recommendations for modification of perioperative or postoperative care can be drawn, the clinical implications of evolving antibiotic resistance are apparent.

J. F. Vander, MD

Primary Treatment of Acute Retinal Necrosis with Oral Antiviral Therapy
Emerson GG, Smith JR, Wilson DJ, et al (Oregon Health & Science Univ, Portland)
Ophthalmology 113:2259-2261, 2006   5–26

Purpose.—To explore the possibility of oral antiviral therapy in lieu of intravenous acyclovir for treating acute retinal necrosis (ARN), a necrotizing retinopathy caused by herpes simplex virus type 1 or 2 or by varicella zoster virus.

Design.—Retrospective, interventional, small case series.

Participants.—Four patients (6 eyes).

Methods.—Patients were treated with oral antiviral therapy. Medications included valacyclovir (1 g 3 times daily), oral famciclovir (500 mg 3 times daily), and topical and oral corticosteroids.

Main Outcome Measures.—Improvement of symptoms, including photophobia, blurred vision, ocular discomfort, and floaters; increase in visual acuity; and resolution of vitreitis, retinitis, and retinal vasculitis, where present.

Results.—Symptoms and visual acuity improved within 2 weeks to 1 month in 3 of 4 patients (75%) treated with oral antiviral medication. One patient required surgical treatment for asymptomatic retinal detachment after 3 weeks of treatment; retinal detachment in the fellow eye was repaired 2 months later. Duration of antiviral therapy ranged from 5 weeks to 3 months.

Conclusions.—For 4 patients with relatively indolent cases of ARN, oral antiviral therapy alone was effective in eliminating signs and symptoms of the disease. In particular, oral valacyclovir and famciclovir appeared to be effective, although further study is necessary to determine whether these drugs are as effective as intravenous acyclovir for initial treatment of ARN.

► In addition to treating infections with IV antibacterial agents, one other situation typically requiring hospitalization has been treatment of ARN. This aggressive retinitis is usually caused by herpes zoster or, occasionally, herpes simplex infection, and the initial method of treatment has been IV acyclovir. After a period of several days of IV therapy and stabilization of infection, one might consider switching to oral treatment. This small case series describes the successful primary use of oral treatment with valacyclovir or famciclovir for controlling patients with ARN. These drugs have better bioavailability with oral administration than acyclovir, making them better candidates for this method of delivery than the older drug. Cases reported were relatively less severe with more peripheral disease, and the authors are careful to point out that severe cases with rapid progression or involvement of the posterior pole may be better treated with an IV drug (or, I would suggest adding an intravitreal drug). Less threatening cases may be treatable with an oral drug alone.

J. F. Vander, MD

Retinal Surgery

Visual Recovery after Scleral Buckling Procedure for Retinal Detachment

Salicone A, Smiddy WE, Venkatraman A, et al (Univ of Miami, Fla)
Ophthalmology 113:1734-1742, 2006 5–27

Purpose.—To evaluate prognostic factors for visual and anatomic outcomes, including complications after scleral buckling procedure (SBP) for primary rhegmatogenous retinal detachments.

Design.—Retrospective, consecutive, nonrandomized, comparative interventional case series.

Participants.—Patients undergoing SBP for primary rhegmatogenous retinal detachment performed by a single surgeon.

Methods.—The patients' medical records were reviewed. Preoperative and intraoperative factors analyzed for their association with visual acuity and anatomic outcomes included macular detachment, duration of macular detachment, preoperative visual acuity, lens status, refractive error, extent of detachment, number of breaks, internal gas tamponade, and drainage of the subretinal fluid. Secondary outcomes included frequency of further surgery, complications, and fellow eye retinal detachment. The fellow eye of the patients was excluded from consideration of prognostic factors.

Main Outcome Measures.—Best-corrected visual acuity at 2 months and at final follow-up examination as well as anatomic factors including retinal reattachment at 1 day, 2 months, and last follow-up examination.

Results.—There were 672 patients studied, including 457 (68%) with macular detachment. The use of gas, drainage of subretinal fluid, and lens status did not influence final anatomic or visual results. Macular detachment was the most important prognostic factor for anatomic ($P = 0.031$) and visual acuity success ($P<0.001$). Better preoperative visual acuity ($P<0.001$), fewer quadrants involved by the detachment (*P*<0.001), and lack of high myopia (*P* = 0.001) were important positive prognostic factors for visual acuity. The duration of macular detachment was not of prognostic value up to 30 days' duration.

Conclusions.—Visual recovery after retinal reattachment was most dependent on macular involvement. Duration of macular detachment had surprisingly little influence on postoperative visual acuity.

▶ Much of the information reported in this large retrospective series is simply a confirmation of older reports, some decades old, concerning the anatomic and vision results of primary scleral buckling surgery. The critical importance of the preoperative presence or absence of macular detachment as the best predictor of final vision after successful repair is not a surprise. The important finding in this study is the minimal effect that small variations in timing of repair had for patients with macula-off detachments. The authors conclude that delaying repair of macular-involving detachments for a few days (at least) will have no appreciable effect on the final vision results. This has practical implications for patients and surgeons alike.

J. F. Vander, MD

Long-Term Outcome of Combined Pars Plana Vitrectomy and Scleral Fixated Sutured Posterior Chamber Intraocular Lens Implantation
Vote BJ, Tranos P, Bunce C, et al (Moorfields Eye Hosp, London)
Am J Ophthalmol 141:308-312, 2006   5–28

Purpose.—To investigate the long-term visual outcome and the complication rate following transscleral suture fixation of posterior chamber intraocular lenses (sutured PC-IOLs).

Design.—A retrospective case-series descriptive study.

Methods.—Records of patients who underwent combined pars plana vitrectomy and sutured PC-IOLs at Moorfields Eye Hospital and who had at least 12 months of follow-up were examined for recorded complications.

Results.—Sixty-one eyes of 48 patients (33 males and 15 females) were identified and included in the analysis, with mean follow-up of 6 years. The mean final best-corrected visual acuity remained at preoperative levels (*P* = .211) and was largely determined by the underlying ocular pathology before sutured PC-IOL. Overall 30 of 61 (49%) eyes, two or more procedures were performed to reverse a significant peri- or postoperative complication. Breakage of polypropylene sutures was the main indication accounting for 17 of 30 (57%) of those reoperations. Subgroup analysis showed that younger patients were more likely to suffer the above complication (*P* = .009). The multivariate analysis also showed that longer follow-up was significantly associated with suture breakage (*P* = .014), with the mean time to breakage approximately 4 years after surgery.

Conclusions.—Long-term follow-up of patients undergoing sutured PC-IOLs appears to be associated with a high rate of postoperative complications and significant need for further surgery, which should be discussed during their informed consent process.

▶ This article provides very important long-term follow-up of a cohort of patients previously reported. It is a retrospective nonconsecutive series of patients, all operated on previously with suturing of a PC-IOL. Nearly half of the patients required additional surgery to remedy complications related to the IOL, primarily breakage of the suture and IOL malposition. The authors point out that there have been many patients lost to follow-up since the earlier report, and so the rate of recurrent problems may be overstated somewhat. Even considering this factor, however, the rate of problems sufficient to require reoperation is 18%. The number is likely higher with longer follow-up. Strong consideration should be given to placement of an open-loop anterior chamber IOL if capsular support is not adequate. If a sutured lens is placed, extensive preoperative counseling about the possibility of late-onset IOL complications must take place.

J. F. Vander, MD

Maintenance of warfarin anticoagulation for patients undergoing vitreoretinal surgery

Dayani PN, Grand MG (Washington Univ, St Louis)
Arch Ophthalmol 124:1558-1565, 2006   5–29

Objective.—To evaluate the risk of hemorrhagic complications associated with vitreoretinal surgery in patients whose warfarin sodium therapy was continued throughout the surgical period.

Methods.—A review of 1737 records of patients undergoing pars plana vitrectomy was conducted. Inclusion criteria included patients receiving warfarin therapy whose international normalized ratios (INRs) were elevated above normal values on the day of surgery. Intraoperative and postoperative hemorrhagic complications were documented.

Results.—Fifty-four patients underwent 57 vitreoretinal surgical procedures with warfarin therapy and were divided into groups as follows: group S with INRs of 1.20 to 1.49, values considered subtherapeutic; group B with INRs of 1.50 to 1.99, values considered borderline therapeutic; group T with INRs of 2.00 to 2.49, values considered therapeutic; and group HT with INRs of 2.50 or greater, values considered highly therapeutic. No patients experienced anesthesia-related or intraoperative hemorrhagic complications. Two (7.7%) of 26 eyes in group S and 2 (16.7%) of 12 eyes in group HT experienced postoperative hemorrhages. All of the patients with vitreous hemorrhages had spontaneous clearing without additional treatment.

Conclusions.—Many patients may safely undergo vitreoretinal surgery while maintaining therapeutic levels of warfarin anticoagulation. We experienced no intraoperative hemorrhagic complications; the 4 postoperative complications resolved spontaneously without persistent visual sequelae or the need for supplemental surgery.

▶ Many patients contemplating vitreous surgery have significant medical conditions, some of which require anticoagulation. Although there are numerous reports describing the maintenance of warfarin anticoagulation during anterior segment surgery, there is little information related to vitrectomy in these patients. Although the number of procedures in this report is still relatively small at 57, this is far more than described in any previous article. It is reassuring that there were no intraoperative complications and that postoperative bleeding was infrequent and self-limited, even for those patients with relatively high levels of anticoagulation at the time of surgery. While there may be selected cases (eg, highly vascularized diabetic epiretinal membranes) where one might consider discontinuing or reversing the drug for surgery, in general, this report reasonably concludes that this is not necessary.

J. F. Vander, MD

6 Oculoplastic Surgery

Are We Doing Our Part to Decrease Antibiotic Resistance?

by Robert B. Penne, MD

The concern over the development of antibiotic resistance has not been a large concern to most ophthalmologists. Ophthalmology is generally an outpatient practice with very little exposure to patients that are in the hospital for long periods of time. In the past, the thought of antibiotic resistance pertained to the institutionalized patients. The article "Ophthalmic manifestations of infections caused by the USA300 clone of community-associated methicillin-resistant Staphylococcus aureus"[1] outlines why this now should be a concern, as the incidence of community acquired methicillin resistant Staphylococcus aureus (CAMRSA) rises. The article also discusses the recognition and treatment of this aggressive organism. What is only briefly mentioned in the article is the emergence of vancomycin resistance in hospital-associated methicillin-resistant Staphylococcus aureus (HAMRSA) and what this could mean in the future. This issue should be a concern for everyone.

Bacteria have an amazing ability to evolve and develop resistance to antibiotics that are used to kill them. We have all been taught to use antibiotics "appropriately" in order to try and lower the chance of development of resistance to these antibiotics. Unfortunately, the bacteria continue to evolve and develop new resistant strains. Looking back at the development of Staphylococcus aureus (SA), resistance to penicillin and methicillin gives some insight into how this happens. With penicillin, the hospital resistance rate rose 25% after 6 years. It took 15-20 years for the community rate of resistance to penicillin to reach 25%. After 30 years the community and hospital rates were similar, with both being greater than 70%. Methicillin was introduced in 1961 and the pattern was similar to that of penicillin, with hospital resistance developing first and then community resistance, and, 37 years (1998) after the discovery of methicillin, both hospital and community resistance rates were over 50%. Vancomycin is the one drug that is still effective against MRSA, but it appears to be proceeding in a similar pattern although in a much slower process. Fortunately it took some 29 years for development of vancomycin resistance by SA, but this resistance is very concerning as there is really no alternative antibiotic to treat these infections with. So far these cases have all been reported in hospital settings, but will this eventually follow the pattern of other antibiotic resistance and migrate to the community? That would be a reason for ophthalmologists to be concerned.

Is there anything an ophthalmologist can do to prevent or slow this process? The answer for all doctors is to stop using prophylactic antibiotics of all kinds—specifically vancomycin. The argument has been made that the total amount of vancomycin ophthalmologists' use is so small (estimated at 0.07% of the total used in medicine[2]) that it really doesn't contribute to the problem. I would argue that any unnecessary use is part of the problem. All of medicine needs to change it's thinking so we responsibly use antibiotics, and we as ophthalmologists need to do our part no matter how small. There is no scientific evidence that vancomycin used prophylactically in the infusion bottle has any effect on the rate of endophthalmitis in cataract surgery. Yet, many ophthalmologists continue to use it. Every time we use an antibiotic of any kind we need to ask, is this effective and necessary therapy?

References

1. Rutar T, Chambers HF, Crawford JB, et al: Ophthalmic manifestations of infections caused by the USA300 clone of community-associated methicillin-resistant Staphylococcus aureus. *Ophthalmology* 113:1455-1462, 2006.
2. Gordon YJ: Vancomycin prophylaxis and emerging resistance: Are ophthalmologists the villains? The heroes? *Am J Ophthalmol* 131:371-376, 2001.

Ophthalmic Manifestations of Infections Caused by the USA300 Clone of Community-Associated Methicillin-Resistant *Staphylococcus aureus*
Rutar T, Chambers HF, Crawford JB, et al (Univ of California San Francisco; San Francisco Gen Hosp)
Ophthalmology 113:1455-1462, 2006   6–1

Purpose.—To report the microbiological, clinical, and pathological characteristics of community-associated methicillin-resistant *Staphylococcus aureus* (CAMRSA) infections of the eye and orbit.

Design.—Prospective case series.

Participants.—Nine patients with CAMRSA infections of the eye and orbit were identified during a 6-month period at 2 tertiary care hospitals in San Francisco.

Methods.—Case identification was by prospective case selection and retrospective laboratory review of 549 MRSA cultures collected in the 2 hospitals. Ophthalmic microbial isolates were analyzed by pulsed-field gel electrophoresis and compared with a control CAMRSA clone (USA300). Clinical characteristics of patients infected with CAMRSA were reviewed, and all surgical specimens underwent pathological examination.

Main Outcome Measures.—Pulsed-field gel electrophoresis banding patterns of MRSA isolates, antibiotic sensitivity profiles, patient demographics, systemic and ocular complications of infection, and posttreatment visual acuities.

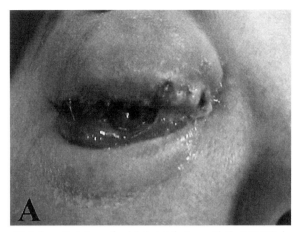

FIGURE 2.—Clinical manifestations of ophthalmic infections with the USA300 clone of methicillin-resistant *Staphylococcus aureus*. **A,** Upper eyelid abscess, lid edema and erythema, and conjunctival chemosis in a 29-year-old female with orbital cellulitis. (Reprinted from iOphthalmology, 113, Rutar T, Chambers HF, Crawford JB, et al: Ophthalmic manifestations of infections caused by the USA300 clone of community-associated methicillin-resistant *Staphylococcus aureus*, pp 1455-1462, Copyright 2006, with permission from Elsevier Science.)

Results.—Nine ophthalmic isolates were CAMRSA clone USA300. The infections included orbital cellulitis, endogenous endophthalmitis, panophthalmitis, lid abscesses (Fig 2), and septic venous thrombosis. Patients were treated with trimethoprim-sulfamethoxazole, rifampin, clindamycin, or vancomycin based on microbial sensitivity studies and severity of infection. Eight of the 9 patients had no history of hospitalization. Seven patients required hospitalization, 3 required surgery, and an additional 4 required invasive procedures. Eight patients had good visual outcomes, but 1 deteriorated to no light perception. Pathological analyses showed extensive necrosis in eyelid and orbital specimens, and disorganized atrophy bulbi in an enucleated eye.

Conclusion.—The USA300 CAMRSA clone, which carries Panton–Valentine leukocidin genes, can cause aggressive infections of the eye and orbit in hospital-naive patients. Treatment of infections often required debridement of necrotic tissues in addition to non–β-lactam class antibiotics. In communities where CAMRSA is prevalent, ophthalmologists should obtain microbial cultures and sensitivity studies to help guide antibiotic therapy for severe ophthalmic infections (Table 2).

▶ Methicillin-resistant *S aureus* (MRSA) is a severe infection that only occurred in patients who were in a hospital or chronic care setting. The goal of this article is to inform the ophthalmic community that MRSA is now present in community-acquired infections. This infection often requires drainage and debridement, unlike most bacterial infections. The organism is not exactly the same strain as the hospital-acquired organism but is a clone, with the USA300 clone being the most common. The good news is that these CAMRSA organisms are sensitive to more antibiotics than the hospital-acquired organism,

TABLE 2.—Clinical Characteristics of Ophthalmology Patients Infected with the USA300 Clone of Community-Associated Methicillin-Resistant *Staphylococcus aureus*

Patient	Age (yrs)	Gender	Coexisting Conditions	Manifestations		Treatment	BCVA	
				Ophthalmic	Systemic		Initial*	Final†
1	29	F	Hypothyroid	Lid abscesses, orbital cellulitis	Multifocal pneumonia	Eyelid debridement, IV vancomycin × 2 wks	20/50	20/30
2	61	M	Diabetes	Lid abscesses, periorbital cellulitis	None	Eyelid debridement, IV vancomycin × 4 days, peroral clidamycin × 10 days	20/30	20/20
3	78	F	Hypertension	Superior ophthalmic vein thrombosis, orbital cellulitis	Sepsis, multifocal pneumonia	IV vancomycin × 4 wks	20/70	20/60
4	61	M	Inmate, IV drug use	Lid abscess, periorbital cellulitis	None	Incision and drainage, peroral trimethoprim–sulfamethoxazole and rifampin × 2 wks	20/30	20/30
5	61	M	Homeless, IV drug use	Panophthalmitis	Bacteremia	Vitrectomy with intravitreal vancomycin, IV vancomycin × 6 wks, enucleation	LP	NLP
6	39	M	Diabetes	Endogenous endophthalmitis	Bacteremia, endocarditis, myositis, pyelonephritis	Intravitreal vancomycin × 2, IV vancomycin × 6 wks	20/60	20/30
7	29	M	None	Lid abscess	None	Peroral clindamycin × 10 days	20/20	20/20
8	39	M	Hemodialysis	Endogenous endophthalmitis	Sepsis, respiratory failure, endocarditis, meningitis, multifocal septic arthritis	Intravitreal vancomycin × 1, IV vancomycin, rifampin, and gentamicin × 6 wks	CF 2 feet	20/40
9	43	M	Homeless, HIV positive	Endogenous endophthalmitis	Bacteremia, endocarditis, multifocal pneumonia, buttocks ulcers	Intravitreal vancomycin × 1, IV vancomycin × 6 wks	20/150	20/30

BCVA = best-corrected visual acuity; CF = counting fingers; F = female; LP = light perception; M = male; NLP = no LP.

*On presentation.

†After completion of treatment.

which is usually only sensitive to vancomycin and linezolid. The concern is that CAMRSA can cause severe infections with necrosis in healthy patients. Although it is responsive to some antibiotics, it is resistant to the commonly used β-lactam antibiotics. Thus, if not suspected, these patients may be receiving antibiotics that are not effective for 24 to 48 hours while their infection gets worse.

With any severe infection that is not responding to antibiotic treatment as expected, CAMRSA should be considered. This is a reason to get cultures whenever possible. CAMRSA infections should be suspected in communities where this organism is more common. Despite cultures and proper antibiotic treatment, these infections can be quite severe and require debridement similar to cases of necrotizing fasciitis.

Six of the 9 patients in this study did have risk factors for more severe infections such as diabetes, IV drug use, dialysis, and being HIV positive. Although these patients acquiring CAMRSA were not in the hospital, they were probably a population at higher risk of getting an infection.

R. B. Penne, MD

Efficacy and Complications of the Transconjunctival Entropion Repair for Lower Eyelid Involutional Entropion
Erb MH, Uzcategui N, Dresner SC (Univ of California at Irvine; Univ of Southern California, Los Angeles)
Ophthalmology 113:2351-2356, 2006   6–2

Purpose.—To evaluate the efficacy of the transconjunctival entropion repair (TCER) for lower eyelid involutional entropion.

Design.—Retrospective, noncomparative, interventional case series.

Participants.—One hundred fifty-one eyelids in 120 patients who underwent TCER for involutional entropion over a 12-year period from February 1991 through January 2003.

Methods.—Surgical technique addressed all 3 anatomic factors underlying the entropion and was performed through a transconjunctival incision. Lateral tarsal strip procedure addressed horizontal eyelid laxity, lower eyelid retractor reinsertion addressed retractor disinsertion, and excision of a strip of the preseptal orbicularis oculi addressed preseptal orbicularis override (Fig 1).

Main Outcome Measures.—Entropion resolution, entropion recurrence, postoperative eyelid retraction, and complication rate.

Results.—Transconjunctival entropion repair resulted in resolution of entropion, with a success rate of 96.7% (146 of 151 eyelids); entropion recurrence rate was 3.3% (5 of 151 eyelids). No patient had postoperative eyelid retraction or scleral show, and there were no overcorrections or secondary ectropions in any of the 151 eyelids. Postoperative complications occurred in 6 of 151 eyelids (4.0%) of 6 of 120 patients (5.0%) and included stitch abscess (1 eyelid, 0.7%), lateral tarsal strip dehiscence (2 eyelids, 1.3%), lat-

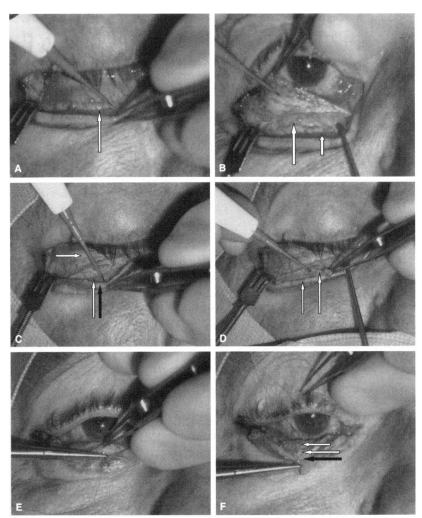

FIGURE 1.—Transconjunctival entropion repair, intraoperative photographs. A, An incision is made with cutting monopolar cautery through the conjunctiva and lower lid retractors, just inferior to the lower tarsal border (arrow), extending from the lateral fornix to the punctum. B, The cautery tip identifies the lower eyelid retractors. Also identified: orbicularis (longer arrow) and tarsal conjunctiva at lower tarsal border (shorter arrow). C, The anterior, inferior surface of the tarsal plate is dissected from orbicularis with monopolar cautery. Also identified: retractors (horizontal arrow), orbicularis (vertical white arrow), and inferior edge of tarsus (vertical black arrow). D, Cutting monopolar cautery is used to excise a thin (1–2 mm) strip of preseptal orbicularis muscles (longer arrow) just inferior to the tarsal border (shorter arrow) along the full length of the incision. Care must be taken to avoid buttonholing the skin, which lies immediately behind the orbicularis muscle in the everted lid. The free edge of retractors is reattached to the tarsus by passing the needle through the retractors E, then through anterior, inferior tarsus with 2 interrupted buried 6-0 polyglactin sutures F. Also identified: anterior surface of tarsus (longer white arrow), inferior edge of tarsus (black arrow), and orbicularis (shorter white arrow). (Reprinted from *Ophthalmology*, 113, Erb MH, Uzcategui N, Dresner SC, Efficacy and complications of the transconjunctival entropion repair for lower eyelid involutional entropion. pp 2351-2356, Copyright 2006, with permission from Elsevier Science.)

eral canthal dystopia (2 eyelids, 1.3%), and conjunctivochalasis (1 eyelid, 0.7%).

Conclusions.—The transconjunctival lower eyelid entropion repair is effective and safe with low recurrence and complication rates. The TCER circumvents the risk of lower eyelid retraction and overcorrections that may occur with the transcutaneous approach.

▶ This article describes another successful approach to the correction of an involutional entropion. This approach, as with other approaches that involve horizontal shortening and addressing the abnormality of the retractors and orbicularis override, shows a success rate of over 95%. This approach is different from many in that it uses a conjunctival approach. Through this conjunctival approach a lateral canthotomy is done, followed by the reattachment of the lower eyelid retractors, and finally, a strip of preseptal orbicularis is excised. The tightening is done via a lateral tarsal strip (Fig 1).

As with many oculoplastic procedures there are multiple ways to successfully treat many of the eyelid problems we deal with. This is a procedure I will keep in mind. However, I still find that 1 or 2 Quickert sutures along with a lateral tarsal strip has similar success in addition to being, at least for myself, a shorter, simpler procedure.

R. B. Penne, MD

Comparing Outcomes of Enucleation and Evisceration

Nakra T, Simon GJB, Douglas RS, et al (Univ of California, Los Angeles)
Ophthalmology 113:2270-2275, 2006   6–3

Purpose.—To compare clinical outcomes of enucleation and evisceration by functional and aesthetic measures.

Design.—Retrospective, nonrandomized, comparative analysis.

Participants.—Eighty-four patients who underwent enucleation or evisceration.

Methods.—The medical records of the participants were retrospectively reviewed. Clinical photographs were graded by blinded observers for qualitative measures.

Main Outcome Measures.—Postoperative eyelid and motility measurements, as well as subjective grades of various aesthetic and functional outcomes.

Results.—There is no statistically significant difference in the overall aesthetic outcome of enucleation and evisceration, although several specific comparisons were found to be significant. Implant motility score is higher in eviscerated eyes (5.58±2.08) than in enucleated eyes (4.35±1.69) ($P = 0.05$). Adduction of the implant is significantly less than abduction in eviscerated eyes (1.34 vs. 1.44; $P = 0.02$). Implant motility is greater than prosthesis motility. Both enucleation and evisceration result in enophthalmos and a sulcus defect. Seven of 32 patients (21.9%) who underwent enucleation experienced a complication, whereas only 7 of 52 patients (13.5%) who under-

TABLE 4.—Postoperative Complications Noted After
Enucleation and Evisceration

	Enucleation	Evisceration
Total no.	32	52
Total complications	7 (21.9%)	7 (13.5%)
Implant exposure	4 (12.5%)	2 (3.8%)
Pyogenic granuloma	1 (3.1%)	2 (3.8%)
Infection	0	1 (1.9%)
Symblepharon	1 (3.1%)	0
Cicatricial entropion	1 (3.1%)	0
Phimosis	0	1 (1.9%)
Lower lid laxity	0	1 (1.9%)

(Reprinted from *Ophthalmology*, 113, Nakra T, Simon GJB, Douglas RS, et al, Comparing outcomes of enucleation and evisceration, pp 2270-2275 Copyright 2006, with permission from Elsevier Science.)

went evisceration experienced a complication ($P = 0.0002$). The 2 most common complications were implant exposure and formation of a pyogenic granuloma (Table 4).

Conclusions.—Although enucleation and evisceration produce aesthetically similar outcomes, eviscerated eyes have better implant motility and experience fewer complications. Both enucleation and evisceration result in enophthalmos, sulcus contour defects, and incomplete transfer of implant motility to the prosthesis.

▶ The debate over long-term outcomes of enucleation versus evisceration continues. It is generally accepted that evisceration is a simple procedure with few complications. The long-term changes in the socket are often thought to be less in an evisceration because it is less invasive in the orbit.

This study was a retrospective chart review of patients undergoing enucleation and evisceration. There were multiple problems with this study that resulted in no conclusive difference; the problems included a small sample size and a large difference in follow-up between the enucleation group (average follow-up, 7 years) and the evisceration group (average follow-up, just over 1 year). The evisceration patients tended to have a better cosmetic result, but nothing was statistically significant. Eviscerated eyes did have better implant motility, but this did not translate into better prosthesis motility. The rate of complications was higher in the enucleation group, but other variables present, such as different implant material being used, make any comparison difficult (Table 4).

There remain certain absolute contraindications to evisceration, such as an intraocular tumor. The other lingering concern for ophthalmologists is the risk of sympathetic ophthalmia occurring after evisceration, although multiple articles have determined this risk to be essentially nonexistent in modern times.

Unfortunately, this article does not offer any conclusion as to which procedure for removing an eye, enucleation or evisceration, gives better long-term aesthetic results. I will continue to favor evisceration for most patients because it is simpler and can usually be done with the patient under local anesthesia. I still do enucleations in patients who are having their eye removed due to recent trauma or those who have so much scarring that an evisceration is not possible. I realize the issue of sympathetic ophthalmia and trauma is probably no longer founded in fact, but when the discussion about sympathetic ophthalmia is brought up, most patients want to proceed with an enucleation no matter how unlikely the occurrence of sympathetic ophthalmia is.

R. B. Penne, MD

▶ Although this study found no statistically significant postoperative functional or aesthetic differences comparing patients treated with evisceration or enucleation, several trends favoring evisceration were identified. Undoubtedly, the results will be used as further justification for eviscerating blind, painful eyes instead of enucleating them. This therapeutic trend has increased markedly in recent years after an article published by Levine et al[1] in 1999 concluded that "evisceration is an effective and safe procedure with a low risk for sympathetic uveitis." In the past, one of the arguments against eviscerating eyes was based on several small series suggesting that evisceration did not prevent sympathetic ophthalmia. The latter risk admittedly does appear to be quite small. I personally have never seen a case of sympathetic ophthalmia that followed ocular evisceration.

Another argument against evisceration (often raised in the past but not mentioned in this article), was the fear of inadvertently eviscerating an eye with an intraocular tumor that was clinically unsuspected. Based on my personal experience, I believe the latter danger is much greater and is definitely real. I have evaluated 3 eyes with unsuspected uveal melanomas that were eviscerated, and am aware of a number of similar cases from other institutions. This is not surprising since it generally was stated that as many as 10% of blind, painful eyes with opaque media were found to contain unsuspected malignant neoplasms, usually uveal melanomas, at pathologic examination, before the availability of modern imaging techniques. This number admittedly is much too high today, but unsuspected tumors still occur and may be present in patients who have confounding inflammatory signs caused by tumor necrosis. Furthermore, necrotic tumors may not enhance with contrast and may not be detected on preoperative imaging studies. Two of the eviscerated eyes with melanoma that I evaluated had had preoperative CT scans.

The effect of inadvertent evisceration of a uveal melanoma on the patient's prognosis is not specifically known, but certainly cannot be good. The physician who eviscerates an unsuspected melanoma is at risk as well. He or she could be found liable for failure to diagnose and properly treat the tumor if the patient subsequently develops metastases and dies. The latter risk certainly is not inconsequential; overall, a patient with a conventionally treated melanoma has about a 50% chance of dying of metastatic melanoma. Therefore, the eviscerating physician has 1 chance in 2 at being blamed whether he or she is truly responsible or not. Is mildly superior cosmesis worth the risk?

R. C. Eagle, Jr, MD

Reference

1. Levine MR, Pou CR, Lash RH: The 1998 Wendell Hughes lecture. Evisceration: Is sympathetic ophthalmia a concern in the new millennium? *Ophthal Plast Reconstr Surg* 15:4-8, 1999.

Prevalence of Floppy Eyelid Syndrome in Obstructive Sleep Apnea–Hypopnea Syndrome

Karger RA, White WA, Park W-C, et al (Mayo Clinic College of Medicine, Rochester, Minn; Univ of Missouri–Kansas City School of Medicine)
Ophthalmology 113:1669-1674, 2006   6–4

Objectives.—To determine the prevalence of floppy eyelid syndrome (FES) in obstructive sleep apnea-hypopnea syndrome (OSAHS) and to develop a method to measure eyelid laxity.

Design.—Masked cross-sectional (prevalence) study examining patients referred to the Mayo Sleep Disorders Center.

Participants and/or Controls.—Fifty-nine subjects were examined before undergoing polysomnography. Forty-four subjects had OSAHS, and 15 did not have it.

Testing.—Subjects underwent slit-lamp examination and eyelid laxity measurements, followed by polysomnography.

Main Outcome Measures.—Presence of FES as defined by subjectively easy eyelid eversion, tarsal papillary conjunctivitis, and lash ptosis; force required to displace the upper lid 5 mm, as measured by a strain gauge device; number of apnea or hypopnea episodes per hour (apnea–hypopnea index [AHI]); presence of OSAHS, as defined by an AHI of ≥ 5; and abnormalities on electrocardiography.

Results.—One patient with OSAHS was found to have FES, yielding a prevalence of 2.3% (95% confidence interval [CI]: 0.1%–12.0%). One patient was referred to the Sleep Disorders Center due to a diagnosis of FES; if this patient were included, the prevalence would be 4.5% (95% CI: 0.5%–15.1%). Subjectively easy lid eversion was more common in OSAHS patients than in non-OSAHS patients. When adjusted for age and body mass index, there was a trend for association between subjectively easy lid eversion and OSAHS, but this did not reach statistical significance. Subjectively easy lid eversion was associated with AHI. Force required to displace the upper lid 5 mm was lower in lids with subjectively easy eversion, but was not associated with OSAHS or AHI. Intraclass correlation among 3 strain gauge measurements was good for both right (82%) and left (83%) lids. There were no statistically significant differences in frequency of electrocardiographic abnormalities among the various groups.

Conclusions.—The prevalence of FES among OSAHS patients is low. Patients with subjectively easy upper lid eversion are at risk for OSAHS. By recognizing the potential for OSAHS in these patients, the ophthalmologist may play an important role in initiating their evaluation and treatment.

▶ There is a high incidence of OSAHS in patients with FES. This study shows that the reverse is not true. The incidence of FES in patients with OSAHS is less than 5%. The value of this article is that it provides ophthalmologists with a perspective on the relationship between OSAHS and FES. We teach that all patients with FES need a workup for OSAHS and my impression is that more than 90% of FES patients have some degree of OSAHS. Because only a small percentage of OSAHS patients have FES, we need to educate the physicians and staff caring for these patients to look for the signs and symptoms of FES. They have to realize that only a minority of their patients will have these symptoms and FES is not a common finding in their population of sleep apnea patients. Those OSAHS patients with chronic ocular irritation and discharge should then be referred to the ophthalmologist to be evaluated for FES.

R. B. Penne, MD

Supramaximal Doses of Botulinum Toxin for Refractory Blepharospasm
Levy RL, Berman D, Parikh M, et al (Johns Hopkins Hosp, Baltimore, Md)
Ophthalmology 113:1665-1668, 2006   6–5

Purpose.—To investigate the response to supramaximal doses of botulinum toxin in patients with refractory blepharospasm.

Design.—Prospective, nonrandomized, open-label interventional case series.

Participants.—Eight consecutive patients with blepharospasm requiring injections every 2 months despite receiving 100 U of botulinum toxin per session (Fig 1).

Intervention.—Increasing the dose of botulinum toxin per session above the conventional maximum.

Main Outcome Measures.—Duration of treatment effect and patients' subjective response to treatment.

Results.—Supramaximal dosages were well tolerated. Seven of 8 patients had a prolonged interval between injections relative to that associated with their previous dosing regimen (Table 1). Four of the patients elected to continue with the new dosage.

Conclusion.—In select patients with essential blepharospasm who are refractory to standard treatment regimens, increasing the dosage of botulinum toxin above 100 U per session may decrease the interval between injections, improve the patient's quality of life, or both.

▶ The exact dose that is optimal for treatment of blepharospasm has never really been studied. This small prospective study looks at the effectiveness of doses greater than 100 U in patients who were requiring Botox (Allergan, Irvine, CA) injections every 2 months. The question is whether or not doses of

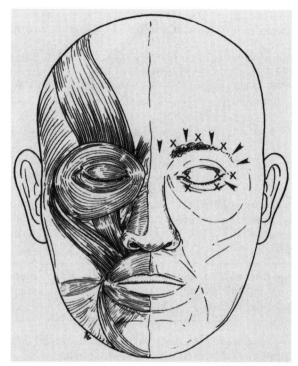

FIGURE 1.—Artist's drawing of standard sites of injection of botulinum. A toxin for blepharospasm (*X*), with additional sites indicated for supramaximal doses (arrowheads). (Reprinted from *Ophthalmology*, 113, Levy RL, Berman D, Parikh M, et al, Supramaximal doses of botulinum toxin for refractory blepharospasm, pp 1665-1668, Copyright 2006, with permission from Elsevier Science.)

125 to 150 U give better effectiveness and duration for these blepharospasm patients. There were only 8 patients and the study's conclusions were confusing. All patients achieved a longer duration between injections with a higher dose of Botox. Four of 8 patients had improvement in symptoms, 2 were unchanged and 2 were worse. Four of 8 patients chose to continue the supramaximal dose and 4 went back to previous dosing.

Even though the results are mixed, the study did not find any increase in the side effects from the higher doses of botulinum toxin. I believe this is worth trying in patients who are not having adequate control with traditional doses of Botox. The other option for these nonresponsive patients is an Anderson procedure, which has variable effectiveness and a definite risk of complications.

Another issue that may be a problem for both patients and physicians is whether or not insurance companies will cover the higher doses. This article should help as a reference when trying to get approval to obtain 2 vials of botulinum toxin for injections instead of 1.

R. B. Penne, MD

TABLE 1.—Patient Demographics, Standard and Increased Doses of Botulinum Toxin A, and Results of Increased Dosing

Patient	Age (yrs)/Gender	Diagnosis	Standard Dose (U)	Supramaximal Dose (U)	Average Interval (Days) (Standard)	Average Interval (Days) (Supramaximal)	Changes to Subjective Disability	Continued Supramaximal Treatment?
A	58/F	Meige's syndrome	115	165	66	83*	No change	No
B	89/F	EB	100	150	63	105	More difficulty shopping	No
C	71/M	EB	100	125	83	98	Improved reading	Yes
D	72/F	EB	100	125	87	85	More difficulty with driving and shopping	No
E	55/F	EB	115	165	70	87	Less aware of blepharospasm	No
F	72/F	Meige's syndrome	100	150	60	88	Improved reading	Yes
G	68/M	Meige's syndrome	100	140	60	92	No change	Yes
H	70/F	Meige's syndrome	115	165	67	83	Less aware of blepharospasm; improvement in all 7 tasks	Yes

EB = essential blepharospasm; F = female; M = male.
*The patient reported she was simply unable to return to the clinic sooner.
(Reprinted from *Ophthalmology*, 113, Levy RL, Berman D, Parikh M, et al, Supramaximal doses of botulinum toxin for refractory blepharospasm, pp 1665-1668, Copyright 2006, with permission from Elsevier Science.)

Management of Complications after Insertion of the SmartPlug Punctal Plug: A Study of 28 Patients

Mauriello JA, and the SmartPlug Study Group (Summit, NJ; et al)
Ophthalmology 113:1859-1862, 2006   6–6

Purpose.—To characterize and describe the management of complications seen in patients who have undergone insertion of the SmartPlug permanent punctal plug.

Design.—Retrospective case series.

Participants.—Patients who experienced complications after SmartPlug insertion and were treated by 1 of 18 ophthalmic plastic and reconstructive surgeons between January 2004 and October 2005.

Methods.—Presenting symptoms and signs and the management of complications were analyzed.

Main Outcome Measures.—Prevalences of canaliculitis and dacryocystitis, tearing at presentation, and outcome of conservative and/or surgical management of the SmartPlug complications.

Results.—Twenty-eight patients were included in the study; 13 had bilateral involvement. On initial presentation, 18 patients had inflammation, including 17 with canaliculitis and 1 with recurrent acute dacryocystitis (Fig 1). Ten patients had little or no inflammation; all 10 had tearing of the involved eye(s). In 5 patients, complications resolved after office irrigation of the lacrimal drainage system; in a sixth patient, silicone intubation was performed as well. Canaliculotomy was performed in 13 patients (bilateral in 3) and combined with silicone intubation (3 patients). Canaliculotomy was

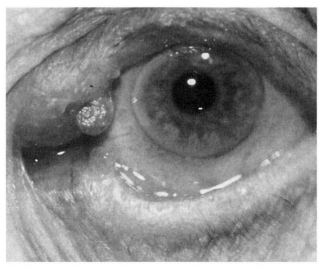

FIGURE 1.—Photograph of a patient with canaliculitis and pyogenic granuloma arising in the puncta of both the left upper and lower lids. (Reprinted from *Ophthalmology*, 113, Mauriello JA, and the SmartPlug Study Group, Management of complications after insertion of the SmartPlug punctal plug, *A study of 28 patients*, pp 1859-1862, Copyright 2006, with permission from Elsevier Science.)

planned in an additional 2 patients. Canaliculitis in 1 patient responded to a course of oral antibiotics; the plug was massaged out of the punctum in a retrograde fashion in another patient. In still another patient, the plugs expressed themselves at the time of planned canaliculotomy. In 4 patients, dacryocystorhinostomy (DCR) with silicone intubation was necessary. Two additional patients refused further treatment including DCR and canaliculotomy; both were lost to follow-up.

Conclusions.—Canaliculitis, acute dacryocystitis, and tearing may be seen in patients who have had SmartPlugs and may be managed by removal of the plug. A trial of topical and oral broad-spectrum antibiotics followed by retrograde massage of the plug through the canaliculus may be helpful should plug removal be deemed appropriate. If conservative measures fail, canaliculotomy with removal of the plug may be considered; DCR may be necessary. Although lacrimal irrigation may resolve the problem, irrigation also may dislodge the plug from its canalicular position and cause permanent obstruction of the lacrimal drainage system.

▶ The use of intracanalicular punctal plugs continues to be a problem. In the 1990s, Herrick intracanalicular plugs caused lacrimal obstructions more commonly in the lacrimal sac. This problem with SmartPlugs has now become the most common cause of canaliculitis in my practice in the last year. This study, conducted between January 2004 and October 2005, identifies 28 patients in 18 practices. The number of patients would be much higher now. The importance of the article is not really the number of patients but to make physicians and patients aware that these intracanalicular plugs do cause problems. The problems in my experience and in the study are almost always in the canaliculus and rarely in the lacrimal sac. Fortunately, simple canaliculotomy usually results in the plug coming out and being curative. Topical and systemic antibiotics may improve the problem temporarily but will not serve as a long-term cure.

It is important to keep an intracanalicular plug in the differential in the case of canaliculitis, and to ask patients with canaliculitis if they have ever had plugs placed. Equally important is to avoid the use of an intracanalicular plug if possible. Punctal cautery and minor procedures on the canaliculus offer effective, alternative ways to close the puncta.

R. B. Penne, MD

Histopathology of Blepharoptosis Induced by Prolonged Hard Contact Lens Wear

Watanabe A, Araki B, Noso K, et al (Kyoto Prefectural Univ of Medicine, Japan; Aichi Med Univ, Japan)
Am J Ophthalmol 141:1092-1096, 2006   6–7

Purpose.—To clarify histopathologically the structural features of blepharoptosis in prolonged hard contact lens wearers.

Design.—Retrospective case-control study.

Methods.—Biopsy specimens from identical sites at the levator aponeurosis and Mueller muscle from 15 long-term hard contact lens wearers were examined histopathologically (group 1). They comprised two men and 13 women with bilateral blepharoptosis ranging in age from 26 to 59 years (mean ± SD, 44.4 ± 10.70 years). The average length of hard contact lens wear was 25.4 years (range 12 to 40 years), and the average spherical equivalent refractive error was −9.100 diopters (range −2.825 to −20.375 diopters). We also examined specimens from 15 patients with involutional blepharoptosis who underwent levator resection; they comprised three men and 12 women ranging in age from 64 to 79 years (mean ± SD, 72.3 ± 4.38 years).

Results.—All patients in group 1 manifested fibrosis and negligible fatty degeneration in Mueller muscle. In group 2, we detected mild fibrosis in Mueller muscle and fatty degeneration of the aponeurosis and Mueller muscle.

Conclusions.—Prolonged hard contact lens wear induces fibrosis in Mueller muscle and may result in contact lens-induced blepharoptosis.

▶ This article found evidence of fibrosis of Mueller's muscle in patients who wore rigid contact lenses and developed ptosis. They were compared to a control group of ptosis patients who did not wear rigid lenses. These patients showed mild fibrosis but more fatty degeneration. The fact that the mean age in the contact lens group was 26 years younger demonstrated that rigid lenses cause early ptosis in some patients. The older age in the nonrigid contact lens group may also explain the fatty degeneration in the levator muscle in the non lens-wearing group.

We have from this article histopathologic evidence that rigid lenses do cause changes in Mueller's muscle and this is likely to be the cause of the ptosis that developed in these patients. Most ophthalmologists accept that rigid lens wearers have ptosis develop at a younger age. The debate whether this was because of daily pulling on the eyelids over years now appears to point to chronic irritation and scarring of Mueller's muscle as the cause.

We as ophthalmologists need to tell our rigid lens patients about this. I doubt many will change lens types as most wear these rigid lenses because soft lenses did not work.

R. B. Penne, MD

Isolated Medial Orbital Wall Fractures With Medial Rectus Muscle Incarceration
Brannan PA, Kersten RC, Kulwin DR (Univ of Cincinnati, Ohio)
Ophthal Plast Reconstr Surg 22:178-183, 2006   6–8

Purpose.—To retrospectively review and analyze cases of isolated medial orbital wall fractures with medial rectus muscle incarceration presenting to a tertiary ophthalmic plastic surgery practice from 1997 to 2005.

Methods.—Retrospective chart review and literature review.

Results.—Nine cases of isolated medial wall fracture with medial rectus muscle incarceration are presented. The most frequently encountered clinical feature was adduction deficit on the affected side. Extraocular motility improved in all patients who underwent surgery, and mean postoperative enophthalmos was minimal.

Conclusions.—Isolated medial orbital wall fractures with medial rectus muscle incarceration are rare. Ocular motility abnormalities were the only indication of underlying fracture in the majority of our cases. Clinicians should be alerted to the anticipated presentation of medial wall fractures with incarceration of the medial rectus muscle, including the possibility of a "white eye" and normal abduction of the traumatized eye.

▶ Isolated medial wall fractures are much less common than orbital floor fractures. This article evaluates 9 cases of isolated medial wall fractures and looks at the motility patterns and presentation of these patients. We have emphasized recognizing a white-eye blow-out fracture (WEBOF) in children where there are minimal signs of trauma, but dysmotility, pain, nausea, and vomiting. Here the emphasis is on the motility pattern. These patients did not seem to have the acute symptoms of pain and nausea, but all of the patients had various patterns of dysmotility. The take-home message of the article is about the motility pattern. Medial wall fracture patients may have a significant adduction deficit but they do not have to have a large abduction deficit.

In my mind it is difficult to separate the temporary rectus muscle paralysis associated with some of these injuries from entrapment. That can be the case with any fracture. What is even more confusing is the fact that in 1 case the forced ductions were termed nearly normal in the operating room before surgery, yet there was entrapment found during surgery.

Medial wall fracture repair has better results when the repair is performed earlier as opposed to floor fractures. This may have something to do with the ethmoid sinus or other unidentified reasons. When a medial wall fracture needs repair, it is not an emergency that needs to be performed in 24 hours, but surgery should not be put off for two weeks if possible.

We can learn from this article the notion that with any trauma to the ocular area a fracture of the orbit must be considered. If this trauma is accompanied by dysmotility, pain, nausea, vomiting, or inability to evaluate the motility, then the patient requires orbital imaging. Similar to the WEBOF, if the medial rectus appears acutely entrapped in the ethmoid sinus, then the timing of the repair is more urgent.

R. B. Penne, MD

Eight-fold Path to Happiness for the Cosmetic Surgery Patient
Silkiss RZ (California Pacific Med Ctr, San Francisco)
Ophthal Plast Reconstr Surg 22:157-160, 2006   6–9

Background.—Patient expectations of cosmetic and reconstructive surgical procedures are unprecedented. As a result, surgeons face an era of unprecedented liability and stress. To identify issues in cosmetic and reconstructive surgery, to treat them more accurately, to avoid problems proactively, and to improve the likelihood of patient satisfaction requires better awareness and communication between surgeon and patient. An 8-step path was identified as a way to manage in this environment.

Method.—Step 1 requires managing the balance of power between doctor and patient. Essentially this means establishing a bilateral and balanced relationship, with each party willing to walk away if indications of imbalance develop.

Step 2 advises that you listen to the patient before surgery. Ask questions to clearly define what the patient wants. Encourage the use of photographs showing the desired or anticipated outcome and openly discuss what is and is not possible. Guide patients to focus on possibilities rather than perfection and document preexisting asymmetries.

In step 3, determine the patient's motivation for the surgery and evaluate whether the patient is an appropriate candidate. Responding to unhappy life situations by having cosmetic surgery can be fraught with peril for the surgeon.

Set realistic surgical goals in step 4. Both surgeon and patient must clearly understand the optimal results a technique can provide as well as its usual results. Never assume patients share your personal esthetics or style. Assess patients for the presence of body dysmorphic syndrome, dysmorphophobia, or heightened narcissism that surgery cannot satisfy. Such patients have unrealistic goals and are unlikely to be happy.

In step 5, assess that patient for the warning signs of difficulties. Such patients may have the psychiatric disorders already noted or be obsessive-compulsive or extremely neurotic. Trust your intuition as well as any objective signs of a difficult patient. Screening questionnaires can effectively evaluate potential patients.

Step 6 is to obtain thorough informed consent. Lay out the specifics of the procedure, potential risks and suboptimal results, and the risk of not meeting expectations. Discuss each topic thoroughly so the consent is truly informed.

In step 7, remind the patient that form follows function. A maximally esthetic result is achieved by managing target tissues appropriately and not overcorrecting. All procedures must consider the patient's age, ethnicity, and preoperative appearance. The current understanding of rejuvenation focused on a youthful fullness of face, not hollowness, a taut appearance of the tissues, or an unnatural frozen look.

The environment is addressed in step 8. Both office and procedure room should express your ability to understand esthetics. Emphasize a clean, comfortable space with a contemporary look. Provide both health and fashion magazines in the waiting room. The staff must be knowledgeable, supportive, and nonjudgmental. Design the procedure room for a calm, controlled, relaxing experience. Send the patient home with items to enhance the experience, such as sunglasses, gel packs, or ointment as well as clearly worded instructions, medications or prescriptions, and a postoperative appointment. Remove sutures with a minimum of discomfort. State your revision policy firmly to avoid conflict.

Conclusions.—Patient selection, communication, expectations, and outcomes can be managed by following the 8 steps outlined and using surgical judgment and skill.

▶ Any physician who deals with patients who undergo elective procedures should read this article. This is even more of a must read for anyone doing cosmetic procedures. In many ways, the thoughts and ideas are common sense, but sometimes in the world of cosmetic surgery what is common sense can be lost. I highly recommend reading this article in its entirety.

R. B. Penne, MD

When Is Enophthalmos "Significant"?

Koo L, Hatton MP, Rubin PAD (Massachusetts Eye and Ear Infirmary, Boston)
Ophthal Plast Reconstr Surg 22:274-277, 2006   6–10

Purpose.—It is currently unknown how many measurable millimeters of enophthalmos may be noticeable to an observer. Identifying the amount of enophthalmos present may help to guide patients and clinicians in regard to surgical management of enophthalmos.

Methods.—The Massachusetts Eye and Ear Infirmary Oculoplastics imaging database was used to select 12 photographs of patients with unilateral enophthalmos whose measurements ranged between 1 mm and 8 mm for the study group and 12 photographs of patients who did not have enophthalmos as the control group. Observers were asked to review each of the photographs from both groups and to comment on whether the appearance was normal or abnormal.

Results.—There was no statistical difference found when observers reviewed photographs from the control group and patients whose measurements ranged between 1 mm and 2 mm (87%, 83% respondents identifying patients as normal, respectively). Twenty-eight percent of observers found patients with 3 mm and 4 mm of enophthalmos as having a normal appearance ($P < 0.001$). Ninety-seven percent of observers commented that patients with measurements of 5 mm and 8 mm had an abnormal appearance ($P < 0.001$).

Conclusions.—Patients with 2 mm and less of measurable enophthalmos had a normal appearance as frequently as those without enophthalmos. Nearly all patients with measurements of 5 mm and greater had abnormal appearances. The point at which enophthalmos becomes detectable lies between 3 mm and 4 mm.

▶ When treating patients with orbital trauma we are often in a situation where an orbital fracture has not caused diplopia but there is enophthalmos. This article attempts to answer the question of when does enophthalmos become noticeable. The study used pictures of patients with various amounts of enophthalmos. Fifty observers (both physicians and ophthalmic support staff) then graded the patients as normal or abnormal. The results showed that patients with 2 mm of enophthalmos were thought to be normal whereas between 3 and 4 mm of enophthalmos is when the enophthalmos became noticeable.

This article is helpful as a guideline to discuss with patients. It is important to remember that these results will not apply to all patients. The fact that this was done from 2-dimensional pictures and not in person may affect the results. Other problems such as globe displacement as well as other facial deformities may make the amount of enophthalmos more or less prominent. Patient expectations are also a big variable. A certain amount enophthalmos may be more bothersome to one patient than another, regardless of what other people's perceptions may be.

I have always considered 2.5 to 3 mm of enophthalmos to be where it becomes clinically significant. This approach is similar to these findings. In clinical practice, what a patient wants to have surgery to correct varies widely and so each patient must be individualized.

R. B. Penne, MD

Efficacy of Botulinum Toxin Type A After Topical Anesthesia
Sami MS, Soparkar CNS, Patrinely JR, et al (Plastic Eye Surgery Associates, PLLC, Houston; Univ of Texas, Houston; Baylor College of Medicine)
Ophthal Plast Reconstr Surg 22:448-452, 2006   6–11

Purpose.—To determine whether the use of topical anesthesia has an impact on botulinum toxin type A (BTX-A) efficacy.

Methods.—Forty patients (20 receiving BTX-A for facial cosmetic rhytid reduction and 20 for benign essential blepharospasm) were evaluated in a double-blind, randomized, triple-crossover study at 2.5- to 4.5-month intervals. The discomfort and efficacy of BTX-A injections after betacaine application to half the face (random assignment) were compared against the discomfort and efficacy of a placebo ointment on the other half of the face. This was followed by cryoanalgesia to the entire face.

Results.—Patients ranged from 27 to 81 years of age (mean, 53 years), and 34 were female. Of the 120 total injection comparisons, a better BTX-A effect on one side of the face was reliably identified by 80% and 77% of blepharospasm and cosmetic patients, respectively, with the placebo-treated side providing better BTX-A effect approximately 90% of the time (p < 0.001). Patients reported a more painful side during injection in just 18 of the 120 trials, and only 1 of 40 patients believed the administration of analgesia was worth the trouble.

Conclusions.—Pretreatment with topical betacaine followed by skin cooling seems to have a deleterious impact on BTX-A effect without a significantly beneficial patient-perceived reduction in injection discomfort.

▶ This is a randomized double-blinded study that looks at the effects of topical anesthesia applied before Botox (Allergan Pharmaceuticals, Irvine, CA) injections. The study looked for any effect the anesthesia had on pain of injection and on the therapeutic effects of the Botox (Allergan Pharmaceuticals, Irvine, Calif.). The results showed that about 80% of patients noted a difference in effect of the BTX-A, and of those 90% noted the side without the topical anesthesia to have the superior effects. The other finding was that in only 18 of the 120 injections did the patient identify one side as more painful than the other. Only 1 of the 40 patients involved thought the process involved in giving the topical anesthesia was worth the trouble.

The results are conclusive that topical anesthesia adversely effects Botox injection (Allergan Pharmaceuticals, Irvine, Calif.). In addition, only a few patients found any beneficial pain relief from the topical anesthesia. I would say this answers any question about the value of using topical anesthesia for Botox injections (Allergan Pharmaceuticals, Irvine, Calif.). I find the simple use of ice compress or pack applied before the injection of Botox (Allergan Pharmaceuticals, Irvine, Calif.) to be very effective in decreasing injection pain without any adverse effect on the Botox (Allergan Pharmaceuticals, Irvine, Calif.).

R. B. Penne, MD

A Permanent and Reversible Procedure to Block Tear Drainage for the Treatment of Dry Eye
DeMartelaere SL, Blaydon SM, Tovilla-Canales JL, et al (Texas Oculoplastic Consultants, Austin; Instituto de Oftalmología, Fundación Conde de Valenciana, UNAM, Mexico)
Ophthal Plast Reconstr Surg 22:352-355, 2006   6–12

Purpose.—To describe a technique of canalicular ligation and report observations on 59 consecutive surgeries.

Methods.—Retrospective, non-comparative case series of canalicular ligation by 3 surgeons over a 7-year period.

Results.—Fifty-nine eyelids of 29 patients (2 men and 27 women) underwent canalicular ligation for the treatment of severe dry eyes. Patient age ranged from 34 to 90 years. Average length of follow-up was 20 months. There were no complications. Ninety-one percent of patients noted an improvement in their symptoms. Two patients developed symptomatic epiphora more than 1 year postoperatively and both underwent successful reversal.

Conclusions.—Canalicular ligation is an effective technique for punctal occlusion in patients with severe dry eyes. It combines surgical ease with excellent cosmetic outcomes.

▶ Punctal plugs have their problems causing canaliculitis or granulomas and can fall out in some patients. This leaves the option of cautery for punctal occlusion. Anyone who has performed enough punctal cautery has found a patient who, despite multiple trials of cautery, has a lacrimal system that continues to reopen. This procedure is perfect for those patients.

This is a simple procedure to occlude the canalicular system. The additional advantage of this procedure is that it creates a localized scar that can be cut out and the canaliculi repaired over a silicone tube if reversal is required. Although the need for this is not often, it is worth remembering for that certain patient whose life will be simplified.

R. B. Penne, MD

Duration of Botulinum Toxin Effect in the Treatment of Crocodile Tears
Nava-Castañeda A, Tovilla-Canales JL, Boullosa V, et al (Instituto de Oftalmología, Fundación Conde de Valenciana, Mexico City)
Ophthal Plast Reconstr Surg 22:453-456, 2006   6–13

Purpose.—To provide clinical evidence of the duration of botulinum toxin type A (BTX-A) effect when applied in the palpebral lobe of the lacrimal gland in patients with gustatory epiphora.

Methods.—Prospective, nonrandomized, nonblinded study. Patients with history of gustatory epiphora were included. A Schirmer test was performed to quantify tearing induced by chewing. Clinical examination included visual acuity, tear-duct syringing, slit lamp examination, corneal staining, and eyelid malpositions. A questionnaire was completed by each patient to asses the severity of hyperlacrimation. A single dose of 2.5 units of BTX-A was injected directly into the lacrimal gland palpebral lobe. Patients were evaluated before and at 1, 4, 12, and 24 weeks after injection. The same person performed the examination and the BTX-A injection. Descriptive statistics, using repeated measures and a paired t test, were used for statistical analysis.

Results.—Fifteen patients were included. Mean age was 63 years. Before BTX-A injection, mean Schirmer test values were 5.47 mm in the unaffected eyes (NAE) and 12.07 mm in the affected eyes (AE). When comparing Schirmer test values in the AE before and after BTX-A injection, there were statistically significant differences ($p < 0.05$). Only 2 patients developed mild transitory ptosis. No other complications were noted.

Conclusions.—The effect of 2.5 units of BTX-A injected into the lacrimal gland lasted 6 months, a duration similar to that reported for other application sites.

▶ There are more and more studies using BTX-A to treat lacrimal hypersecretion or even to try and decrease normal secretion in patients with untreatable lacrimal obstruction. This study shows success in treating crocodile tears in 15 patients. This has been demonstrated before but these authors did it with a low dose of BTX-A requiring only 2.5 U, in a simple and reproducible way. They did note 2 patients with a transient ptosis but no other side effects.

Their success was both objectively measured with Schirmer testing and the patients all had subjective improvement, which lasted at least 6 months. This convinces me that this technique is useful for crocodile tears and I will be more likely to try it in patients with a scarred lacrimal system who have either failed all lacrimal surgery or do not want to have surgery.

This is a simple procedure with low risk. Having said that, it must be emphasized here, and to the patient, that this is an off label use of BTX-A. That information may influence whether patients and physicians are willing to use it. The other issue is paying for the BTX-A. Insurance companies may not pay for this because it is off-label. For physicians who do not use BTX-A for other reasons, this would mean buying a 100-U bottle costing more than $500, which is not practical. For physicians using BTX-A cosmetically the patient would be responsible for the cost of 2.5 U of BTX-A.

R. B. Penne, MD

Implant Infection in Porous Orbital Implants
Karslioğlu Ş, Serin D, Şimşek i, et al (Şişli Etfal Research Hosp, Istanbul, Turkey; Abant Izzet Baysal Univ, Istanbul, Turkey)
Ophthal Plast Reconstr Surg 22:461-466, 2006   6–14

Purpose.—To analyze implant infection in patients with porous orbital implants.

Methods.—A retrospective analysis of 212 patients with one of five types of porous orbital implants (bone-derived hydroxyapatite [HA], coralline HA, synthetic HA, porous polyethylene, and aluminium oxide) was conducted. Reasons for surgery, type of surgery, type of implant, peg system used, time of pegging, problems before and after pegging, treatment, and follow-up duration were recorded for all patients, along with additional data including time of onset of infection, microorganism cultured, antibiotics used, patient response to antibiotic therapy, additional interventions, and final status for patients with infection.

Results.—Of the 212 patients with porous orbital implants, 116 (54.72%) were pegged. Implant infection was observed in 11 of 116 patients (9.48%) with pegs, whereas 0% of unpegged implants was infected ($p = 0.001$). The interval between pegging and the onset of infection was 3 to 83 months (average, 36.27 ± 29.12 months). Implant exposure was noted in 5 of the 11 patients with infection. Symptoms resolved completely with antibiotic treatment in 7 patients. One patient required implant removal as the result of frequent exacerbations. The remaining 3 patients presented with hemorrhagic, purulent discharge and/or pyogenic granuloma on their last visits after being free of symptoms for 5 to 6 months.

Conclusions.—Implant infection is a serious problem that requires additional patient visits, intensive antibiotic therapy, surgery, or some combination of these. Existence of a peg system appears to play a role in implant infection. Infection may develop as late as 6 to 7 years after pegging, and the patient should be cautioned about potential late-onset problems. It is possible to control the infection with appropriate antibiotic therapy; removal should be reserved for refractory cases.

▶ Implant infections are a more frequent and difficult problem with a porous implant, which is what most patients have implanted. This study found a nearly 10% infection rate in the porous implants that had peg placement. This is a higher rate than previously reported, but these authors also have a very high rate of peg placement (54.72%). They had no incidence of implant infection in the nonpegged implants, which is also different from previous studies. What is impressive is that 7 of the 11 patients with infected implants were treated successfully with a 2-week course of antibiotics and their symptoms were resolved. In the past, we often thought that an infected porous implant was a lost implant. These findings give hope for saving an infected implant with systemic antibiotics.

It make sense that any conjunctival defect, whether spontaneous as in implant exposure or induced as in peg placement, creates the risk of bacterial exposure and infection of the implant. Their rate of 10% infections seems high but is another reason to think long and hard about placing pegs. Pegs definitely improve motility but the problems they bring have me concluding that they are often not worth it.

There have been recent attempts to give improved motility without a peg sticking out of the conjunctiva through the use of magnets. This is a good idea, but thus far the motility improvement obtained has been minimal and there have been problems with conjunctival breakdown over the magnets. Time will tell if this will become useful. In the meantime, we are left with peg placement being the only reliable way to improve prosthetic movement, but we also continue to find more complications with the pegs.

R. B. Penne, MD

Stepwise Treatment Paradigm for Congenital Nasolacrimal Duct Obstruction

Casady DR, Meyer DR, Simon JW, et al (Albany Med College, NY)
Ophthal Plast Reconstr Surg 22:243-247, 2006   6–15

Purpose.—To compare the outcomes achieved by a series of patients treated in a stepwise fashion who presented with congenital nasolacrimal duct obstruction.

Methods.—In this retrospective interventional case series, 127 patients, ranging in age from 1 month to 81 months, with 173 lacrimal systems diagnosed with congenital nasolacrimal duct obstruction, were treated in a stepwise fashion. A treatment paradigm was evaluated that prescribed probing as an initial procedure regardless of age. Those who failed probing received balloon catheter dilation. Those who failed probing and balloon catheterization received silicone intubation. Dacryocystorhinostomy was reserved for patients failing the above treatments. Clinical success was defined as complete resolution of symptoms. Success rates at each step were evaluated, and a cost analysis was performed.

Results.—Lacrimal probing was successful in 134 of 173 (76.9%) cases. Of the 39 probing failures, 32 (82.1%) were cured with balloon catheterization. All 7 cases (100%) that failed probing and balloon catheterization were cured with silicone intubation. No patient in this series required dacryocystorhinostomy.

Conclusions.—A stepwise approach to the treatment of congenital nasolacrimal duct obstruction is a clinically and financially effective model for treatment.

▶ This stepwise approach to congenital nasolacrimal duct obstruction (CNLDO) was 100% successful, cost efficient, and provides a logical simple approach to CNLDO. It simply involves probing first, if that fails, a balloon dacryoplasty, and finally, if needed, silicone tubes. It must be emphasized that this is not the only approach that works, and different doctors and patients may have their individualized approach that work as well or even better. This is an approach that mimics what many people already do, and the statistical results show the logic and efficiency of this approach.

This stepwise approach is attractive to patients because it is successful and gives them a mapped out approach so they can understand what is involved if the first procedure does not work, and to providers because the cost is predictable. The approach is important for physicians because it offers a straightforward approach that works and should make both patients and providers happy.

R. B. Penne, MD

Longitudinal Correlation of Thyroid-Stimulating Immunoglobulin With Clinical Activity of Disease in Thyroid-Associated Orbitopathy
Dragan LR, Seiff SR, Lee DC (Colorado Permanente Med Group; Univ of California, San Francisco)
Ophthal Plast Reconstr Surg 22:13-19, 2006   6–16

Purpose.—To investigate the possible correlation between the changes in inflammatory active phase of thyroid-associated orbitopathy (TAO) with measured changes in thyroid-stimulating immunoglobulin (TSI) levels over time. This study was undertaken to evaluate the potential usefulness of measured TSI values in following and treating patients with TAO.

Methods.—A retrospective chart analysis was performed on 23 patients who had been referred to a tertiary care oculoplastics service between July of 2002 and April of 2004 with suspected TAO. The activity status of patients with TAO was graded by using the TAO activity scale (TAOS), created to distinguish between the active and cicatricial phases of TAO. Laboratory values of TSI reported during the course of the study period were compiled for each study patient.

Results.—Linear regression analysis revealed a statistical correlation between the changes in activity of TAO, as measured by the TAOS score, and changes in measured values of TSI over time. A statistically significant correlation was also found between the activity of TAO (measured by the TAOS score) and TSI value.

Conclusions.—It was found that changes in inflammatory phase of TAO, as measured by the TAOS score, statistically correlate with changes in measured TSI. An additional correlation was also found between the absolute score of TAO activity and measured level of TSI. These findings suggest that serial TSI measurements may be an adjunct in assessing clinical inflammatory activity of TAO and may help direct clinical decision making regarding treatment decisions in TAO.

▶ TAO continues to be a disease entity that has more aspects we do not understand as opposed to aspects that we do. We have many theories and know the broad range of clinical manifestations of TAO. The ability to have any test to confirm the disease early or to tell when the disease is no longer active remains elusive. This article looks at the correlations between disease activity in TAO and the levels of TSI. This was a retrospective study and, as with any study on TAO, the ability to assess disease activity in an objective way is a challenge. The results suggest a correlation between the levels of TSI and the disease activity.

I think this is a good start and I would encourage physicians who take care of TAO patients to follow TSI levels. I am not convinced yet that this is the total answer to knowing when TAO has become inactive, but it is a start. If everyone uses this, we will obtain a larger pool of data to better determine the usefulness of TSI in assessing disease activity in TAO.

R. B. Penne, MD

7 Pediatric Ophthalmology

Retinopathy of Prematurity Challenges

by Kammi B. Gunton, MD

Retinopathy of prematurity (ROP) presents many challenges to the medical community. The spectrum of disease has changed in the last decade, and screening and treatment criteria have also been updated to address the improvements in extension of survival in these young infants. The medicolegal risks to those physicians involved in the treatment of ROP have been known to be high for some time.[1] Recently, physicians have been forced to re-evaluate their decision to provide this care because of the high indemnity cost associated with screening for ROP. Several factors contribute to the medicolegal risk presented by these young infants. The adherence to screening guidelines, proper communication between parents, neonatologists, and the ophthalmologist in these children with multiple medical issues, and the diligence required for follow-up present unique and taxing challenges in the care of patients with ROP.

The current screening guidelines adovated by the American Academy of Pediatrics (AAP), the American Association of Pediatric Ophthalmology and Strabismus (AAPOS), and the American Academy of Ophthalmology (AAO) recommend screening of infants with a birth weight of ≤1500 g or with a gestational age of 28 weeks or less, and those infants more than 1500 g with an unstable clinical course felt to be at high risk by the pediatrician or neonatologist. The prescribed follow-up schedule requires re-examination based on the findings at the first exam using the International Classification of ROP with meticulous follow-up.[2]

Most studies have proven the efficacy of these guidelines,[3,4] although a recent study evaluating children with a birth weight between 1500 and 2000 g found that 10% of these larger infants had any stage of ROP and 5.2% required cryotherapy for ROP.[5] The detection of ROP in infants with birth weight >1500g can be increased by screening those infants with the following risk factors: sepsis, necrotizing enterocolitis, intraventricular hemorrhage >stage I, pneumothorax, direct transfusions, and mechanical ventilation >96 hours.[4] Additionally, larger, more mature infants are more likely to develop severe ROP when born in countries with low to moderate levels of development.[6] To further complicate matters, another study has suggested that screening infants with birth weight <1251g and gestational age <30 weeks detected all infants at that institution with ROP requiring treatment.[7] Using this criteria, 44% fewer infants were screened, resulting in savings in time, screening costs, and stress to these young infants. The need to balance detecting all cases of ROP with cost containment strategies further complicates the treatment of ROP. In general, the identification of at-risk infants and referral of screening for ROP is the responsibility of the neonatologist or pediatrician involved in the care of the infant.

The care provided by the ophthalmologist while the child is hospitalized can be coordinated with the hospital staff with routine weekly visits to the neonatal unit. Nevertheless, diligent follow-up requires coordination with other medical team members when infants are transferred to other institutions, discharged from the hospital, or miss scheduled in-hospital appointments due to conflicting scheduling issues such as radiologic exams, surgical procedures or other tests.[8] Without assignment of responsibility to ensure follow-up, there is liability exposure, which results in extra cost to screening. Most estimates of the cost of screening are based on the mean Medicaid reimbursement rates, which estimate reimbursement for screening to be $230 and treatment of ROP as $2000.[4] The physician's cost of treatment must also factor in extra staffing required to ensure follow-up with adequate written notification of parents of missed appointments, loss of income while traveling to the hospital setting to screen infants, and reduced reimbursement in some patients because of the cost of their overall medical stay in the intensive care unit and limits of the medical insurance reimbursement. An additional cost of screening for ROP is the liability exposure. The main factor affecting the liability is failure of communication resulting in unexpected results or failure to ensure follow-up.[9]

Factors that affect non-compliance for follow-up in premature infants have been studied.[10] The majority of parents stated that inaccessibility and refusal for care in scheduling follow-up visits were the main reasons for non-compliance. Other factors increasing non-compliance were a higher rate of multiple births, short paternal education years, mothers as housewives, and a lower incidence of being the first child. Interestingly, the occurrence of other neonatal diseases did not impact compliance with follow-up in this study. Efforts in parental education while infants are hospitalized are needed to improve their understanding of ROP to improve their efforts in compliance. An approach that includes verbal and written information presented by both the ophthalmologist and neonatologist is more likely to be effective.

Claims against ophthalmologists for mismanagement of ROP are not frequent. In the experience of a medical ophthalmology expert reviewing cases, those involving ROP were 5.5% of the total, compared to 22% of the total involving cataract management.[9] Nationally, ROP case settlements are very substantial, usually over $1 million.[8] The high indemnity payments are occasionally shared between the hospital, the neonatologist, the pediatrician, and the ophthalmologist, but there is a 20-year statute of limitations during which physicians are liable for malpractice suits by minors. There are reports of loss of malpractice coverage or higher premium for physicians undertaking screening and treatment of children with ROP, which has caused some physician to eliminate ROP screening from their practice.[11]

In contrast to the difficulties physicians encounter in the screening and treatment of ROP, many studies have proven the cost-effectiveness of the current screening strategy.[4,12] These analyses factor in the lifetime estimated cost of a legally-blind individual due to ROP compared to the cost of screening and treatment. Using the previously mentioned Medicare figures, this estimates the overall cost of screening and treating infants as approximately $5.2 million annually in the United States. Based on published data on the effectiveness of treatment and impact on vision, the cost/benefit of screening for ROP with the current guidelines is $326.[4] Overall, ROP screening and treatment is favorable, especially compared with other categories of medical treatments. Other studies have also shown that children with ROP who experience a more favorable visual outcome have less functional disability when evaluating motor disability, self-care disability, and continence disability,[13] and the need for special education placement.[14] With regression of ROP, poor visual outcome is relatively rare.[15]

Several factors combine to result in challenges in the care of children with ROP. The screening guidelines need to be constantly reviewed for efficiency and safety. Policies for communication between medical personnel to ensure follow-up of infants when transfer of care to other institutions occurs are required. In addition, methods to ensure that scheduled exams occur are needed. Follow-up practices require diligence, parental education to identify potential risk factors for non-compliance, and most importantly a communication strategy with built-in checks to prevent loss of follow-up with the potential for sight-threatening disease and associated increased liability. Also, factors affecting malpractice coverage and changes in policies regarding screening and treatment of ROP need to be addressed so that physicians can continue to provide this valuable care. Screening of ROP has been proven to be cost-effective. Qualified physicians need the opportunity to continue to provide this valuable service.

References

1. Kraushar MF. Legal implications of retrolental fibroplasias. *Arch Ophthal* 88:86, 1972.
2. Joint Statement of the American Academy of Pediatrics, the American Association for Pediatric Ophthalmology and Strabismus, and the American Academy of Ophthalmology. Screening Examination of Premature Infants for Retinopathy of Prematurity, 2002.
3. Wright K, Anderson ME, Walker E, et al. Should fewer premature infants be screened for retinopathy of prematurity in the managed care era? *Pediatrics* 102:31-34, 1998.
4. Yanovitch TL, Siatkowski RM, McCaffree M, et al. Retinopathy of prematurity in infants with birth weight ≥1250 grams–Incidence, severity, and screening guideline cost-analysis. *J AAPOS* 10:128-134, 2006.
5. Flores-Santos R, Hernandez-Cabrera MA, Henandez-Herrera RJ, et al. Screening for retinopathy of prematurity: Results of a 7-year study of underweight newborns. *Arch Med Res* 38:440-443, 2007.

6. Gilbert C, Fielder A, Gordillo L, et al. Characteristcs of infants with severe retinopathy of prematurity in countries with low, moderate, and high levels of development: Implications for screening programs. *Pediatrics* 115:e518-525, 2005.
7. Ho SF, Mathew MRK, Wykes W, et al. Retinopathy of prematurity: An optimum screening strategy. *J AAPOS* 9:584-588, 2005.
8. Demorest BH. Retinopathy of prematurity requires diligent follow-up care. *Surv Opthalmol* 41:175-178, 1996.
9. Bettman JW. Seven hundred medicolegal cases in ophthalmology. *Ophthalmol* 97:1379-1384, 1990.
10. Tsou KI, Hsu CH, Fang LJ, et al. Factors affecting the non-compliance for follow-up in very low birth weight children. *Acta Paediatr Taiwan* 47:284-292, 2006.
11. Wagner RS. A potential retinopathy of prematurity crisis. *J Pediatr Opthalmol Strabismus* 39:325, 2002.
12. Quinn GE, and the Cryo-ROP Cooperative Group. Health-related quality of life at age 10 years in very low-birth-weight children with and without threshold retinopathy of prematurity. *Arch Ophthalmol* 122:1659-1666, 2004.
13. Msall ME, Phelps DL, DiGaudio KM, et al. Severity of neonatal retinopathy of prematurity is predictive of neurodevelopmental functional outcome at age 5.5 years. Behalf of the Cyrotherapy for Retinopathy of Prematurity Cooperative Group. *Pediatrics* 106:998-1005, 2000.
14. Msall ME, Phelps DL, Hardy RJ, et al. Educational and social competencies at 8 years in children with threshold retinopathy of prematurity in the CRYO-ROP multicenter study. *Pediatrics* 113:790-799, 2004.
15. Siatkowski RM, Dobson V, Quinn GE, et al. Severe visual impairment in children with mild or moderate retinal residua following regressed threshold retinopathy of prematurity. *J AAPOS* 11:148-152, 2007.

Controlling Contagious Bacterial Conjunctivitis

Lichtenstein SJ, Dorfman M, Kennedy R, et al (Univ of Illinois at Chicago; Joe DiMaggio Children's Hosp, Hollywood, Fla; North Texas Ophthalmic Plastic Surgery, Fort Worth, Tex; et al)
J Pediatr Ophthalmol Strabismus 43:19-26, 2006   7–1

Background.—Recent outbreaks (epidemics) of *Streptococcus pneumoniae* conjunctivitis, involving hundreds of patients, underscore the importance of following recommended guidelines to minimize disease transmission. These include the use of antimicrobial agents capable of minimizing patients' symptoms and the duration of the infectious period when disease can be transmitted to others.

Purpose.—To compare the amount of time required for various antibiotic solutions to kill *S. pneumoniae*, a common cause of bacterial conjunctivitis.

Materials and Methods.—Isolates of *S. pneumoniae* from three patients were exposed to selected ophthalmic antibiotic products: moxifloxacin 0.5%, tobramycin 0.3%, gentamicin 0.3%, and polymyxin B 10,000 IU–trimethoprim 1.0%. The products were diluted 1:100 and 1:1000 for testing. At 15, 30, 60, 120, and 180 minutes after exposure, aliquots of broth were withdrawn, the cells were separated and cultured, and the viable cell count was determined.

Results.—Moxifloxacin killed actively growing *S. pneumoniae* faster and to a greater extent than did the other three antibiotic products when tested at concentrations corresponding to tear film concentrations 5 to 10 minutes and 30 to 60 minutes after instillation of the products.

Conclusions.—Moxifloxacin killed *S. pneumoniae* in vitro faster than did the other antibiotics. Consequently, its use should complement other generally accepted measures for minimizing patients' symptoms and limiting the contagiousness of bacterial conjunctivitis. Also, this is consistent with the recommendations of other investigators to prescribe the most recent generation of fluoroquinolone antibiotics for the specific purpose of limiting the spread of bacterial resistance.

▶ Traditionally, gram-negative pathogens have been the major course of bacterial conjunctivitis. However, more recently, gram-positive pathogens have assumed a more prominent role in causing bacterial conjunctivitis in children. Although most symptoms are self-limiting and bacterial conjunctivitis will eventually resolve itself, it is important to stop the spread of bacterial conjunctivitis to others by killing as many pathogens as quickly as possible. Therefore, the goal of treating bacterial conjunctivitis is to kill both gram-positive and gram-negative pathogens quickly to stop possible spread and resolve infection. The eye drops should be as comfortable as possible, especially when treating children. Also, the antibiotic should have a realistic dosing schedule. The authors confirm that moxifloxacin kills pathogens in vitro faster than other antibiotics do. Not only does moxifloxacin prevent the spread of bacterial conjunctivitis more efficiently than other antibiotics, but it has been suggested by some investigators that a schedule of 2 times a day for 3 to 4 days is just as effective.

L. B. Nelson, MD, MBA

Effect of Adult Strabismus on Ratings of Official U.S. Army Photographs
Goff MJ, Suhr AW, Ward JA, et al (Brooke Army Med Ctr, San Antonio, Tex; Darnall Army Community Hosp, Ft Hood, Tex; Univ of California, Davis, Sacramento)
J AAPOS 10:400-403, 2006   7–2

Purpose.—To determine if strabismus affects the ratings of official U.S. Army photographs.

Methods.—Photographs of seven women and seven men officers (subjects) were digitally altered to give the impression of strabismus. Four photographs of each subject were obtained: two in an orthotropic state; one in a left exotropic state; and one in a left esotropic state. The photographs were presented randomly to a panel of 38 raters. Masked to the study design, the raters rated every photograph on a 1 to 10 Likert scale. The results were grouped according to eye alignment: two orthotropic groups, one exotropic group, and one esotropic group. Comparisons of the mean ratings were made between each eye alignment group and based on the subject's gender.

Results.—The mean rating for each orthotropic group was 5.4 and 5.5 Likert scale units with a SD of 0.8 and 0.9, respectively (group 1 and group

2). The mean rating for the exotropic group was 5.4 Likert scale units with a SD of 0.7. The mean rating for the esotropic group was 5.1 Likert scale units with a SD of 0.8. Significantly lower ratings were obtained for the esotropic group compared with the orthotropic group ($p = 0.028$). Women received significantly lower ratings regardless of eye alignment ($p = 0.044$).

Conclusions.—This study indicates that the presence of esotropia negatively affects the rating of an official U.S. Army photograph; furthermore, female gender negatively affects ratings.

▶ The psychosocial effects of strabismus have been previously described. It has also been reported that individuals with strabismus are judged more negatively with respect to communication skills, intelligence, and leadership ability. Finally, the negative influence of strabismus on gaining employment has been studied. This study demonstrates that esotropia may negatively affect the careers of soldiers in the United States Army. It is interesting that women would be more affected by the strabismus. Only a small number of the raters were female, which may have biased the results.

L. B. Nelson, MD, MBA

The Cost Utility of Strabismus Surgery in Adults

Beauchamp CL, Beauchamp GR, Stager DR Sr, et al (Univ of Texas, Dallas; Ctr for Evidence Based Medicine, Flourtown, Pa; Wills Eye Hosp, Philadelphia; et al)

J AAPOS 10:394-399, 2006   7–3

Purpose.—Cost-utility analysis evaluates the cost of medical care in relation to the gain in quality-adjusted life years (QALYs). Our purpose was to develop a cost model for surgical care for adult strabismus, to estimate the mean cost per case, to determine the associated gain in QALYs, and to perform cost-utility analysis.

Methods.—A cost model incorporated surgery, pre- and postoperative care, and a mean of 1.5 procedures per patient. The gain in QALYs was based on the improvement of utility on a scale from 0 (death) to 1 (perfect health). Utility was measured through physician-conducted interviews employing a time tradeoff question (seeking to estimate the portion of life expectancy a patient would be willing to trade for being rid of disease and associated effects). The interviews were conducted before and 5 to 8 weeks after surgery in 35 strabismic patients (age 19-75 years).

Results.—The cost model resulted in an estimated total cost of $4,254 per case. A significant improvement of utility was found: 0.96 ± 0.11 postoperatively versus 0.85 ± 0.20 preoperatively ($p = 0.00008$). Based on the mean life expectancy (36.0 years) of these patients, and discounting outcomes and costs by 3% annually, this resulted in a mean value gain of 2.61 QALYs after surgery and a cost-utility for strabismus surgery of $1,632/QALY.

Conclusions.—In the United States, treatments <$50,000/QALY are generally considered "very cost-effective." Strabismus surgery in adults falls well within this range.

▶ Cost-utility analysis is one way of measuring the value of medical treatment. It is not surprising that adult strabismus has a negative impact on the quality of life of the affected individual. Not only is there a significant improvement in utility after strabismus surgery, but it is very cost-effective. While there is the concern that bias may have been introduced into the study because the patient actually desired strabismus surgery, it cannot be denied that improving an adult's strabismus has a positive impact on the psychosocial effects of a manifest deviation.

L. B. Nelson, MD, MBA

The Course of Intermittent Exotropia in a Population-Based Cohort
Nusz KJ, Mohney BG, Diehl NN (Mayo Clinic, Rochester, Minn)
Ophthalmology 113:1154-1158, 2006   7–4

Purpose.—To evaluate the change in the angle of deviation in an incidence cohort of pediatric patients diagnosed with intermittent exotropia during a 20-year period.

Design.—Retrospective, population-based observational study.

Participants.—All pediatric (<19 years old) residents of Olmsted County, Minnesota diagnosed with intermittent exotropia (≥10 prism diopters) from January 1, 1975 through December 31, 1994.

Methods.—The medical records of all potential patients identified by the resources of the Rochester Epidemiology Project were reviewed.

Main Outcome Measures.—The change in the angle of deviation and its association with treatment were reviewed for each patient.

Results.—A total of 184 pediatric patients were diagnosed during the study period, of which 138 patients (75.0%) had ≥2 examinations. The deviation resolved in 5 of the 138 patients (3.6%) during a median follow-up of 9.2 years, while the Kaplan–Meier rate of increasing by 10 or more prism diopters (PD) was 23.1% at 5 years and 52.8% at 20 years. The distance deviation increased by a median of 5 PD during the preoperative period in the 55 patients who underwent surgery during a mean follow-up of 3.2 years compared with a zero PD median change in the 83 patients who avoided surgery during a mean follow-up of 7.1 years. The Kaplan–Meier probability of undergoing surgery within 20 years after diagnosis was 74.0% in this population. We were unable to detect a significant association between nonsurgical treatments and a change in the angle of deviation.

Conclusions.—In this population-based cohort of pediatric patients with intermittent exotropia, the deviation resolved in 4%, and more than half of the patients were expected to have an increase of 10 or more PD within 20 years of their diagnosis. Children who received surgery in this population were significantly more likely to have demonstrated an increase in their deviation during the preoperative period.

▶ When an exo-deviation is intermittent, eliminated with a blink, and occurs only with fatigue, observation is warranted. If the condition occurs during periods when the child is alert and lasts through a blink or change in fixation, surgery may be indicated to prevent further development of a suppression scotoma. Also, if a child shows signs of diplopia by covering one eye on a regular basis, surgery may be required. While the majority of patients with intermittent exotropia did not improve, with any retrospective study, the fixation patterns were not available.

L. B. Nelson, MD, MBA

Parental Understanding of the Role of Trainees in the Ophthalmic Care of Their Children
Zeller M, Perruzza E, Austin L, et al (Univ of Toronto; Hosp for Sick Children, Toronto)
Ophthalmology 113:2292-2297, 2006   7–5

Objective.—To examine parental knowledge and expectations regarding the roles of trainees involved in their child's ophthalmic care.

Design.—Prospective survey.

Participants.—Parents of 128 children attending outpatient pediatric ophthalmology clinics at The Hospital for Sick Children in Toronto.

Methods.—A questionnaire was given prospectively to parents (and 1 custodial grandparent). They were asked to identify, using a checklist, the roles and responsibilities of medical students, residents, and fellows and to explore their expectations regarding trainee participation using a multiple choice questionnaire.

Main Outcome Measures.—Parental knowledge and expectations regarding the roles and participation of medical trainees in the ophthalmic care of their children as measured by survey questionnaire.

Results.—Parental knowledge about the roles of trainees was very limited with one exception: more than 95% knew that medical students are learning to be doctors and most had a good knowledge of the medical student role. More than 76% wanted to be asked specifically if they would allow trainees involved in their child's care. Seventy-five percent were happy to have capable trainees involved, provided that the trainees discuss all decisions with the responsible staff doctor. Parents wanted health care providers to identify themselves by name (77%) and position (86%). Only 3% did not want trainees involved in any part of their child's care.

Conclusions.—Although parental knowledge regarding the relative roles of trainees is poor, parents generally are willing to have trainees involved in their child's medical and surgical care, provided they are adequately supervised and that the parent is aware of their participation.

▶ It is important for ophthalmologists in an academic setting where residents and medical students are commonly involved in patient care to inform parents of the responsibilities of the trainees. Most parents are willing to have medical trainees participate in the care of their children as long as they are informed ahead of time and are assured that they are under the direct supervision of an attending. Even though medical trainees assume an important role in the overall care of patients, staff physicians must respect and understand the feelings of the few parents who do object to medical students and residents involved in their children's care.

L. B. Nelson, MD, MBA

Recurrence of Amblyopia after Occlusion Therapy
Bhola R, Keech RV, Kutschke P, et al (Univ of Iowa, Iowa City)
Ophthalmology 113:2097-2100, 2006   7–6

Purpose.—To determine the stability of visual acuity (VA) after a standardized occlusion regimen in children with strabismic and/or anisometropic amblyopia.

Design.—Retrospective, population-based, consecutive observational case series.

Participants.—Four hundred forty-nine patients younger than 10 years who underwent an occlusion trial for amblyopia and were observed until there was a recurrence of amblyopia or for a maximum of 1 year after decrease or cessation of occlusion therapy.

Methods.—We performed a retrospective chart review of all patients treated by occlusion therapy for strabismic and/or anisometropic amblyopia at our institution over a 34-year period. Of the 1621 patients identified in our database, 449 met the eligibility criteria and were included in this study. Patients having at least a 2 logarithm of the minimum angle of resolution (logMAR)–level improvement in VA by optotypes or a change from unmaintained to maintained fixation preference during the course of occlusion therapy were included. A recurrence of amblyopia was defined as ≥ 2 logMAR levels of VA reduction or reversal of fixation preference within 1 year after a decrease or cessation of occlusion therapy.

Main Outcome Measure.—Recurrence of amblyopia after a decrease or cessation of occlusion therapy and its relationship with patient age and VA of the amblyopic eye at the time of decrease or cessation of occlusion therapy.

Results.—Of 653 occlusion trials, 179 (27%) resulted in recurrence of amblyopia. The recurrence was found to be inversely correlated with patient age (Table 2). There was no statistically significant association between the recurrence of amblyopia and VA of the amblyopic eye at the end of maximal occlusion therapy.

TABLE 2.—Percentage of Amblyopia Recurrence and 95% Confidence Intervals (CIs) by Age Using Optotype Visual Acuity Assessment

Age (mos)	Occlusion Trials	Recurrence [n (%)]	95% CI
24-36	25	8 (32)	17%-52%
36-48	67	20 (30)	20%-42%
48-60	87	26 (30)	21%-40%
60-72	99	27 (27)	19%-37%
72-84	83	19 (23)	15%-33%
84-96	51	9 (18)	9%-31%
96-108	38	4 (11)	4%-25%
108-120	9	1 (11)	2%-50%

There was a significant trend with the percentage of recurrence decreasing with increasing age (P = 0.03).

(Reprinted from *Ophthalmology*, 113, Bhola R, Keech RV, Kutschke P, et al, Recurrence of amblyopia after occlusion therapy, pp 2097-2100, 2006, Copyright 2006, with permission from Elsevier Science.)

Conclusions.—There is a clinically important risk of amblyopia recurrence when occlusion therapy is decreased before the age of 10 years. The risk of recurrence is inversely correlated with age ($P<0.0001$).

▶ The goal of amblyopia treatment is to obtain normal and equal vision in each eye. This goal, unfortunately, is not always reached. The younger the age at which treatment is instituted, the more likely it is to be successful. An improvement in acuity must be maintained until the child reaches visual maturity, generally considered to be 9 years of age. As the authors showed, discontinuation of patching before 9 years of age results in a substantial recurrence of amblyopia. This recurrence rate is particularly higher the younger the child. Therefore, ophthalmologists must be diligent in expressing the importance of consistent patching to parents of children with amblyopia.

L. B. Nelson, MD, MBA

Atropine for the Treatment of Childhood Myopia
Chua W-H, Balakrishnan V, Chan Y-H, et al (Singapore Natl Eye Centre; Singapore Eye Research Inst; Natl Univ of Singapore)
Ophthalmology 113:2285-2291, 2006   7–7

Purpose.—To evaluate the efficacy and safety of topical atropine, a nonselective muscarinic antagonist, in slowing the progression of myopia and ocular axial elongation in Asian children.

Design.—Parallel-group, placebo-controlled, randomized, double-masked study.

Participants.—Four hundred children aged 6 to 12 years with refractive error of spherical equivalent −1.00 to −6.00 diopters (D) and astigmatism of −1.50 D or less.

Intervention.—Participants were assigned with equal probability to receive either 1% atropine or vehicle eye drops once nightly for 2 years. Only 1 eye of each subject was chosen through randomization for treatment.

Main Outcome Measures.—The main efficacy outcome measures were change in spherical equivalent refraction as measured by cycloplegic autorefraction and change in ocular axial length as measured by ultrasonography. The primary safety outcome measure was the occurrence of adverse events.

Results.—Three hundred forty-six (86.5%) children completed the 2-year study. After 2 years, the mean progression of myopia and of axial elongation in the placebo-treated control eyes was -1.20 ± 0.69 D and 0.38 ± 0.38 mm, respectively. In the atropine-treated eyes, myopia progression was only -0.28 ± 0.92 D, whereas the axial length remained essentially unchanged compared with baseline (-0.02 ± 0.35 mm). The differences in myopia progression and axial elongation between the 2 groups were -0.92 D (95% confidence interval, -1.10 to -0.77 D; $P<0.001$) and 0.40 mm (95% confidence interval, 0.35–0.45 mm; $P<0.001$), respectively. No serious adverse events related to atropine were reported.

Conclusions.—Topical atropine was well tolerated and effective in slowing the progression of low and moderate myopia and ocular axial elongation in Asian children.

▶ Myopia is one of the most common ocular conditions treated by ophthalmologists. One of the inherent problems in evaluating progression of myopia in children is that the refractive error change is variable. The authors' study protocol of randomization using only one eye for treatment and finally comparing atropine-treated eyes with placebo-treated eyes attempted to overcome the obstacles of other studies in evaluating the progression of myopia in children. While atropine seemed to slow the progression of myopia, the duration of treatment was only 2 years. It is unclear whether the effects of atropine could continue.

L. B. Nelson, MD, MBA

Attainment of Educational Levels in Patients with Leber's Congenital Amaurosis

Apushkin MA, Fishman GA (Univ of Illinois at Chicago)
Ophthalmology 113:481-482, 2006   7–8

Purpose.—To assess the educational level attained by patients legally blind with Leber's congenital amaurosis (LCA).

Design.—Cross-sectional assessment.

Intervention.—None.

Main Outcome Measure.—Highest educational level attained by 55 patients with LCA.

Results.—A total of 55 patients with LCA were included in the study. Of the 55, 54 finished high school. In addition, 36 patients (65%) completed a college education and received a bachelor's degree, and 5 additional patients (9%) were recently accepted to college, whereas 3 others (5%) were currently attending college classes. Further, 18 patients were either pursuing (n = 3) or had attained (n = 15) an educational level beyond a bachelor's degree.

Conclusions.—Compromised visual function does not preclude the successful attainment of an academic education in patients with LCA who are substantially visually impaired from birth. These data have clinically relevant implications for the parents of children with LCA and for the patients themselves in providing a tone of optimism for their potential of attaining competitive academic achievements.

▶ As pediatric ophthalmologists, we are often faced with the challenge of examining and treating children with severe visual impairment. We not only must explain to parents the circumstances surrounding the ocular condition, but encourage these children and their parents to pursue educational opportunities and activities similar to other children with normal visual potential. The fact that a majority of these patients with a severe visual impairment either were accepted to college, attending college, or graduating from college is clear evidence of the educational potential of these individuals.

L. B. Nelson, MD, MBA

Factors Associated with Childhood Strabismus: Findings from a Population-Based Study
Robaei D, Rose KA, Kifley A, et al (Westmead Millennium Inst, Sydney; Univ of Sydney)
Ophthalmology 113:1146-1153, 2006   7–9

Purpose.—To describe strabismus prevalence and associated factors in a representative sample of 6-year-old Australian children.

Design.—Population-based cross-sectional study.

Participants.—One thousand seven hundred thirty-nine predominantly 6-year-old children resident in Sydney examined in 2003 and 2004.

Methods.—Cover testing was performed at near and distance fixation, and with spectacles if worn. Logarithm of the minimum angle of resolution visual acuity was measured in both eyes before and after pinhole correction, after correcting any cylindrical refraction >0.50 diopters and with spectacles, if worn. Cycloplegic autorefraction (cyclopentolate) and detailed dilated fundus examination were performed. Each child's medical and perinatal histories were sought in a detailed parental questionnaire.

Main Outcome Measures.—Strabismus was defined as any heterotropia at near or distance fixation, or both, on cover testing. Microstrabismus was defined as a deviation of fewer than 10 prism diopters.

Results.—Strabismus was diagnosed in 48 children (2.8% of the population), 5 of whom had previously undergone surgical correction; 26 children (54%) had esotropia, 14 (29%) had exotropia, 7 (15%) had microstrabismus, and 1 child had VIth cranial nerve palsy (Table 3). Prematurity was associated with a 5-fold increase in the risk of esotropia (odds ratio, 5.0; 95% confidence interval, 1.8–14.1). Visual impairment (with presenting correc-

TABLE 3.—Proportion of Strabismus by Type

Category	n (%)
Esotropia	26 (54.2)
Constant	
Basic nonaccommodative	10
Refractive (full) accommodative	3
Refractive (partial) accommodative	3
Mixed accommodative	3
Intermittent	
Convergence excess	4
Divergence insufficiency	2
Basic	1
Exotropia	14 (29.2)
Constant	1
Intermittent	
Basic	6
Convergence insufficiency	4
Divergence excess	3
Microtropia	7 (14.6)
Microexotropia	6
Microesotropia	1
Vertical deviations	11 (22.9)
In isolation	0
In combination with esotropia	8
In combination with exotropia	3
Incomitant strabismus	
VIth cranial nerve palsy	1 (2.1)

(Reprinted from *Ophthalmology*, 113, Robaei D, Rose KA, Kifley A, et al, Factors associated with childhood strabismus: Findings from a population-based study, pp 1146-1153, Copyright 2006, with permission from Elsevier Science.)

tion) was significantly more common in children with (22.9%) than without (1.3%) strabismus ($P<0.0001$). The presence of strabismus was significantly associated with hyperopia, astigmatism, anisometropia, and amblyopia ($P<0.0001$).

Conclusions.—This report documents the prevalence of strabismus and its relation to other ocular signs and visual impairment in a representative sample of Australian school children. Presence of strabismus was significantly associated with prematurity.

▶ While the incidence of strabismus in the study population was lower (2.8%) than that reported in other epidemiologic studies, the authors did not include developmentally delayed children. Children with neurologic abnormalities are well known to have a higher-than-normal incidence of strabismus. Even though the incidence of strabismus in low birth weight children is quite significant, the authors found that among the children who were breast-fed, the incidence is much lower. It is unclear what potential role breast-feeding may play in reducing the incidence of strabismus in low birth weight children. Further research in this area needs to be done.

L. B. Nelson, MD, MBA

Visual Acuity in Children with Glaucoma

Kargi SH, Koc F, Biglan AW, et al (Univ of Karaelmas, Zonguldak, Turkey; SSK Ankara Eye Hosp, Turkey; Univ of Pittsburgh, Pa)
Ophthalmology 113:229-238, 2006   7–10

Purpose.—To investigate the risk factors that influence outcome of visual function in children with glaucoma.

Design.—Retrospective noncomparative interventional case series.

Participants.—One hundred twenty-six patients (204 eyes) who had childhood glaucoma observed over 30 years, with a mean follow-up of 11.6 years.

Interventions.—Full ophthalmologic examination, including measurement of corrected visual acuity (VA), slit-lamp and fundus examinations, intraocular pressure (IOP) measurement, and gonioscopic evaluation; periodic cycloplegic refraction and perimetry; and treatment of amblyopia.

Main Outcome Measures.—Type of glaucoma; final best-corrected VA of good (6/6–6/12), fair (6/15–6/30), or poor (≤6/60); patient age at time of development of glaucoma complications; and percentage of IOP measurements of ≤19 mmHg, perimetry results, and cup-to-disc (C/D) ratio during follow-up.

Results.—The most recently measured VAs of children treated for glaucoma were good in 29%, fair in 24%, and poor in 47%. The most favorable outcome was for patients with primary infantile glaucoma followed by secondary glaucoma. Amblyopia and optic nerve damage due to glaucoma were the most frequent complications affecting VA. Patients with an IOP of ≤19 mmHg on 80% of determinations had stable optic nerve C/D ratios and visual fields.

Conclusions.—Vision sufficient to qualify for a motor vehicle driving license was attainable in almost 30% of affected eyes. Visual acuity achieved at 6 years of age remained stable over the study period. Treatment of amblyopia is important to achieve this result.

▶ Once the IOP is controlled in children with glaucoma, amblyopia often becomes an important sequela that requires diligent treatment. Even when there is no residual corneal cloudiness, significant refractive errors commonly cause anisometropia amblyopia in childhood glaucoma. I was surprised that the authors included patients with aniridia in the study since a majority of these patients never attain better then 20/200 acuity even if glaucoma does not occur. I would have thought that more than half the eyes with aphakic glaucoma had amblyopia.

L. B. Nelson, MD, MBA

Age-Related Distance Esotropia

Mittelman D (Advocate Lutheran Gen Hosp, Park Ridge, Ill)
J AAPOS 10:212-213, 2006   7–11

Purpose.—To describe a form of acquired esotropia occurring in older adults, which here is termed age-related distance esotropia.

Methods.—A retrospective consecutive case series of 26 patients with this condition was reviewed.

Results.—The patients ranged in age from 62 to 91 years old with a median age of 77 years. The distance deviation varied from 4 prism diopters (PD) ET (esotropia) to 20 PD ET, with a median angle of 9 PD ET. At near fixation, the measurements ranged from 9 PD ET' to 10 PD X' (exophoria), with a median deviation of 3 PD ET'. Ductions and versions were full, with no evidence of lateral rectus paresis. None of these patients had an obvious underlying neurologic disorder, such as tumor or stroke. Treatment consisted of prescribing the minimum prismatic correction that eliminated distance diplopia, which was then incorporated into the patients' current spectacles. This treatment successfully eliminated the symptoms in all patients. No patient in this study required surgery.

Conclusion.—A distinctive form of strabismus occurs in older adults that is characterized by esotropia greater at distance than near fixation. The etiology of this disorder is unknown, but it is likely secondary to anatomical changes in the orbit and/or muscles associated with aging. Most patients are readily corrected by prisms but, surgical correction might be required in some cases.

▶ Even though the author coined the term age-related distance esotropia as a new condition, it seems to me the patients described have the same clinical findings as divergence insufficiency. Fewer than half the patients had imaging studies before the author's evaluation. I believe that any adult who presents with recent-onset diplopia and esotropia greater at distance than near fixation should still have imaging studies. Occasionally a patient with the findings presented in this article could have an intracranial abnormality that needs treatment and can affect the well-being of the patient.

L. B. Nelson, MD, MBA

Combined Strabismus and Lens Surgery

Ticho BH, Ticho KE, Kaufman LM (Christ Hosp and Med Ctr, Oak Lawn, Ill; Hope Children's Hosp, Oak Lawn, Ill; Univ of Illinois, Chicago)
J AAPOS 10:430-434, 2006   7–12

Background.—Simultaneous eye muscle and lens surgery in patients with strabismus and lens abnormalities offers the advantage of avoiding staged surgery.

Methods.—Thirty-three combined strabismus and lens surgeries were performed on 30 patients who ranged in age from 22 months to 91 years.

Fifteen of the strabismus procedures were performed for esotropia, 12 for exotropia, 4 for vertical deviations, and 2 for combined vertical-horizontal deviations. Surgical amounts often were reduced to lessen the risk of overcorrection, to minimize anesthetic requirements (when using topical rather than general anesthesia), or to avoiding additional surgery on the contralateral or ipsilateral eye. The intraocular surgeries included cataract extraction without or with posterior chamber intraocular lens, secondary intraocular lens implantation, and YAG laser posterior capsulotomy. In 28 cases, muscle and intraocular surgery was performed on the same eye, and in 5 cases the strabismus surgery was performed on the eye opposite the intraocular surgery.

Results.—The average length of postoperative follow-up was 23.2 months (range, 1-94 months). Surgical, anesthetic, and postoperative complications, other than unsatisfactory ocular alignment, were limited to one retinal detachment in a patient with persistent fetal vasculature. Strabismic undercorrections (>12$^\Delta$ of horizontal deviation or >5$^\Delta$ of vertical deviation) occurred in 11 cases (37%). There were no overcorrections. A poor visual response (<20/50) to the intraocular surgery was encountered in 6 patients, all as the result of amblyopia or preexisting vitreoretinal pathology.

Conclusions.—Simultaneous extraocular muscle and lens surgery is an option for patients with strabismus and lens abnormalities. Standard strabismus surgical amounts are recommended.

▶ While simultaneous strabismus and lens surgery is an option, I have a number of concerns about this procedure. With the added manipulation of strabismus surgery to lens surgery, is there a greater chance of endophthalmitis? Once the lens is removed and improved vision results, it is possible that the magnitude of the strabismus may change. This could affect the outcome of the strabismus surgery. While the authors did not report any overcorrections, they reduced the strabismus surgery amounts in many patients. This seemed to be a questionable compromise since only 67% of patients had a strabismus surgical success. While the authors suggested that simultaneous surgery could be cost saving, I believe this type of surgery may compromise the outcome.

L. B. Nelson, MD, MBA

Prevalence and Development of Strabismus in 10-Year-Old Premature Children: A Population-Based Study
Holmström G, Rydberg A, Larsson E (Uppsala Univ, Sweden; Karolinska Institutet, Stockholm)
J Pediatr Ophthalmol Strabismus 43:346-352, 2006   7–13

Purpose.—To evaluate the prevalence and development of strabismus, at 10 years, in children born prematurely.

Methods.—This population-based study included 216 premature and 217 full-term children from the same geographic area.

Results.—Strabismus was noted in 16.2% (35 of 216) premature and in 3.2% (7 of 217) full-term children. The most important risk factors for strabismus at 10 years were anisometropia at 6 months, spherical equivalent refractive errors (i.e., > +3 D or < −3 D) at 2.5 years, and various neurologic conditions.

Conclusion.—At 10 years, children born prematurely have a greater risk of strabismus than children born at term.

▶ While retinopathy of prematurity is the ophthalmologic condition that has the most potential for serious visual impairment in premature infants, myopia and strabismus are common late ocular sequelae. It is not surprising that the authors found strabismus to be 5 times more common in 10-year-old premature children than in full-term children. Previous severe retinopathy of prematurity seems to be an important risk factor for the development of strabismus. It is important that premature infants not only receive regular ophthalmologic follow-up care for years, but the parents need to be made aware that strabismus and myopia are common ophthalmologic conditions that might affect their children.

L. B. Nelson, MD, MBA

Factors Affecting Sensory Functions After Successful Postoperative Ocular Alignment of Acquired Esotropia
Kassem RR, Elhilali HM (Cairo Univ)
J AAPOS 10:112-116, 2006   7–14

Purpose.—We sought to evaluate the sensory status of patients with acquired esotropia who were able to re-establish stable alignment by optical correction and surgery and to determine the possible predictors of the different sensory outcomes.

Methods.—Thirty-four successfully aligned esotropic patients were included in the study. Preoperative evaluation comprised history taking, measurement of visual acuity, evaluation of the sensory status (using the Worth 4-Dot test, and the Titmus Stereo test), measurement of ocular deviation, cycloplegic refraction, and fundus examination. All patients underwent successful surgical alignment to within 10 prism diopters (Δ) of orthotropia. At each postoperative follow-up visit, the sensory functions and ocular alignment were assessed. Statistical analysis of the results was performed.

Results.—Among the 34 patients included in the study, 62% achieved fusion, 17% had diplopia, 15% had suppression, and 6% had a variable response to the Worth 4-Dot test at 6 months after surgery. Stereopsis was achieved in 32% as determined by the Titmus Stereo test. Statistical analysis revealed a significant relationship between the sensory status and the duration of strabismus ($P = .00002$), the age at surgery ($P = .00289$), and postoperative ocular alignment ($P = .02211$).

Conclusion.—Early surgical and optical ocular alignment of strabismic patients is advisable to achieve fusion and stereopsis.

▶ The most important factor to determine the reestablishment of binocular visual function in acquired esotropia is the duration of the misalignment. If an acquired nonaccommodative esotropia can be corrected while it is intermittent or less than 4 months' duration, excellent binocular function can result. Even with a much longer duration of acquired esotropia, a smaller but yet possible postoperative fusion potential can be achieved. Therefore, adults with acquired strabismus of long duration can possibly achieve even rudimentary binocular function.

L. B. Nelson, MD, MBA

Long-term Outcomes of Photorefractive Keratectomy for Anisometropic Amblyopia in Children
Paysse EA, Coats DK, Hussein MAW, et al (Baylor College of Medicine, Houston)
Ophthalmology 113:169-176, 2006   7–15

Purpose.—To evaluate the long-term visual acuity (VA) and refractive error responses to excimer laser photorefractive keratectomy (PRK) for treatment of anisometropic amblyopia in children.

Design.—Prospective interventional case–control study.

Participants.—Eleven children, 2 to 11 years old, with anisometropic amblyopia who were noncompliant with conventional therapy with glasses or contact lenses and occlusion therapy were treated with PRK. A cohort derived retrospectively of 13 compliant and 10 noncompliant children with refractive errors similar to those of the PRK group who were treated with traditional anisometropic amblyopia therapy served as control groups.

Intervention.—Photorefractive keratectomy for the eye with the higher refractive error.

Main Outcome Measures.—(1) Refractive error reduction and stability in the treated eye, (2) cycloplegic refraction, (3) VA, (4) stereoacuity, and (5) corneal haze up to 3 years after PRK. Compliant and noncompliant children with anisometropia amblyopia were analyzed as controls for refractive error and VA.

Results.—Preoperative refractive errors were -13.70 diopters (D) (± 3.77) for the myopic group and $+4.75$ D (± 0.50) for the hyperopic group. Mean postoperative refractive errors at last follow-up (mean, 31 months) were -3.55 D (± 2.25) and $+1.41$ D (± 1.07) for the myopic and hyperopic groups, respectively. At last follow-up, cycloplegic refractions in 4 (50%) of 8 myopes and all hyperopes (100%) were within 3 D of that of the fellow eye. Five (63%) of 8 myopic children achieved a refraction within 2 D of the target refraction. Two (67%) of 3 hyperopic patients maintained their refractions within 2 D of the target. Refractive regressions (from 1 year after surgery to last follow-up) were 0.50 ± 1.41 D (myopes) and 0.60 ± 0.57 D (hyperopes). Seven children (77%) were able to perform psychophysical VA testing preoperatively and postoperatively. Five (71%) of the 7 children had uncorrected VA improvement of at least 2 lines, and 4 (57%) of 7 had best spectacle-corrected VA improvement of at least 2 lines, with 1 improving 7 lines. Five (55%) of 9 children had improvement of their stereoacuity at last follow-up. Subepithelial corneal haze remained negligible. The mean final VA of the PRK group was significantly better than that of the noncompliant control group ($P = 0.003$). The mean final refractive error for both myopic and hyperopic groups was also significantly better that that of the control groups ($P = 0.007$ and $P < 0.0001$, respectively).

Conclusions.—Photorefractive keratectomy for severe anisometropic amblyopia in children resulted in long-term stable reduction in refractive error and improvement in VA and stereopsis, with negligible persistent corneal haze.

▶ What the authors showed was that refractive surgery can be performed on children. However, this pilot study did not demonstrate that refractive surgery improves VA in noncompliant patients with anisometropia amblyopia. Refractive surgery is not appropriate for most children with anisometropia amblyopia because they can usually be treated with glasses. However, the patients in this study all were selected because of poor VA, recalcitrant amblyopia, and noncompliance. Therefore, it is not surprising that there was not a significant improvement in VA after refractive surgery. Further studies with refractive surgery for children with anisometropia amblyopia prior to amblyopia becoming recalcitrant need to be performed.

L. B. Nelson, MD, MBA

8   Neuro-ophthalmology

Traditional Beliefs Fall With Neurodegenerative Diseases in Neuro-Ophthalmology

by Robert C. Sergott, MD

This year's selections in neuro-ophthalmology highlight how skeptical we must be about traditional ideas in neuro-ophthalmology that are accepted as dogma. We now read how patients with Alzheimer's disease and Parkinson's disease may have significant visual problems that need to be addressed diagnostically and therapeutically by neuro-ophthalmologists.

A theme has been developing subtly with neuro-degenerative diseases and neuro-ophthalmology. First, the traditional theory that multiple sclerosis (MS) almost completely spared axons has been disproved. At approximately the same time the academic neuro-ophthalmology world realized that MS was not a disease of relapses and complete remissions, but one of chronic disease activity between attacks.

Realizing the critical nature of axonal transaction in MS coincided with the development of optical coherence tomography (OCT).[1] Suddenly, we had a non-invasive, accurate method to directly and serially measure axonal thickness in MS. OCT now promises to be a reliable measure of disease activity in MS and to be a clinical biomarker not only to aid in the care of the individual patient but also to determine the efficacy of established and new pharmaceutical agents.

As cited in the ensuing articles, OCT changes in the retinal nerve fiber layer thickness may correlate well with the cognitive impairment in Alzheimer's disease. Similar to the clinical and research situation with MS, OCT may provide us with an invaluable method to quantitate axonal preservation for Alzheimer's treatments and trials.

Parkinson's disease is one of the most common and most devastating neurological diseases. Traditional teaching had invariably emphasized that Parkinson's does not affect the afferent visual system. But once again, careful investigators have found that Parkinson's patients may have significant issues with visual processing.[2] Once again, the visual system may provide the substrate to follow various therapeutic interventions in this major public health problem.

Therefore, clinicians and researchers alike must always remain skeptical about so-called established facts. New technology for the evaluation of the structure of the visual system such as OCT have thrust neuro-ophthalmology into the forefront of the clinical care and research initiatives in MS. I predict that we will see similar developments in Alzheimer's and Parkinson's disease.

References

1. Iseri PK, Altinas O, Tokay T, et al: Relationship between cognitive impairment and retinal morphological and visual functional abnormalities in Alzheimer's Disease. *J. Neuroophthalmol* 26:18-24, 2006.
2. Uc EY, Rizzo M, Anderson SW, et al: Impaired visual search in drivers with Parkinson's Disease. *Ann Neurol* 60:407-413, 2006.

Optic pathway gliomas in neurofibromatosis-1: controversies and recommendations
Listernick R, Ferner RE, Liu GT, et al (Northwestern Univ, Chicago)
Ann Neurol 61:189-198, 2007 8–1

Optic pathway glioma (OPG), seen in 15% to 20% of individuals with neurofibromatosis type 1 (NF1), account for significant morbidity in young children with NF1. Overwhelmingly a tumor of children younger than 7 years, OPG may present in individuals with NF1 at any age. Although many OPG may remain indolent and never cause signs or symptoms, others lead to vision loss, proptosis, or precocious puberty. Because the natural history and treatment of NF1-associated OPG is different from that of sporadic OPG in individuals without NF1, a task force composed of basic scientists and clinical researchers was assembled in 1997 to propose a set of guidelines for the diagnosis and management of NF1-associated OPG. This new review highlights advances in our understanding of the pathophysiology and clinical behavior of these tumors made over the last 10 years. Controversies in both the diagnosis and management of these tumors are examined. Finally, specific evidence-based recommendations are proposed for clinicians caring for children with NF1.

► This excellent review updates the recent advances in the treatment and research of OPGs in NF1. This review updates the progress during the last 10 years since a major review article was last published in 1997.

NF1 is not an insignificant problem as it affects 1 in 3500 people worldwide with an autosomal dominant inheritance pattern. OPGs affect 15% to 20% of children with NF1, with a highly variable natural history characterized by aggressive behavior in two thirds of patients. The current review not only defines the current understanding of the pathogenesis of these disorders but also reviews the clinical history, natural history, and controversies concerning treatment.

The "take-home" messages from the review are:

1. No widely accepted definition of "progressive disease" exists. Probably the best measurement for progression is a combination of increasing visual dysfunction and neuroradiologic growth.
2. Chemotherapy with carboplatin and vincristine should be the initial treatment with progressive OPGs.
3. Because of the risk of secondary malignancies and radiation necrosis, radiation therapy is not recommended except in the case when all chemotherapeutic options have been utilized.
4. Surgical removal is recommended only in the case of a blind or nearly blind eye when the degree of proptosis threatens chronic corneal exposure.

This article is a "must read" for any ophthalmologist involved in the care of patients with NF1.

R. C. Sergott, MD

Ophthalmic Management of Facial Nerve Palsy: A Review
Rahman I, Sadiq SA (Manchester Royal Eye Hosp, England)
Surv Ophthalmol 52:121-144, 2007   8–2

Facial nerve palsy affects individuals of all ages, races, and sexes. Psychological and functional implications of the paralysis present a devastating management problem to those afflicted, as well as the carriers. Since Sir Charles Bell's original description of facial palsy in 1821, our understanding and treatment options have expanded. It is essential that a multidisciplinary approach, encompassing ophthalmologists; Ear, Nose, and Throat surgeons; plastic surgeons; and psychologists work closely to optimize patient management in a staged approach. Although the etiology remains unknown, strong histological, cerebral spinal fluid, and radiological evidence suggests a possible association with herpes simplex virus in idiopathic facial nerve palsy (Bell's palsy). The use of steroids has been suggested as a means of limiting facial nerve damage in the acute phase. Unfortunately, no single randomized control trial has achieved an unquestionable benefit with the use of oral steroid therapy and thus remains controversial. In the acute phase, ophthalmologists play a pivotal role in preventing irreversible blindness from corneal exposure. This may be successfully achieved by using intensive lubrication, medical therapy (botulinum toxin), or surgery (upper lid weighting or tarsorraphy). Once the cornea is adequately protected and recovery deemed unlikely, longer term planning for eyelid and facial reanimation may take place in an individualized manner. Onset is sudden and management potentially lengthy. Physician empathy, knowledge, and experience are essential in averting long-term lifestyle and psychological discomfort for patients.

▶ The acute onset of a unilateral paralysis of the face always prompts immediate medical attention, often to an ophthalmologist. After the clinician has established the unilateral, isolated, and lower motor neuron nature of this problem, attention must be directed at protecting the cornea and improving the chances for functional recovery. Systemic causes such as sarcoidosis and Lyme disease must be excluded before concluding that the paralysis is "idiopathic" (most data now suggest that a herpes simplex infection is responsible for the majority of cases).

For treatment, the best clinical trial reports that treatment initiated within 3 days of symptoms with acyclovir (400 mg 5 times daily) and prednisone (minimum of 30 mg twice daily) results in a superior recovery compared with only prednisolone or placebo. The treatment should continue for 10 days.

The article also provides an impartial, unbiased assessment of the various surgical procedures available for any long-term anatomic sequelae of an acute facial palsy. This review should be mandatory reading for all ophthalmology residents and is an excellent update for all active practitioners.

R. C. Sergott, MD

Mutations in *FRMD7*, a newly identified member of the FERM family, cause X-linked idiopathic congenital nystagmus
Tarpey P, Thomas S, Sarvananthan N, et al (Wellcome Trust Sanger Inst, Hinxton, Cambridge, England)
Nature Genet 38:1242-1244, 2006   8–3

Background.—The prevalence of idiopathic congenital nystagmus (ICN) is estimated to be 1 in 1000. Visual function in patients with ICN can be significantly reduced because of constant eye movement, but the degree of visual impairment varies. ICN is likely a result of abnormal development of areas in the brain controlling eye movements and gaze stability. It is usually inherited as an X-linked trait with incomplete penetrance in females. Most families map to Xq26–q27, and the locus (known as *NYSI*) has previously been mapped to a ~12-Mb interval between markers DXS9909 and DXS1211.

Overview.—This study included 16 families with X-linked ICN using 17 markers extending from Xq26–q27. ICN was fully penetrant in males in these families and ~50% penetrant in females. The phenotype was variable even within families. In all 16 families, marker haplotypes were compatible with linkage to Xq26–q27. Recombinant events in affected males in family N1 refined the location of *NYSI* to a ~7.5-Mb interval between markers DXS1047 and DXS1041. The candidate interval contained more than 80 genes. High-throughput DNA sequence analysis was performed on all coding exons of all genes within this interval. Mutations were detected in *FRMD7* (FERM domain–containing 7, previously known as *LOC90167*) at Xq26.2 in 15 of the 16 linked families after screening > 40 genes by sequence analysis. All mutations in identified in *FRMD7* cosegregated with disease in the linked families and were absent from 300 male control chromosomes. Screening of 42 singleton cases of ICN yielded 3 mutations (7%). Restricted expression of *FRMD7* was found in human embryonic brain and in developing neural retina. These findings are suggestive of a specific role for *FRMD7* in the control of eye movement and gaze stability.

Conclusions.—Mutations in *FRMD7* are a major cause of familial X-linked congenital motor nystagmus. It is hypothesized that null mutations in *FRMD7*, as found in families with X-linked congenital motor nystagmus, alter the neurite length and degree of branching of developing neurons in the midbrain, cerebellum, and retina, thereby causing disease.

▶ Every resident and most clinicians dread the evaluation of a nystagmus patient. The examination is extremely difficult and the ability to understand the entire subject is complicated by a lack of understanding of the biological basis of these syndromes.

While this article does not contain material that you will use next week, it offers new, exciting genetic information that some day may allow for rational treatment of this problem. This group describes the presence of a mutated gene in 15 of 16 families in which every man and half of the women had nystagmus.

How the mutation and its resulting aberrant gene product(s) may cause the nystagmus is unknown, but this discovery is of potentially landmark proportions for many congenital eye movement syndromes. Similar proteins influence neurite branching in utero in some mammals, leading to the hypothesis that neurite branching could be affected in the midbrain and cerebellum in X-linked idiopathic congenital nystagmus.

R. C. Sergott, MD

Resolution of homonymous visual field loss documented with functional magnetic resonance and diffusion tensor imaging
Yoshida M, Ida M, Nguyen TH, et al (Tokyo Metropolitan Ebara Hosp)
J Neuroophthalmol 26:11-17, 2006   8–4

A 68-year-old man developed right homonymous hemianopic paracentral scotomas from acute infarction of the left extrastriate area. He was studied over the ensuing 12 months with visual fields, conventional MRI, functional MRI (fMRI), and diffusion tensor imaging (DTI). As the visual field defect became smaller, fMRI demonstrated progressively larger areas of cortical activation. DTI initially showed that the lesioned posterior optic radiations were completely interrupted. This interruption lessened in time and had disappeared by one year after onset. fMRI and DTI are innovative measures to follow functional and structural recovery in the central nervous system. This is the first reported application of these imaging techniques to acute cerebral visual field disorders.

▶ MRI technologies are rapidly advancing into the "functional realm." Because of the precise anatomic and physiologic localization of the afferent visual system, reports like the current case report provide excellent verification about the accuracy of these techniques.

fMRI and DTI are 2 of the most promising applications. fMRI indirectly evaluates local blood oxygenation that is associated with neural activity. By quantitating diffusion anisotropy (directional distribution of free water), DTI produces a fiber tract map closely resembling axonal fibers.

This case report describes a patient with an acute stroke involving the left extrastriate area, resulting in a right hemianopic paracentral scotoma. As the visual field defect became smaller, fMRI demonstrated larger areas of cortical activation. At first, DTI demonstrated complete interruption of the optic radiations. However, as the visual field defect improved, the DTI deficits resolved.

Both fMRI and DTI will be utilized much more in the future, especially for evaluating treatments for acute stroke syndromes as well as possible attempts at rehabilitation.

R. C. Sergott, MD

Relationship between cognitive impairment and retinal morphological and visual functional abnormalities in Alzheimer disease

Iseri PK, Altinas O, Tokay T, et al (Kocaeli Univ, Turkey)
J Neuroophthalmol 26:18-24, 2006   8–5

Background.—There is conflicting evidence as to whether Alzheimer disease (AD) is accompanied by loss of retinal ganglion cells. To evaluate this issue, we have used optical coherence tomography (OCT) to assess the thickness and volume of the retina. We have also sought to correlate our findings with visual function and cognitive impairment.

Methods.—We evaluated 28 eyes of 14 patients with AD and 30 eyes of 15 age-matched control subjects. In these two groups, we measured retinal nerve fiber layer (RNFL) thickness, macular thickness, and macular volume with OCT, visual function through latency of the pattern visual evoked potential (VEP) signal, and cognitive impairment through the Mini-Mental State Examination (MMSE).

Results.—The parapapillary and macular RNFL thickness in all quadrants and positions of AD patients were thinner than in control subjects. The mean total macular volume of AD patients was significantly reduced as compared with control subjects ($P < 0.05$). Total macular volume and MMSE scores were significantly correlated. No significant difference was found in the latency of the VEP P100 of AD patients and control subjects.

Conclusions.—Our study confirms some other studies in showing that in AD patients there is a reduction of parapapillary and macular RNFL thickness and macular volume as measured by OCT. The reduction in macular volume was related to the severity of cognitive impairment.

▶ In many diseases, such as multiple sclerosis and optic neuritis, and papilledema and pseudotumor cerebri or brain tumors, the neuro-ophthalmologic process and examination represent a microcosm of the pathology occurring in the larger context of the entire brain and CNS.

Previous studies had provided conflicting information about a potential relationship between RNFL thickness and AD. The current study does report a statistically significant reduction of the mean total macular volume in patients with AD, as well as a significant association between the total macular volume and the MMSE score. This finding is extremely important because it provides another possible metric for therapeutic trials for AD. Also, ophthalmologists and neuro-ophthalmologists must more carefully define the visual symptoms and findings in these patients.

R. C. Sergott, MD

Impaired visual search in drivers with Parkinson's disease
Uc EY, Rizzo M, Anderson SW, et al (Univ of Iowa, Iowa City)
Ann Neurol 60:407-413, 2006   8–6

Objective.—To assess the ability for visual search and recognition of roadside targets and safety errors during a landmark and traffic sign identification task in drivers with Parkinson's disease (PD).

Methods.—Seventy-nine drivers with PD and 151 neurologically normal older adults underwent a battery of visual, cognitive, and motor tests. The drivers were asked to report sightings of specific landmarks and traffic signs along a four-lane commercial strip during an experimental drive in an instrumented vehicle.

Results.—The drivers with PD identified significantly fewer landmarks and traffic signs, and they committed more at-fault safety errors during the task than control subjects, even after adjusting for baseline errors. Within the PD group, the most important predictors of landmark and traffic sign identification rate were performances on Useful Field of View (visual speed of processing and attention) and Complex Figure Test-Copy (visuospatial abilities). Trail Making Test (B-A), a measure of cognitive flexibility independent of motor function, was the only independent predictor of at-fault safety errors in drivers with PD.

Interpretation.—The cognitive and visual deficits associated with PD resulted in impaired visual search while driving, and the increased cognitive load during this task worsened their driving safety.

▶ Except for decreased blinking and slowing of saccadic eye movements, the neuro-ophthalmologic manifestations of PD have been largely ignored. The present article is of tremendous importance for patients, their families, ophthalmologists, and public policy agencies.

The authors utilized a variety of visual, cognitive, and motor tests. The patients with PD and age-matched controls identified sighting of specific landmarks and traffic signs along a 4-lane commercial strip during an experimental drive in a vehicle simulator. The patients with PD demonstrated impaired visual search while driving, which ultimately worsened their ability to drive safely. Previous epidemiologic studies have demonstrated impaired driver safety in these patients. A subset of patients with PD did perform quite well without safety errors, suggesting that the impairment is not universal but does occur in a substantial number of patients with this condition.

I believe that in the future, testing the driving abilities of patients with PD will be mandatory.

R. C. Sergott, MD

Driving with Parkinson's Disease: More Than Meets the Eye
Newman NJ (Emory Univ School of Medicine, Atlanta, Ga)
Ann Neurol 60:387-388, 2006   8–7

Background.—Driving is one of the critical features of daily living because it often defines a person's independence and competence. Driving cessation has been associated with depression and social isolation. The act of driving an automobile is complex and requires the performance of multiple competing tasks, attendance to objects and ongoing events, and simultaneous monitoring of traffic with central and peripheral vision. Good vision is not the only physical criterion for safe driving. However, in most of the United States, the only testing requirements for legal driving after initial licensing relate to visual acuity and visual field. Most neurologists, particularly those who care for patients with Parkinson's disease, do not systematically test visual acuity and visual fields on their patients. Although simple tests of visual function are available, they are not adequate for determining a patient's ability to safely operate a motor vehicle. The issue of driving safety in neurologically impaired persons has been a concern among patients with progressive degenerative diseases, such as Parkinson's disease and Alzheimer's disease. A report described in this editorial provided important data regarding the ability of patient's with Parkinson's disease to safely operate a motor vehicle.

Overview.—A battery of visual, cognitive, and motor tests were performed in 79 drivers with Parkinson's disease and 151 neurologically normal older adults to determine whether patient driving performance and safety errors could be predicted independently. The drivers with Parkinson's disease identified significantly fewer landmarks and traffic signs and committed more at-fault safety errors. The most important predictors of landmark and traffic sign identification rate were performances on Useful Field of View and Complex Figure Test–Copy. Trail Making Test (B-A), which measures cognitive flexibility independent of motor function, was the only independent predictor of at-fault safety errors in drivers with Parkinson's disease. Impairments in attentional control, working memory, executive functions, and visuospatial ability are present early in the course of Parkinson's disease. The cognitive and visual deficits associated with this disease result in impaired visual search and object recognition while driving, and the increased cognitive load that results from this visual search task degrades the driving safety of these patients. There was a subset of drivers with Parkinson's disease that performed relatively well on the identification task, and about 17% of patients made no safety errors. However, the study confirmed that drivers with Parkinson's disease are significantly less safe than age-matched control drivers.

Conclusions.—Drivers with Parkinson's disease are significantly less safe than neurologically normal older adult drivers. Certain standardized neuropsychological and visual tests can provide indices of some of the key functional abilities in these patients that are important for driving. However, the question remains whether early identification and application of rehabilitation targeted to those aspects of driving most troublesome for these patients would improve their driving performance and prolong their independence without risking their safety and the safety of others.

▶ This insightful and practical editorial provides clinicians with the necessary perspective to care for the visual needs of Parkinson's patients. Testing visual acuity, visual fields, and color vision is clearly insufficient.

Ophthalmologists and neurologists must inquire about how the patient is functioning visually in a variety of environments, especially those that require motor, memory, cognitive, and visual processing involvement.

To insure the safety of these patients as well as that of other drivers and pedestrians, physicians need to educate not only the patients but also the families about the increased danger involved in operating a motor vehicle. We must aim to strike a fine balance so that the independence of many of these patients is not compromised while we work to provide a policy to make our highways as safe as possible.

R. C. Sergott, MD

Association between parasite infection and immune responses in multiple sclerosis
Correale J, Farez M (Raul Carrea Inst for Neurological Research (FLENI), Buenos Aires, Argentina)
Ann Neurol 61:97-108, 2007   8–8

Objective.—To assess whether parasite infection is correlated with a reduced number of exacerbations and altered immune reactivity in multiple sclerosis (MS).

Methods.—A prospective, double-cohort study was performed to assess the clinical course and radiological findings in 12 MS patients presenting associated eosinophilia. All patients presented parasitic infections with positive stool specimens. In all parasite-infected MS patients, the eosinophilia was not present during the 2 previous years. Eosinophil counts were monitored at 3- to 6-month intervals. When counts became elevated, patients were enrolled in the study. Interleukin (IL)-4, IL-10, IL-12, transforming growth factor (TGF)-beta, and interferon-gamma production by myelin basic protein-specific peripheral blood mononuclear cells were studied using enzyme-linked immunospot (ELISPOT). FoxP3 and Smad7 expression were studied by reverse-transcriptase polymerase chain reaction.

Results.—During a 4.6-year follow-up period, parasite-infected MS patients showed a significantly lower number of exacerbations, minimal variation in disability scores, as well as fewer magnetic resonance imaging changes when compared with uninfected MS patients. Furthermore, myelin basic protein-specific responses in peripheral blood showed a significant increase in IL-10 and TGF-beta and a decrease in IL-12 and interferon-gamma-secreting cells in infected MS patients compared with noninfected patients. Myelin basic protein-specific T cells cloned from infected subjects were characterized by the absence of IL-2 and IL-4 production, but high IL-10 and/or TGF-beta secretion, showing a cytokine profile similar to the T-cell subsets Tr1 and Th3. Moreover, cloning frequency of CD4+CD25+ FoxP3+ T cells was substantially increased in infected patients compared with uninfected MS subjects. Finally, Smad7 messenger RNA was not detected in T cells from infected MS patients secreting TGF-beta.

Interpretation.—Increased production of IL-10 and TGF-beta, together with induction of CD25+CD4+ FoxP3+ T cells, suggests that regulatory T cells induced during parasite infections can alter the course of MS.

▶ No disease in neuro-ophthalmology remains as enigmatic as MS. While the immunologic nature of MS is well established, no unifying viral, immunologic, or degenerative hypothesis has emerged.

While the current article does not report a clear pathogenesis, it does provide enchanting data revealing that patients with MS who harbor a parasitic infection demonstrated a lower number of exacerbations, stable disability scores, and fewer MRI changes. The parasitic infection and protection were associated with induction of T regulatory cells secreting immunosuppressive cytokines, IL-10, and TGF-beta.

These observations may be valuable in explaining the relationship of MS to various environmental factors as well as aiding in the rational design of pharmaceutical agents to mimic the immune response to parasitic infections.

R. C. Sergott, MD

Vitrectomy and Release of Presumed Epipapillary Vitreous Traction for Treatment of Nonarteritic Anterior Ischemic Optic Neuropathy Associated with Partial Posterior Vitreous Detachment
Modarres M, Sanjari MS, Falavarjani KG (Rasool Akram Med Ctr, Tehran, Iran; Iran Univ of Med Sciences, Tehran)
Ophthalmology 114:340-344, 2007   8–9

Objective.—To study the results of vitrectomy and release of epipapillary vitreous adhesions for the treatment of nonarteritic anterior ischemic optic neuropathy (NAION) associated with partial posterior vitreous detachment (PVD).

Design.—Prospective noncomparative interventional case series.

Participants.—A series of 16 patients with clinical picture of NAION and small discs associated with partial PVD, diagnosed clinically and confirmed by optical coherence tomography and B-scan ultrasonography.

Intervention.—All patients underwent standard pars plana vitrectomy with meticulous removal of epipapillary vitreous adhesions within 1 month from the onset of visual symptoms.

Main Outcome Measures.—Best-corrected visual acuity (BCVA), mean deviation of visual fields, and color vision testing.

Results.—In 15 patients BCVA improved (93.7%), mean preoperative BCVA was 6/38 (0.82±0.53 logarithm of the minimum angle of resolution [logMAR]), which improved to 6/18 (0.49±0.37 logMAR) postoperatively at 3 months. Nine eyes (56%) had ≥3 lines of visual improvement. Visual fields improved in 4 patients and color vision improved in 1 patient.

Conclusion.—Vitreous traction from partial PVD may have a causative role in some cases of NAION associated with small discs. In these cases, vitrectomy and removal of epipapillary vitreous may result in improvement of visual acuity.

▶ No disease in neuro-ophthalmology has been more resistant to treatment than NAION. Over the years, promising, but unfulfilled, therapeutic efforts have included corticosteroids, phenytoin, optic nerve sheath decompression (a personal favorite), transvitreal optic neurotomy, antiglaucoma medications, hyperbaric oxygen, and medications used primarily to treat Parkinson's disease.

Now, Dr Modarres and his colleagues report that vitrectomy surgery to release presumed vitreous traction on the optic disc may have some promise. There is no doubt, as first reported by Professor William Hoyt, that some patients with NAION will report vitreoretinal traction symptoms before the development of disc edema and ischemia. Optical coherence tomography (OCT) certainly demonstrates attachment of the vitreous to an elevated optic disc in some patients with NAION.

Of course, we will need an independent randomized trial to answer whether this approach is viable. The last such trial produced a completely different natural history for NAION than had been previously described. As of now, many neuro-ophthalmologists still adhere to the "traditional" rather than the "revisionist" natural history. Therefore, a vitrectory NAION study must have a natural history arm and also must be acutely attentive to the level of skill and experience of the operating surgeons.

R. C. Sergott, MD

Depression and Anxiety in Visually Impaired Older People
Evans JR, Fletcher AE, Wormald RPL (London School of Hygiene and Tropical Medicine; Moorfields Eye Hosp, London)
Ophthalmology 114:283-288, 2007   8–10

Purpose.—To investigate the association between visual impairment and depression and anxiety in older people in Britain.

Design.—Population-based cross-sectional study.

Participants.—Thirteen thousand nine hundred people aged 75 years and older in 49 family practices in Britain.

Methods.—Vision was measured in 13 900 people aged 75 years and older in 49 family practices taking part in a randomized trial of health screening that included depression (Geriatric Depression Scale [GDS-15]) and anxiety (General Health Questionnaire [GHQ-28]). Cause of visual impairment (binocular acuity less than 6/18) was assessed from medical records. Analysis was by logistic regression (odds ratio [OR] and 95% confidence interval [CI]), taking account of potential health and social confounders.

Main Outcome Measures.—Levels of depression and anxiety.

Results.—Visually impaired people had a higher prevalence of depression compared with people with good vision. Of visually impaired older people, 13.5% were depressed (GDS-15 score of 6 or more) compared with 4.6% of people with good vision (age- and gender-adjusted OR, 2.69; 95% CI, 2.03–3.56). Controlling for potential confounding factors, particularly activities of daily living, markedly attenuated the association between visual impairment and depression (OR, 1.26; 95% CI, 0.94–1.70). There was little evidence for any association between visual impairment and anxiety. On the GHQ-28 scale, 9.3% of visually impaired people had 2 or more symptoms of anxiety compared with 7.4% of people with good vision.

Conclusions.—Although cause and effect cannot be established in a cross-sectional study, it is plausible that people with visual impairment are more likely to experience problems with functioning, which in turn leads to depression.

▶ Depression accompanying visual loss may occur in almost every patient who is unfortunate to experience permanent impairment of sight. Yet, most ophthalmologists and neuro-ophthalmologists (myself included) too often fail to address this vitally important part of a patient's disease process.

In this very large study from Britain, depression in visually impaired older patients (defined as 75 years and older) occurred in 13.5% of the group compared with 4.6% of people with good vision (age and sex adjusted). This study proves that Britain is no different from the rest of the world (maybe that was true to some staunch Britishers before the end of the Empire). In fact, similar results have been obtained from Asia, North America, and Europe.

No correlation was found with the cause of the visual loss and the levels of depression.

Ophthalmologists and family physicians must be aware of this strong association and refer patients to psychiatrists to provide proper medical attention for all their needs.

R. C. Sergott, MD

Sino-orbital Fistula: A Complication of Exenteration

Limawararut V, Leibovitch I, Davis G, et al (Univ of Adelaide, Australia; South Australian Inst of Ophthalmology, Adelaide; David Geffen School of Medicine at UCLA, Los Angeles)
Ophthalmology 114:355-361, 2007   8–11

Purpose.—To report the incidence, characteristics, and management of sino-orbital fistulas, a complication of orbital exenteration.

Design.—Retrospective interventional case series.

Participants.—One hundred ten patients who underwent orbital exenteration at 2 orbital units.

Methods.—Retrospective chart review of all cases of orbital exenteration between 1993 and 2005 at one orbital unit and between 1999 and 2005 at a second orbital unit.

Main Outcome Measures.—Incidence of sino-orbital fistulas.

Results.—Seventy-three and 37 orbital exenterations were performed at the first and second orbital units, respectively. Five patients developed sino-orbital fistulas, 1 of whom developed 2 fistulas at separate sites. In the first unit, 4 fistulas developed in 3 of 73 (4.1%) patients who underwent orbital exenteration. In the second unit, 2 fistulas developed in 2 of 37 (5.4%) exenterated orbits. The majority (5/6) of fistulas occurred medially to the ethmoid sinus, whereas 1 occurred superiorly to the frontal sinus. Risk factors that may have contributed to fistula formation include radiotherapy (3/6), sinus disease (3/6), intraoperative penetration into a sinus (3/6), and immunocompromise (1/6). Management was tailored to the individual case and ranged from conservative socket hygiene to surgical repair with grafts or flaps. Four of the 6 fistulas recurred after repair. Three of these subsequently were closed successfully. Only 1 fistula persisted until the patient died from malignant disease.

Conclusions.—Sino-orbital fistulas are uncommon but not rare complications of orbital exenteration that may be predicted by several risk factors. Bothersome symptoms may necessitate treatment, which can range from conservative management to surgical repair with various grafts or flaps. Despite repair, fistulas may be difficult to eradicate.

▶ Orbital exenteration surgery is required to treat potentially life-threatening problems such as extensive malignancies and infections. Because the entire orbital contents are removed, patients are at risk for fistulas between the orbit to the nose and sinuses.

Risk factors for these problems include diabetes mellitus and an immunocompromised state that contribute to deficient wound healing. Surgical repair of the fistulas is indicated if foul-smelling discharge, breakdown, difficulty with nose blowing, or inability to wear an exenteration prosthesis develops.

While these problems are rare, ophthalmologists need to recognize them so that the fistulas can be treated properly.

R. C. Sergott, MD

The American Society of Anesthesiologists Postoperative Visual Loss Registry: analysis of 93 spine surgery cases with postoperative visual loss
Lee LA, Roth S, Posner KL, et al (Univ of Washington, Seattle)
Anesthesiology 105:652-659, 2006   8–12

Background.—Postoperative visual loss after prone spine surgery is increasingly reported in association with ischemic optic neuropathy, but its etiology is unknown.

Methods.—To describe the clinical characteristics of these patients, the authors analyzed a retrospectively collected series of 93 spine surgery cases voluntarily submitted to the American Society of Anesthesiologists Postoperative Visual Loss Registry on standardized data forms.

Results.—Ischemic optic neuropathy was associated with 83 of 93 spine surgery cases. The mean age of the patients was 50 ± 14 yr, and most patients were relatively healthy. Mayfield pins supported the head in 16 of 83 cases. The mean anesthetic duration was 9.8 ± 3.1 h, and the median estimated blood loss was 2.0 l (range, 0.1-25 l). Bilateral disease was present in 55 patients, with complete visual loss in the affected eye(s) in 47. Ischemic optic neuropathy cases had significantly higher anesthetic duration, blood loss, percentage of patients in Mayfield pins, and percentage of patients with bilateral disease compared with the remaining 10 cases of visual loss diagnosed with central retinal artery occlusion ($P < 0.05$), suggesting they are of different etiology.

Conclusions.—Ischemic optic neuropathy was the most common cause of visual loss after spine surgery in the Registry, and most patients were relatively healthy. Blood loss of 1,000 ml or greater or anesthetic duration of 6 h or longer was present in 96% of these cases. For patients undergoing lengthy spine surgery in the prone position, the risk of visual loss should be considered in the preoperative discussion with patients.

▶ No event in neuro-ophthalmology is more guaranteed to produce malpractice litigation than loss of vision in the immediate postoperative time frame. Rarely in the past have patients ever been warned about such a possibility during the informed consent process. In addition, the loss of vision is often profound and permanent, laying the foundation for an accusation of care below the standard.

In this report, two thirds of the patients underwent spine surgery in the prone position and 89% were associated with ischemic optic neuropathy. Ninety-six percent of these individuals had an estimated blood loss of 1 liter or greater or an anesthetic duration of 6 hours or longer.

Previous studies had indicated that low hematocrits and significant decreases in mean systolic blood pressure were also important factors.

For the ophthalmologist evaluating these patients, the clinical challenge is always great. I advocate immediate transfusion with at least 2 units of blood as well as optimization of all hemodynamic parameters.

R. C. Sergott, MD

Most cases labeled as "retinal migraine" are not migraine

Hill DL, Daroff RB, Ducros A, et al (Emory Univ, Atlanta, Ga)
J Neuroophthalmol 27:3-8, 2007   8–13

Background.—Monocular visual loss has often been labeled "retinal migraine." Yet there is reason to believe that many such cases do not meet the criteria set out by the International Headache Society (IHS), which defines "retinal migraine" as attacks of fully reversible monocular visual disturbance associated with migraine headache and a normal neuro-ophthalmic examination between attacks.

Methods.—We performed a literature search of articles mentioning "retinal migraine," "anterior visual pathway migraine," "monocular migraine," "ocular migraine," "retinal vasospasm," "transient monocular visual loss," and "retinal spreading depression" using Medline and older textbooks. We applied the IHS criteria for retinal migraine to all cases so labeled. To be included as definite retinal migraine, patients were required to have had at least two episodes of transient monocular visual loss associated with, or followed by, a headache with migrainous features.

Results.—Only 16 patients with transient monocular visual loss had clinical manifestations consistent with retinal migraine. Only 5 of these patients met the IHS criteria for definite retinal migraine. No patient with permanent visual loss met the IHS criteria for retinal migraine.

Conclusions.—Definite retinal migraine, as defined by the IHS criteria, is an exceedingly rare cause of transient monocular visual loss. There are no convincing reports of permanent monocular visual loss associated with migraine. Most cases of transient monocular visual loss diagnosed as retinal migraine would more properly be diagnosed as "presumed retinal vasospasm."

▶ Transient loss of vision is always a diagnostic and therapeutic challenge for ophthalmologist. On one hand, the events may be benign and self-limited, while on the other hand they may predict bilateral permanent blindness as in giant cell arteritis or a devastating hemispheric stroke as in a hemodynamically significant internal carotid artery occlusion.

The authors provide an invaluable historical perspective about the terms ophthalmic and retinal migraine as well as educating the reader about the criteria for migraine as devised by the International Headache Society.

Since migraine affects approximately 20% of the population, ophthalmologists encounter this possible diagnosis on an almost daily basis. The study found that, when the International Headache Society criteria are applied, "retinal migraine" is an exceedingly rare entity.

On the basis of this review, retinal migraine is a diagnosis best made only after a thorough, exhaustive investigation and cardiac, carotid, ocular, hematologic, and intracranial causes of transient visual loss are excluded. Even after that, the diagnosis may be provisional at best.

R. C. Sergott, MD

Pediatric Horner Syndrome: Etiologies and Roles of Imaging and Urine Studies to Detect Neuroblastoma and Other Responsible Mass Lesions

Mahoney NR, Liu GT, Menacker SJ, et al (Univ of Pennsylvania, Philadelphia; Children's Hosp of Philadelphia)
Am J Ophthalmol 142:651-659, 2006   8–14

Purpose.—To evaluate the frequency of etiologies of Horner syndrome in children and suggest an imaging and laboratory diagnostic protocol to evaluate for neuroblastoma and other lesions in a child presenting with Horner syndrome and no known cause.

Design.—Retrospective chart and data review.

Methods.—A retrospective review of all children seen at a large pediatric neuro-ophthalmology referral center with a diagnosis of Horner syndrome between 1993 and 2005 with particular attention to underlying etiologies and the results of imaging and urine catecholamine studies.

Results.—Fifty-six children met criteria for Horner syndrome and further review. Twenty-eight children (50%) had no previously identified cause for Horner syndrome. Of these children, 24 (85.7%) had urine catecholamine metabolite studies, and all had negative results. Twenty (71.4%) had complete modern imaging of the brain, neck, and chest. Of the 18 children who had complete imaging and urine studies, responsible mass lesions were found in six (33%). Four had neuroblastoma, one had Ewing sarcoma, and the other had juvenile xanthogranuloma. Of all patients (diagnosis known and unknown), neoplasm was the etiology in 13 of 56 (23%) of patients.

Conclusions.—We confirm that Horner syndrome in a child of any age without a surgical history requires a complete examination to exclude a mass lesion. In such patients, we recommend brain, neck, and chest magnetic resonance imaging (MRI) with and without contrast as well as urinary catecholamine metabolite testing. However, imaging is more sensitive than urine testing in this setting.

▶ Horner syndrome in a child always requires extensive, careful evaluation unless unequivocal evidence exists to confirm a congenital etiology.

The authors provide a logical approach to this clinical problem on the basis of their experience at a large urban referral center. The authors found that magnetic resonance imaging of the head, neck, and chest were the best diagnostic procedures to discover a mass lesion responsible for the Horner syndrome. Previously, 24-hour urine collection for catecholamine levels was thought to be sufficient to exclude a neuroblastoma. However, in this study, 4 patients with normal urinary catecholamines were found to have a neuroblastoma with gadolinium-enhanced MRI scans.

I also believe that the same approach is necessary in adults, but in addition adults require magnetic resonance angiography to exclude a carotid artery dissection.

R. C. Sergott, MD

NovaVision: vision restoration therapy
McFadzean RM (Univ of Glasgow, Scotland)
Curr Opin Ophthalmol 17:498-503, 2006   8–15

Purpose of Review.—The aim of this article is to review the controversial findings for NovaVision's vision restoration therapy.

Recent Findings.—It has been claimed that NovaVision's computerized therapy results in expansion of the visual field in optic nerve and occipital lesions, but the outcome has been challenged on the grounds of unsatisfactory perimetric control of central fixation and disputed mechanisms.

Summary.—In clinical practice NovaVision's therapy should not currently gain acceptance in view of unacceptable perimetric standards and equivocal results. Possible effects on a relative scotoma at the edge of a lesion have not been adequately explored. In the interim, research should also be focused on compensatory eye movement strategies.

Capturing the benefit of vision restoration therapy
Glisson CC (Michigan State Univ, East Lansing)
Curr Opin Ophthalmol 17:504-508, 2006   8–16

Purpose of Review.—Vision restoration therapy has shown promise as a treatment strategy to improve visual field deficits in patients with lesions of the brain or optic nerve. Objective measures of its efficacy, however, have remained controversial. A review of the current theories supporting the reported benefits of vision restoration therapy, and the dissenting opinions, reconsiders vision restoration therapy as an emerging therapy.

Recent Findings.—The benefits of vision restoration therapy have been challenged by a study suggesting that no improvement exists with careful control of fixation. Alternatively, others suggest that eye movements are not induced by vision restoration therapy. Functional imaging studies demonstrate the potential role of plasticity in vision restoration therapy. While the exact mechanism remains to be elucidated, subjective improvement in daily functioning is reported in a significant percentage of patients.

Summary.—Vision restoration therapy is a noninvasive, home-based strategy for the rehabilitation of patients with visual field loss caused by structural or ischemic damage. While subjective benefits in functional status have been reported by patients following completion of the program, debate centers around the inadequacy of the methods used to document its efficacy. Until such a method is validated by carefully controlled studies, subjective improvement in visual function stands alone as evidence of vision restoration therapy's benefit.

Neuro-ophthalmology

Sergott RC (Wills Eye Hosp, Philadelphia)
Curr Opin Ophthalmol 17:497, 2006   8–17

Background.—Visual restoration therapy (VRT) has become an increasingly controversial topic in neuro-ophthalmology during the past 5 years.

Overview.—There have been claims in the literature that VRT can somewhat expand visual field defects in patients with optic nerve and homonymous hemianopias. The public debate has been intense and impassioned as to whether or not VRT is a tremendous breakthrough and whether the findings in support of the effectiveness of VRT are the result of poorly controlled clinical trials. The 2 articles in *Current Opinion in Ophthalmology* referenced here are presented in an attempt to provide some perspective on this debate by presenting the independent opinions of well-respected authorities in both the United States and Europe. Neither author has any financial ties to the VRT technology.

Conclusions.—Visual restoration therapy is the most controversial topic in neuro-ophthalmology. Clinicians involved in the care of patients with permanent severe visual defects should be aware of this therapy and the controversy surrounding it.

▶ VRT is now the most controversial topic in neuro-ophthalmology. These eye exercises are alleged to improve scotomas caused by optic nerve disorders as well as from multiple disease processes affecting the posterior afferent visual system.

These 3 articles (Abstracts 8–15 to 8–17) in *Current Opinion in Ophthalmology* attempt to provide some perspective in this intensely emotional anatomical, physiological, and financial debate. The advocates and skeptics remain as harshly divided as the Hatfields and McCoys of the legendary West Virginia family feud.

Drs McFadzean and Glisson provide separate, independent analyses of this technique, its results, and need for future independent, randomized, blinded studies. Patients are becoming more aware of this alleged therapy and are more than willing to pay the $6000 fee in the hopes that their visual deficits will improve, allowing them to return to a more nearly normal life.

For additional perspective, readers are also referred to a well-researched, unbiased set of articles in *Eyenet*, a monthly publication of the American Academy of Ophthalmology. The articles by senior editor Denny Smith are: "Hemianopia: A Treatment Attracts Turmoil, Part 1" (February 2007, pp 31-33) and "Hemianopia: A Treatment Attracts Turmoil, Part 2 (March 2007, also pp 31-33).

Every ophthalmologist, neurologist, and neurosurgeon who cares for patients with permanent, severe visual loss needs to be educated about this debate before prescribing VRT for their patients.

R. C. Sergott, MD

9 Ocular Oncology

Chromosomal Mutations in Uveal Melanoma - The Good, The Bad, and The Ugly

by Carol L. Shields, MD

Some movies are legendary. Sergio Leone's dramatic, widescreen Western entitled "The Good, The Bad, and The Ugly" is an ageless piece of work. This three hour movie was released in 1966, starring Clint Eastwood as Blondie and Eli Wallach as Tuco. These two dudes are not particularly best friends, but through their combined knowledge they work together in a treasure hunt for $200,000 dollars, which was a large sum of money during the time. The setting is during the Civil War and the plot has endless, unexpected twists and turns in their search for the money. They are lucky and unlucky. They face good guys and bad guys. They are funny and serious. They are friends and competitors in their search for their treasure.

In some ways, the hunt for the origin of uveal melanoma has been the same. It has been a long haul over the past decades with numerous investigations into host and environmental factors. Many previous reports were contradictory and unrevealing. This past year, Weis et al provided a meta-analysis of 132 published reports on host factors important in the development of melanoma.[1] They found light eye color, fair skin color, and inability to tan to be risks. Also this past year, Shah et al provided a meta-analysis of 133 published reports on environmental factors for development of uveal melanoma and found only arc welding to be a risk factor.[2] So we now have an idea of the group of people at greatest risk for uveal melanoma.

The most difficult aspect of uveal melanoma is not the local ocular treatment, but it is prevention of metastatic disease. Clinical and histopathologic prognostic factors have been identified. Some of the clinical factors include ciliary body location, diffuse tumor configuration, extrascleral extension, and large tumor size. Some of the histopathological factors include epithelioid cell type, high mitotic activity, infiltrating tumor lymphocytes, and vascular networks. But that is not enough. We need to better understand the chromosomal aberrations that lead to the development of uveal melanoma.

So the treasure hunt began about 15 years ago. In 1992, Horsthemke and coworkers from Germany found loss of chromosome 3 alleles and multiplication of chromosome 8 alleles in uveal melanoma.[3] Later, Prescher and coworkers from the same laboratory in Germany published in Lancet the prognostic implications of monosomy 3.[4] They evaluated 54 patients enucleated for uveal melanoma and found monosomy 3 in 30 tumors and disomy 3 in 24 tumors. Those patients with monosomy 3 showed 50% metastasis by 3 years whereas those with disomy 3 showed no metastatic disease. They concluded that monosomy 3 was a significant predictor of poor prognosis.

Meanwhile, across the English Channel in England, similar results were generated. In 1990, Sisley et al published the cytogenetic findings in six eyes with posterior uveal melanoma that showed monosomy 3 and 8q abnormalities in 3 cases, chromosome 1 abnormality in 2 cases and chromosome 6 abnormality in 4 cases.[5] Two years later, this same team presented 10 cases of uveal melanoma and only one had normal chromosome complement.[6] The remaining nine cases showed abnormalities of chromosomes 3, 6, and 8 in five cases, chromosome 11 in three cases, and chromosome 13 in two cases. In 1997, they found that monosomy 3 and additional copies of 8q statistically correlated with reduced patient survival.[7] In 2000, Sisley and associates found that the amount of chromosomal abnormalities increased with increasing tumor size.[8] Each contribution added one more facet to our understanding of uveal melanoma.

Meanwhile, across the Atlantic Ocean, Onken and associates from the United States showed in 2004 that gene expression microarray analysis allowed reliable separation of uveal melanoma into two classes, class 1 (low grade) and class 2 (high grade).[9] They found significant clusters of down-regulated genes of chromosome 3 and up-regulated genes of chromosome 8q. This molecular classification was predictive of tumor metastasis.

The secrets of uveal melanoma are slowly unfolding as we diligently work apart in competition and work together to achieve a unified goal. Like Blondie and Tuco, we search for the hidden treasure that reveals the secrets of melanoma. Blondie knew a little bit of this and Tuco knew a little of that, but together they were able to fight villians, escape in a wink, and find the treasure.

References

1. Weis E, Shah CP, Lajous M, et al: The association between host susceptibility factors and uveal melanoma: A meta-analysis. *Arch Ophthalmol* 124:54-60, 2006.
2. Shah CP, Weis E, Lajous M, et al: Intermitttent and chronic ultraviolet light exposure and uveal melanoma: A meta-analysis. *Ophthalmology* 112:1599-1607, 2005.
3. Horsthemke B, Prescher G, Bornfeld N, et al. Loss of chromosome 3 alleles and multiplication of chromosome 8 alleles in uveal melanoma. *Genes Chromosomes Cancer* 4:217-221, 1992.
4. Prescher G, Bornfeld N, Hirche H, et al: Prognostic implications of monosomy 3 in uveal melanoma. *Lancet* 347;1222-1225, 1997.
5. Sisley K, Rennie IG, Cottam DW, et al: Cytogenetic findings in six posterior uveal melanomas: Involvement of chromosomes 3,6,and 8. *Genes Chromosomes Cancer* 2:205-209, 1990.
6. Sisley K, Cottam DW, Rennie IG, et al: Non-random abnormalities of chromosomes 3,6,and 8 associated with posterior uveal melanoma. *Genes Chromosomes Cancer* 5:197-200, 1992.

7. Sisley K, Rennie IG, Parsons MA, et al: Abnormalities of chromosomes 3 and 8 in posterior uveal melanoma correlate with prognosis. *Genes Chromosomes Cancer* 19:22-28, 1997.
8. Sisley K, Parsons MA, Garnham J, et al: Association of specific chromosome alteration with tumour phenotype in posterior uveal melanoma. *Br J Cancer* 82:330-338, 2000.
9. Onken MD, Worley LA, Ehlers JP, et al: Gene expression profiling in uveal melanoma reveals two molecular classes and predicts metastatic death. *Cancer Research* 64:7205-7209, 2004.

Monosomy 3 Predicts Death but Not Time until Death in Choroidal Melanoma

Sandinha MT, Farquharson MA, McKay IC, et al (Tennent Inst of Ophthalmology, Glasgow, England; Royal Infirmary, Glasgow, England; Univ of Glasgow, England; et al)

Invest Ophthalmol Vis Sci 46:3497-3501, 2005   9–1

Purpose.—To study whether monosomy 3 can predict time until death caused by metastatic melanoma, whether life expectancy can be predicted in patients after surgical excision of a melanoma displaying monosomy 3, and to confirm the prognostic value of monosomy 3 and its correlation with tumor histology.

Methods.—Archival specimens from 71 patients who died of metastatic melanoma and 40 patients who were living or had died of other causes were identified. The number of copies of chromosome 3 was assessed by chromosome in situ hybridization, and monosomy 3 was compared with clinicopathologic features.

Results.—Monosomy 3 was detected in 47 of 71 metastasizing melanomas (66.1%) and was significantly associated with metastasis-related death ($P < 0.0001$). All 40 nonmetastasizing tumors were balanced for chromosome 3 (two copies). In 70% of cases, epithelioid cells and vascular loops in combination predicted the presence of monosomy 3 ($P < 0.0001$). Among the 71 patients who had died of metastasizing melanoma, there was no difference in time until death between monosomic and balanced tumors. However, a survival curve corrected for age of the patients at the time of surgery suggested that very-long-term survival with monosomy 3 is probably rare.

Conclusions.—Monosomy 3 is an important predictor of death in melanoma and is in some cases predicted by histology. However, death of metastatic disease occurs in a significant number of patients without monosomy 3. There is no significant difference in time until death between metastatic melanomas, with and without monosomy 3. However, survival of patients with tumors displaying monosomy 3 is generally short.

▶ Monosomy 3 has been shown by many investigators to be associated with death from uveal melanoma metastasis. Sandinha et al found that monosomy 3 was present in 66% of tumors that lead to death of the patient, but 34% of patients who died had disomy 3. This indicates that there may be other mutations contributing to this malignancy. Of those patients who survived without metastasis, all demonstrated disomy 3. There were no patients with mono-somy 3 mutation who survived.

Monosomy 3 has been found in 50% to 73% of choroidal melanomas, based on several investigations. It is currently the most important factor related to metastatic disease. Sandinha et al found that even though it is a predictor of death, it does not predict the time until death.

The interest in monosomy 3 mutation in melanoma has currently changed our approach to this tumor. We offer testing that uses microarray analysis to all patients. Patients who undergo enucleation or local tumor resection have fresh tissue harvested for cytogenetic analysis. Patients who undergo plaque radiotherapy have a needle aspiration performed and sent for cytogenetic analysis. Those patients without monosomy 3 might be reassured to know of the lack of this mutation. Those patients with monosomy 3 are encouraged to consider therapeutic chemotherapy, immunotherapy, or other trials to prevent metastasis.

C. L. Shields, MD

The Association Between Host Susceptibility Factors and Uveal Melano-ma: *A Meta-analysis*
Weis E, Shah CP, Lajous M, et al (Harvard School of Public Health, Boston; Univ of Alberta, Edmonton, Canada; Univ of Rochester, NY; et al)
Arch Ophthalmol 124:54-60, 2006   9–2

Objective.—To conduct a meta-analysis, using observational studies, to examine the association between host susceptibility factors and uveal mela-noma.

Methods.—A review of 132 published reports on risk factors for uveal melanoma revealed 10 case-control studies that provided enough informa-tion to calculate odds ratios (ORs) and standard errors for host susceptibil-ity factors. Data from these studies were extracted and categorized. Sum-mary statistics were calculated for all risk factors reported by at least 4 independent studies.

Results.—Summary statistics using meta-analysis are presented as ORs and their 95% confidence intervals (CIs). Statistically significant risk factors include light eye color (OR, 1.75 [95% CI, 1.31-2.34]), using 10 studies (1732 cases); fair skin color (OR, 1.80 [95% CI, 1.31-2.47]), using 5 studies (586 cases); and ability to tan (OR, 1.64 [95% CI, 1.29-2.09]), using 6 stud-ies (1021 cases). Blond or red hair color, using 7 studies (1012 cases), was not a statistically significant independent risk factor (OR, 1.02 [95% CI, 0.82-1.26]).

Conclusion.—This meta-analysis yielded strong evidence associating the host susceptibility factors of iris color, skin color, and ability to tan with uveal melanoma.

▶ It is well established that host susceptibility factors increase the risk for de-velopment of certain subtypes of cutaneous melanoma. These characteristics include blonde or red hair, fair skin color, light eye color, skin freckling, presence of cutaneous nevi, and sensitivity to sunlight. Furthermore, the risk increases with the number and pathologic severity of cutaneous nevi. The incidence rate of cutaneous melanoma is 17 times higher in white men in comparison with black men.

There have been several observational studies to assess the host factors for the development of uveal melanoma. Except for eye color, the impact of other factors has been inconsistent. In this analysis, Weis et al reviewed 132 publications on the topic of host factors and uveal melanoma. Only 10 studies were appropriate for meta-analysis. They found that significant host risk factors were light eye color, fair skin color, and inability to tan. Surprisingly, blond or red hair color was not a risk factor, but they explain that this might be misleading as most recorded hair color was based on the date of visit as an adult and might more accurately be recorded as hair color during childhood.

These results confirm that fair-skinned white persons with blue or green eyes are at greatest risk for the development of uveal melanoma. It is established that white people have an 8 times greater risk for uveal melanoma than black people. Despite these odds, each month we examine and manage black patients with uveal melanoma. The clinician should be suspicious of any pigmented choroidal mass in any patient, no matter the skin color, especially if the tumor is over 2 mm in thickness, with overlying subretinal fluid, or with orange pigment on the tumor surface. It could be a melanoma.

C. L. Shields, MD

Intermittent and Chronic Ultraviolet Light Exposure and Uveal Melanoma: *A Meta-analysis*
Shah CP, Weis E, Lajous M, et al (Harvard School of Public Health, Boston; Univ of Rochester, NY; Univ of Alberta, Edmonton, Canada; et al)
Ophthalmology 112:1599-1607, 2005   9–3

Objective.—To examine the association between ultraviolet light exposure and uveal melanoma.

Design.—Meta-analysis.

Methods.—A review of 133 published reports on risk factors for uveal melanoma revealed 12 studies that provided sufficient information to calculate odds ratios (ORs) and standard errors for ultraviolet light exposure factors. Data from these studies were extracted and categorized into intermittent ultraviolet exposure factors (welding, outdoor leisure, photokeratitis) and chronic ultraviolet exposure factors (occupational sunlight exposure, birth latitude, lifetime ultraviolet exposure index). Summary statistics were calculated for all risk factors reported by ≥4 independent studies.

Main Exposure Measures.—Welding, outdoor leisure, photokeratitis, occupational sunlight exposure, birth latitude, and lifetime ultraviolet exposure index.

Results.—For intermittent ultraviolet exposure, welding was found to be a significant risk factor (5 studies, 1137 cases; OR, 2.05 [95% confidence interval [CI], 1.20–3.51]). Outdoor leisure was found to be nonsignificant (4 studies, 1332 cases; OR, 0.86 [95% CI, 0.71–1.04]). Photokeratitis conferred susceptibility in 3 reports studying this variable, but there were too few studies to validate meta-analyses. For chronic ultraviolet exposure, meta-analysis found occupational sunlight exposure to be a borderline nonsignificant risk factor for development of uveal melanoma (4 studies, 572 cases; OR, 1.37 [95% CI, 0.96–1.96]). Latitude of birth was found to be nonsignificant (5 studies, 1765 cases; OR, 1.08 [95% CI, 0.67–1.74]).

Conclusion.—This meta-analysis yielded inconsistent results associating ultraviolet light with development of uveal melanoma. There was evidence implicating welding as a possible risk factor for uveal melanoma.

▶ It is well established that UV light is the most important modifiable risk factor for certain subtypes of cutaneous melanoma. The prevalence of cutaneous melanoma increases with proximity to the equator, known as latitude gradient, and with higher altitudes. It is also known that there is a critical period of UV light susceptibility during childhood that confers a greater risk for cutaneous melanoma. Lastly, the pattern of UV exposure is important. Intermittent exposure confers greater risk than chronic exposure. That is, a 1-week trip to the Caribbean might be of greater risk for cutaneous melanoma than working outdoor construction full time.

The environmental risks for uveal melanoma are not well understood. Some reports show no effect and others report harmful effects. Shah et al reviewed 133 published reports on the topic of UV light exposure and uveal melanoma. There were only 12 studies that had sufficient data for the meta-analysis. They found that welding was a risk factor in 5 published studies and was the only significant risk factor in their meta-analysis. There was no risk conferred by outdoor leisure, photokeratitis, occupational sunlight exposure, birth latitude, and lifetime UV exposure index.

I still advise UV block sunglasses and a wide-brimmed hat for all people who spend time in the sun. It could protect from cutaneous actinic keratosis, squamous cell carcinoma, basal cell carcinoma, and cutaneous melanoma. Shah et al informs us that it has no effect on the development of uveal melanoma.

I will now advise that welders minimize direct focus on the welding arc and that protective UV block glasses might be of benefit. Better yet, why not let a remote controlled machine do the welding.

C. L. Shields, MD

Whole Body Positron Emission Tomography/Computed Tomography Staging of Metastatic Choroidal Melanoma

Kurli M, Reddy S, Tena LB, et al (New York Eye Cancer Ctr; Saint Vincent's Comprehensive Cancer Ctr, New York; New York Eye and Ear Infirmary; et al)

Am J Ophthalmol 140:193-199, 2005   9–4

Purpose.—To evaluate whole-body positron emission tomography (PET)/computed tomography in staging of patients with metastatic choroidal melanoma.

Design.—Interventional non-randomized clinical study.

Methods.—Twenty patients were referred for whole-body 18-fluoro-2-deoxy-D-glucose (FDG) PET/computed tomography imaging because of suspected metastatic choroidal melanoma. PET/computed tomography images were studied for the presence and distribution of metastatic melanoma. Subsequent biopsies were performed to confirm the presence of metastatic disease.

Results.—Twenty patients underwent PET/computed tomography. Eighteen were imaged because of abnormal clinical, hematologic, or radiographic screening studies during the course of their follow-up after plaque brachytherapy or enucleation. Two were imaged before treatment of their primary tumor. PET/computed tomography revealed or confirmed metastatic melanoma in eight (40%) of these 20 patients. The mean time from initial diagnosis to metastasis was 47 months (range 0 to 154). The most common sites for metastases were the liver (100%), bone (50%), lung (25%), lymph nodes (25%), and subcutaneous tissue (25%). Cardiac, brain, thyroid, and posterior abdominal wall lesions (12.5%) were also noted. Six patients (75%) had multiple organ involvement. No false positives were noted. PET/computed tomography imaging also detected benign lesions of the bone and lymph nodes in three patients (15%). All patients had hepatic metastases and liver enzyme assays were abnormal in only one (12.5%) of eight patients.

Conclusions.—PET/computed tomography imaging is a sensitive tool for the detection and localization of hepatic and extra-hepatic (particularly osseous) metastatic choroidal melanoma.

▶ Whole body PET scanning has become a popular method to image metabolically active parts of the body. With regard to tumors, this technique has been found useful for staging lymphoma, cutaneous melanoma, and gastrointestinal malignancies. PET scanning requires the patient to avoid carbohydrates the evening before the test and to fast for 4 to 6 hours immediately before the test. This minimizes physiologic glucose utilization and reduces serum insulin levels to baseline and allows for a more sensitive PET scan. The technique involves the injection of a radioactive glucose FDG with the dose calculated on the basis of body weight to achieve a target dose of 5 mCi in the system which then accumulates in the more metabolically active cells. The patient is imaged with simultaneous PET scanner and CT scanner. The PET scan detects the metabolically active points in the body, but with poor anatomic resolution. The overlying CT scan allows for accurate anatomic localization of the PET activity. PET reaches up to 4 mm resolution. Glucose uptake above levels of the surrounding tissue and above the standardized value unit (SUV) of 2.5 are considered suggestive of malignancy.

In this analysis, Reddy et al used PET/CT to image 20 patients with choroidal melanoma (18 treated; 2 untreated) for evidence of metastatic disease. Eighteen of the patients were imaged because of suspected metastasis based on abnormal liver function studies, radiographs, or clinical findings. Eight of the 20 patients showed hepatic metastasis despite liver function tests being abnormal in only 1 patient. However, CT or MRI showed a mass in 5 of the 8 patients. The remaining 2 patients did not have previous testing and the PET/CT was part of their initial staging. Thus, PET/CT appears to be more sensitive than liver function tests, but its sensitivity compared with MRI, standard CT, or chest x-ray (CXR) for this disease is not known. There were 14 patients with abnormalities on MRI, CT, or CXR and PET/CT detected hypermetabolic activity in 5. The remaining 9 patients were negative on PET/CT. I wonder if they had metastases that were not detected on PET/CT as further evaluation was not revealed by the authors. It would have been more scientific if the authors performed needle aspiration liver biopsy in these 9 patients, as this would have been allowed a comparative sensitivity of the imaging methods. The authors claim that PET/CT is 100% sensitive compared with liver function tests, a common test that is known to be somewhat insensitive.[1] The overall sensitivity of PET/CT should be compared with liver biopsy in all patients for an accurate comparison.

PET/CT is an expensive test. However, it is difficult to weigh its costs with hopefully earlier detection of metastasis against the costs of late detection of metastasis. If effective systemic therapy were available for treatment of patients with metastatic disease, then the costs would become trivial. Unfortunately, longevity is poor despite early detection of melanoma metastasis.

In summary, PET/CT has been introduced as yet another testing method for the evaluation of metastatic disease in patients with choroidal melanoma. Its role is not clearly defined, but based on this report, it appears that PET/CT may be a valuable asset in patient management.

C. L. Shields, MD

Reference

1. Hicks C, Foss AJE, Hungerford JL: Predictive power of screening tests for metastasis in uveal melanoma. *Eye* 12:945-948, 1998.

Clinical Analysis of the Effect of Intraarterial Cytoreductive Chemotherapy in the Treatment of Lacrimal Gland Adenoid Cystic Carcinoma

Tse DT, Benedetto P, Dubovy S, et al (Univ of Miami, Fla)
Am J Ophthalmol 141:44-53, 2006   9–5

Purpose.—To determine the effect of intraarterial cytoreductive chemotherapy (IACC) as an adjunct to conventional surgery and radiation therapy for lacrimal gland adenoid cystic carcinoma (ACC).

Design.—A retrospective, comparative, interventional case series.

Methods.—Setting: Institutional.

Patient Population.—Nine consecutive patients with lacrimal gland ACC were treated with IACC, followed by orbital exenteration and chemoradiotherapy. This case series was compared with a series of seven patients treated by conventional local therapies in the same institution.

Intervention Procedure.—Clinical records, imaging studies, histologic sections, and archival specimens from all 16 patients were reviewed. Information analyzed included site of disease, histologic characteristics, extent of disease, incidence of locoregional recurrence or distant metastases, and disease-free survival and overall survival time.

Main Outcome Measure.—The effect of IACC was assessed by the radiographic and histologic response and survival outcome in comparison to a historical cohort of patients managed by conventional local therapies.

Results.—The difference between the carcinoma cause-specific death rate of the study group versus conventional treatment was significant ($P = .029$, log rank test). The cumulative 5-year carcinoma cause-specific death rate in the IACC treated group was 16.7% compared with 57.1% in the conventional treatment group. The cumulative 5-year recurrence rate in the IACC treated group was 23.8% compared with 71.4% in the conventional treatment group.

Conclusions.—The preliminary data suggest that IACC as an integral component of a multimodal treatment strategy is potentially effective in improving local disease control and overall disease-free survival in lacrimal gland adenoid cystic carcinoma.

▶ Adenoid cystic carcinoma of the lacrimal gland is a rare malignancy that carries a grim prognosis. There is controversy regarding optimal treatment for this cancer and most surgeons agree that exenteration plus external beam radiotherapy is the most common approach. Because of its rarity, it is difficult to appreciate the best therapeutic modality. A review of 94 adult patients from 4 major tertiary centers found distant metastasis in 50% of patients by 5 years.

Tse et al evaluated the effect of presurgical intraarterial cis-platinum and doxorubicin on patient outcome. They used 2 or 3 cycles then performed exenteration 1 month later, followed by radiotherapy. They found a significant reduction in local recurrence and related deaths. These results are impressive. However, it should be realized that the cohort groups were small with only 9 patients in the chemotherapy group and 7 patients in the control group. In addition, the groups were not adequately compared for differences. The authors did show that there were no differences in age, sex, race, eye, and follow-up time by using the t test and χ^2 test. However, they did not assess differences in the duration of symptoms, tumor size or extent, bone involvement, previous surgeries, and other factors. For example, 2 of the 7 control patients did not receive radiotherapy, but all 9 of the chemotherapy patients did. This factor alone could make a difference in patient outcome.

I agree with Tse et al that occult disease is the reason for failure in adenoid cystic carcinoma and systemic chemotherapy is warranted. However, the toxicities of such treatment should be realized. Intraarterial injection should only be performed at an experienced center. Accuracy of injection into the external carotid artery to reach the lacrimal gland rather than the internal carotid artery, which perfuses the brain, is critical as these medications are toxic.

C. L. Shields, MD

Amniotic Membrane Transplantation in Acute Phase of Toxic Epidermal Necrolysis with Severe Corneal Involvement

Kobayashi A, Yoshita T, Sugiyama K, et al (Kanazawa Univ, Japan; Ocular Surface Ctr, Miami, Fla)
Ophthalmology 113:126-132, 2006   9–6

Objective.—To report successful management of acute stage toxic epidermal necrolysis (TEN) by amniotic membrane transplantation.

Design.—Interventional case report.

Method/Intervention.—A 6-year-old boy who had convulsions and fever due to encephalitis was treated by oral phenobarbital. Two weeks later, he developed a high fever and skin rashes involving >40% of the body, with a positive Nikolsky sign and oral blisters. Examination under general anesthesia performed 5 days after the onset of eye symptoms showed severe inflammation and ulceration on the lid margin and the tarsal conjunctiva in both eyes, a total corneal epithelial defect in the right eye, and a geographical corneal epithelial defect in the left eye. Amniotic membrane was transplanted in both eyes as a patch to cover the entire ocular surface, including upper and lower lid margins.

Results.—Fourteen days after amniotic membrane transplantation, complete corneal and conjunctival epithelialization was observed in the left eye. However, a second amniotic membrane transplantation was performed in the right eye, which still had a total corneal and conjunctival epithelial defect, and resulted in complete epithelialization 14 days later. Corrected visual acuity improved to 20/16 without any superficial punctate keratitis in both eyes 6 months postoperatively. Minimal symblepharon and peripheral scarring were observed only in the right eye.

Conclusions.—Amniotic membrane transplantation performed at the acute phase of TEN is highly effective not only in reducing inflammation and preventing scarring in the conjunctival surface, but also in restoring corneal epithelial integrity in eyes with both corneal and conjunctival ulceration. As a result, in this case it prevented sight-threatening cicatricial complications at the chronic stage.

▶ TEN, also known as Lyell's disease, is the most severe form of Stevens-Johnson syndrome (SJS) and manifests with extensive necrosis of the skin and mucous membranes. The skin detachment extent is <10% in classic SJS and >30% in TEN. The mortality rate in TEN can reach 70%, because of sepsis or organ failure. Unfortunately, TEN usually occurs in children or AIDS patients.

TEN can cause substantial long-term damage to the ocular surface. Patients with TEN are usually managed in burn units or ICUs. Typically, the ocular measures included topical lubrication with artificial tears and ointments, prophylactic topical antibiotics, and lysis of symblepharon. Despite good ophthalmic care, most patients with TEN have severe ocular surface failure and poor vision develop.

Kobayashi et al attempted novel therapy for a child with TEN who had bilateral sloughing of the corneal epithelium and large conjunctival epithelial defects. They applied a single, large amniotic graft (5 × 5 cm) to the entire ocular surface of each eye. First, the cilia were trimmed flush to the eyelid. The graft was sutured with 10-0 nylon to the external eyelid margin of the lower eyelid, then tucked into the inferior fornix with two 6-0 polypropylene sutures tied externally to bolsters, then similarly tucked into the superior fornix with sutures and bolsters, and finally sutured to the upper eyelid external surface with 10-0 nylon. The graft rested on the entire conjunctival–corneal surface like a large sheet. It was secured around the cornea with 10-0 nylon running purse string suture. A bandage lens was applied. Topical antibiotics and corticosteroids were applied 4 times daily and topical autologous serum was applied 5 times daily. The patient was on systemic steroids for extensive cutaneous blistering. The grafts were surgically removed 14 days later and a second graft was applied to the right eye for nonhealed cornea. The results were remarkable with complete healing of the ocular surface and return of vision to 20/16 in each eye. There was minimal symblepharon formation.

This technique might be applicable for rehabilitation of the ocular surface in many conditions such as corneal burns, SJS, and after resection and reconstruction of large conjunctival malignancies. The amniotic membrane acts like a bandage, keeps the ocular surface moist, and permits the epithelium to grow underneath it without the microtrauma of dryness and eyelid blinking.

C. L. Shields, MD

Natural Killer/T-cell Lymphoma with Ocular and Adnexal Involvement
Woog JJ, Kim YD, Yeatts RP, et al (Mayo Clinic, Rochester, Minn; Samsung Med Ctr, Seoul, Korea; Wake Forest Univ, Winston-Salem, NC; et al)
Ophthalmology 113:140-147, 2006   9–7

Purpose.—To review the clinical, radiological, and histopathologic features in 8 patients with natural killer/T-cell lymphoma (NKTL) involving the orbit and/or ocular adnexa, and to describe the responses of these patients to various treatment regimens.

Design.—Retrospective observational case series.

Participants.—Eight patients (5 male, 3 female) with NKTL involving the orbit and/or ocular adnexa were identified from 1999 through 2005. The mean age at presentation was 45 years (range, 26–65).

Methods.—We retrospectively identified patients with NKTL of the ocular adnexa treated in the authors' medical centers from 1999 through 2004 using computerized diagnostic index retrieval. The clinical records and radiologic studies were analyzed to define modes of presentation and progression, response to therapy, and areas of anatomic involvement. Histopathologic findings, including the presence of CD3, CD56, and Epstein–Barr virus–encoded mRNA in each patient, were reviewed.

Main Outcome Measurements.—Time of survival from presentation to last known follow-up and tumor-related death.

Results.—Four of the 8 patients (50%) with NKTL involving the orbit or ocular adnexa had systemic involvement at presentation. Five of the 8 patients (62.5%) had concurrent sinonasal involvement, whereas 3 (37.5%) had orbital involvement alone. All lesions demonstrated CD3, CD56, and/or Epstein–Barr virus positivity on immunopathology studies. Therapy consisted of various chemotherapeutic regimens typically employed in the treatment of non-Hodgkins lymphoma, steroids, surgical intervention, and radiation. Seven (87.5%) patients died 5 weeks to 13 months after presentation, and 1 (12.5%) is alive without disease (5-year follow-up).

Conclusions.—Natural killer/T-cell orbital lymphoma is a rare Epstein–Barr virus–associated neoplasm that may occur with or without associated sinonasal involvement. Our series, the largest cohort reported to date, demonstrates the high lethality of this condition despite aggressive conventional therapy, suggesting that new treatment options should be considered early in the course of treatment of patients with this disorder.

▶ Natural killer (NK) cells are normal circulating lymphocytes capable of mounting cytotoxic reactant without antigen priming. Natural killer lymphoma (NKTL) is a form of lymphoma comprised of NK cells and or cytotoxic T lymphocytoes. This aggressive lymphoma is deadly and classically involves the nasal cavity and paranasal sinuses in Asian or Central American patients. Rarely is orbital involvement described.

In review, there are 3 basic specialized lymphocytes, the antibody-producing (B) lymphocytes, thymus-derived (T) lymphocytes, and NK lymphocytes. T lymphocytes are further subdivided into T helper and cytotoxic T lymphocytes. The latter are involved in immune response and proliferate after exposure to foreign cells, tumor cells, or infectious agents. NK cells are active against many tumor cell lines and pathogens without prior exposure to antigens, and are part of the rapid immune response. NK cells can produce cytokines, including interferon and tumor necrosis factor, that can stimulate neutrophils and macrophages into action.

According to the World Health Organization, NKTL is composed mostly of NK cells and a smaller population of T cells. In addition, Epstein–Barr virus infection is noted. This tumor has also been termed "lethal midline granuloma" and "angiocentric T cell lymphoma." The nasal cavity is the most common site of this malignancy.

Most ocular adnexal lymphomas are B cell in origin and most patients display a low-grade chronic course with fairly good long-term prognosis. In this report, Woog et al collaborate and report on 8 patients with NKTL of the orbit and adnexa. All of the patients had ocular symptoms of facial or periocular swelling and 4 manifested nasal symptoms. They illustrate the aggressiveness of this malignancy in that nearly 90% of the patients were dead by 1 year follow-up.

C. L. Shields, MD

Orbital Eosinophilic Angiocentric Fibrosis: *Case Report and Review of the Literature*
Leibovitch I, James CL, Wormald PJ, et al (Univ of Adelaide, Australia; Adelaide Pathology Partners, Australia)
Ophthalmology 113:148-152, 2006   9–8

Objectives.—To report a patient with a rare case of orbital eosinophilic angiocentric fibrosis (EAF) and to review the literature.

Design.—Interventional case report.

Methods.—A 61-year-old man presented with a 6-week history of right periorbital edema and painless proptosis. Examination revealed a nonaxial proptosis, lateral globe displacement, and mild limitation in right eye adduction.

Main Outcome Measures.—Clinical course and radiological and histological findings.

Results.—Orbital imaging revealed a right medial orbital mass with involvement of middle ethmoidal air cells. An orbital biopsy of the mass demonstrated an inflammatory infiltrate with a marked eosinophilic component, onion skinning of vessels, and surrounding fibrosis. The diagnosis of orbital EAF was made. There was no response to a 3-month treatment course with systemic steroids, but the patient did not want any further surgical interventions.

Conclusion.—Although orbital EAF is rare, ophthalmologists need to be aware of this entity, as it may invade the orbit from the sinonasal tract or present as a localized orbital mass. The presence of even minimal sinus involvement and the characteristic histopathology are useful in establishing the correct diagnosis.

▶ EAF is a disease usually managed by otolaryngologists, not ophthalmologists. This benign condition typically involves the upper respiratory tract mucosa. It is characterized by an indolent, but progressive inflammatory process that usually appears in the fifth and sixth decades. Some authors believe this disease falls under the umbrella of allergic or atopic disorders, but the lack of response to immunosuppressives does not support that theory. The exact pathophysiology remains unclear.

Radiologic findings typically reveal soft tissue swelling of the septum and lateral nasal walls and opacification of the sinuses, sometimes with bone destruction. There have been only a few reports to find erosion of the medial orbital wall with soft tissue swelling within the orbit. Leibovitch et al reported similar findings in their case, but the orbital findings were far more predominant than the minor ethmoidal opacification.

The diagnosis is established by histopathology with features of eosinophilic vasculitis without fibrinoid necrosis, occurring in a patchy fashion and involving groups of capillaries and/or venules. A mixture of plasma cells, lymphocytes, and fibroblasts are notes. There are no epithelioid cells or multinucleated giant cells. Late in the disease, fibrous thickening of the stroma and obliterative perivascular onionskin whirling of collagen fibers and reticulin is noted, whereas the inflammatory component becomes scanty and only eosinophils remain. There is not cellular atypia.

The differential diagnosis includes Wegener's granulomatosis, Churg-Strauss syndrome, sarcoidosis, Sjögren's disease, Kimura's disease, erythema elevatum diutinum, granuloma faciale, and infection. Hence, all patients should be evaluated for these simulating systemic conditions. Eosinophilic angiocentric fibrosis shows little response to corticosteroids or immunosuppression so that surgical resection is the treatment of choice. There have been no cases of malignant transformation or death from this condition.

C. L. Shields, MD

Localized Orbital Amyloidosis Involving the Lacrimal Sac and Nasolacrimal Duct
Marcet MM, Roh JH, Mandeville JT, et al (Tufts Univ, Boston; Kosin Univ, Pusan, Korea; Eye Health Services, Quincy, Mass; et al)
Ophthalmology 113:153-156, 2006   9–9

Purpose.—To report the case of a 70-year-old man who presented with tearing in his left eye and a firm palpable lump in the area overlying his left lacrimal sac.

Design.—Retrospective interventional case report.

Methods.—Noninvasive diagnostic evaluation followed by external dacryocystorhinostomy, histopathologic studies, and systemic evaluation.

Results.—The patient was found to have idiopathic localized amyloidosis limited to the lacrimal sac and nasolacrimal duct.

Conclusion.—The localized form of amyloidosis is rare, typically involves the head and neck without systemic manifestations, and carries an excellent prognosis. Previous reports of orbital amyloidosis have described involvement of the lacrimal gland, extraocular muscles, and the cranial nerves. To our knowledge, this is the first report of a patient with nasolacrimal duct obstruction secondary to amyloid deposition in the lacrimal sac and fossa.

▶ Amyloidosis is an idiopathic disorder in which extracellular deposits of amorphous, proteinaceous material is found in connective tissue. Amyloidosis is categorized into 2 types: systemic and localized. Systemic amyloidosis is usually fatal from amyloid deposition in multiple organ systems leading to loss of structure and function. The localized form of amyloidosis has a good prognosis and is usually nonfatal. Localized amyloidosis is rare and often involves the head and neck region without systemic manifestations.

In general, orbital and ocular adnexal amyloidoisis is typically in the localized form without systemic disease, and it classically occurs in an older patient. Involvement of the lacrimal gland, extraocular muscles, cranial nerves, and orbital soft tissues have been described. Marcet et al report the additional localized involvement of the lacrimal sac and nasolacrimal duct. In their case, a 70-year-old man had unilateral epiphora develop and was found to have a lump just below the lacrimal sac. CT revealed a bone-destructive mass and histopathology confirmed amyloidosis.

Both types of amyloidosis can be either primary or secondary. Immunoperoxidase staining can reveal the protein amyloid AA or AL. Protein AA is believed to represent secondary amyloidosis, whereas AL represents primary amyloidosis. Nevertheless, all patients should have systemic evaluation to rule out an underlying inflammatory process such as tuberculosis, leprosy, rheumatoid arthritis, or osteomyelitis, and to rule out underlying neoplasia such as a plasma cell disorder (multiple myeloma, Waldenström's macroglobulinemia) or lymphoma.

Orbital amyloidosis is generally of the localized, primary variant, but lifelong systemic monitoring by a hematologist–oncologist is advised. Management of the orbital condition involves conservative observation or cautious debulking. Because of its infiltrative nature, complete resection is difficult. Recurrence of amyloidosis is not uncommon.

C. L. Shields, MD

Immunotherapy With Imiquimod 5% Cream for Eyelid Nodular Basal Cell Carcinoma

Blasi MA, Giammaria D, Balestrazzi E (Univ of L'Aquila, Italy; Università Cattolica del Sacro Cuore, Rome)
Am J Ophthalmol 140:1136-1139, 2005   9–10

Purpose.—To evaluate the efficacy and safety of topical imiquimod 5% cream for the treatment of eyelid basal cell carcinoma.

Design.—Two interventional case reports.

Methods.—Imiquimod 5% cream was applied topically once daily, 3 days a week for 8 to 12 weeks, in two patients affected by eyelid nodular basal cell carcinoma. Patients were followed up clinically with slit-lamp examination for evidence of tumor disappearance or recurrence, and local and systemic side effects.

Results.—Complete clinical response was obtained in both patients. No severe local side effects were observed. Patients did not show any local recurrence after 1 year.

Conclusions.—Topical imiquimod 5% cream seems to be a useful treatment for eyelid nodular basal cell carcinoma in selected cases, but further long-term studies are needed to assess the efficacy and safety of this approach.

▶ Basal cell carcinoma is the most common malignancy of the eyelid in white people. This tumor tends to present along the lower lid margin as an ulcerated nodule with loss of cilia and superficial telangiectasia. It can also manifest as a diffusely infiltrating morpheaform mass. If neglected, basal cell carcinoma can invade the orbit, sinus, and brain, leading to the rare case of tumor-related death.

The classic treatment of basal cell carcinoma has been complete surgical excision with histopathologic confirmation of tumor-free margins by frozen sections or Mohs surgery. Advanced cases with orbital invasion require exenteration. In this report, Blasi et al inform us of a novel treatment that uses immunotherapy with imiquimod 5% (Aldara, 3M Pharmaceuticals, Minneapolis, MN).

Imiquimod 5% (Aldara, 3M Pharmaceuticals) has revolutionized the treatment of cutaneous tumors. This medication was approved by the Food and Drug Administration in 1997 for treatment of anogenital warts. Subsequently, Imiquimod 5% (3M Pharmaceuticals) has been found efficacious for many more cutaneous conditions, including actiic keratosis, lentigo maligna, cutaneous melanoma metastasis, superficial basal cell carcinoma, and others.

Imiquimod 5% (3M Pharmaceuticals) works through Toll-like receptor 7 to stimulate monocytes, macrophages, and antigen-presenting cells to produce interferon alpha and other cytokines. This medication stimulates the body's own cutaneous immune system to fight malignancy. It is typically applied daily for 8 hours for a total of approximately 12 weeks.

Application to the periocular region should be cautious as Blasi et al indicated that conjunctival hyperemia and corneal epithelial dryness occurred in 1 of their 2 patients. In both patients, the tumor showed a central ulceration during treatment that gradually healed as the tumor regressed completely to a flat scar over 2 to 3 months.

C. L. Shields, MD

Orbital Cellulitis: A Rare Complication After Orbital Blowout Fracture
Simon GJB, Bush S, Selva D, et al (Royal Victorian Eye and Ear Hosp, Melbourne, Australia)
Ophthalmology 112:2030-2034, 2005   9–11

Purpose.—To report the incidence of orbital cellulitis after orbital blowout fracture.

Design.—Retrospective, noncomparative, interventional case series.

Participants.—All patients with orbital cellulitis and a history of recent orbital fracture.

Methods.—A medical record review of clinical history, imaging studies, and surgical and treatment outcome was performed.

Main Outcome Measures.—Resolution of orbital cellulitis and surgical and imaging findings.

Results.—Four patients (3 male; mean age, 30 years [range, 4.5–58]) were treated for orbital cellulitis complicating orbital fracture. All patients had evidence of paranasal sinusitis before or after the orbital injury, and 2 also reported forceful nose blowing after sustaining orbital trauma. Although 3 patients received prophylactic oral antibiotics after the fracture, this failed to prevent infection. Sinusitis commenced 1 to 2 weeks before and as late as 5 weeks after orbital injury. All patients were treated with IV antibiotics. Two developed an orbital abscess that required surgical drainage; 1 patient improved after an endonasal maxillary antrostomy. One patient improved on IV antibiotics alone and underwent fracture repair at a later stage. These 4 patients represent 0.8% of all cases of orbital fractures treated in the study period.

Conclusions.—Orbital cellulitis is a rare complication of orbital fracture, and seems to be more common when paranasal sinus infection preexists or occurs within several weeks of the injury. Oral antibiotics given after the orbital injury may not prevent orbital cellulitis or abscess formation. Surgery may be required to drain orbital abscess or in nonresolving cellulitis to drain the paranasal sinuses. Fracture repair, if indicated, should be delayed, particularly if an alloplastic implant is used.

▶ Orbital exenteration is a procedure in which the entire orbit is removed. This is typically performed for malignancies that are not radiosensitive or chemosensitive. Occasionally, exenteration for life-threatening infections, such as mucormycosis, is sometimes necessary. From my perspective there are 2 types of exenteration, including eyelid-sacrificing exenteration and eyelid-sparing exenteration. In the former, the entire orbit with eyelids is removed; in the latter, the entire orbit is removed, but the anterior lamella of the eyelids is spared. Our group has previously reported that the latter provides faster healing within 2 weeks as opposed to many months or years using granulation with the latter.[1,2] Patient satisfaction and cosmetic appearance is more favorable with eyelid-sparing exenteration.

In the report of Ben Simon and coworkers, an evaluation of the 2 types of exenteration would have been ideal, but in my opinion, the scientific design of the analysis was flawed with far too many variables. They included many different surgical techniques or levels of exenteration and then made comments on the entire group regarding "clear margins." This information would have been more informative if expressed as a result of the specific surgical technique. Additionally, terminology such as "partial or subtotal exenteration" and "extended exenteration" added to confusion in the results. Furthermore, the definition of "subtotal exenteration" was foggy. Subtotal exenteration could include an area as small as a quarter of the orbit up to nearly the entire orbit. By definition, maybe some of those with "subtotal exenteration" would have been better classified as "orbitotomy," especially if the eye was salvaged. Lastly, the authors calculated Kaplan-Meier survival analysis for the entire group, but unfortunately, they included many different conditions with various diagnoses and known variable prognoses, lending to uninformative Kaplan-Meier results.

On the other hand, the procedure of exenteration is not commonly performed by ophthalmologists, and only a few ophthalmic centers nationwide have experience as mentioned in this article. These authors have had extensive experience, and I credit them with their desire to draw some conclusions from such a complex subject. There are a few points to take away from this report, the most reliable being that most patients prefer to wear an eye patch rather than prosthesis after exenteration.

C. L. Shields, MD

References

1. Shields JA, Shields CL, Suvarnamani C, et al: Orbital exenteration with eyelid sparing: Indications, technique and results. *Ophthalmic Surg* 22:292-297, 1991.
2. Shields JA, Shields CL, Demirci H, et al: Experience with eyelid-sparing orbital exenteration. The 2000 Tullos O. Coston Lecture. *Ophthal Plast Reconstr Surg* 17:355-361, 2001.

10 Pathology

New Developments in Retinoblastoma

by Ralph C. Eagle, Jr, MD

There have been a number of new developments in the field of retinoblastoma in recent years. These include major new trends in therapy, a new clinical classification of retinoblastoma that predicts therapeutic success, a new study sponsored by the Children's Oncology Group that is investigating histopathologic prognostic factors in a prospective fashion, and interesting research involving the molecular genetics of retinoma/retinocytoma. We will discuss these new developments in this introduction.

New Trends in Therapy

There have been major changes in the treatment of retinoblastoma in developed countries during the last decade. In the past, external beam radiotherapy (EBRT) was a mainstay of retinoblastoma treatment. There is no question that EBRT is a highly successful method of tumor control. Unfortunately, it does have major complications. These include disfiguring facial deformities and, most importantly, the production of secondary malignant neoplasms in the field of radiation such as soft tissue sarcomas. [1,2] The latter typically develop in patients who carry germline mutations and have bilateral tumors, who are at high risk for the development of secondary neoplasms. Such secondary neoplasms are now the major cause of mortality in retinoblastoma patients, since the cure rate of primary tumors now approaches 100% in many centers. For this reason there has been a concerted effort to avoid the use of external beam radiotherapy.

Many infants with retinoblastoma, particularly those with bilateral tumors spawned by germline mutations are being treated with systemic chemotherapy.[3,5] In many instances chemotherapy is used to shrink tumors so they are amenable to additional treatment or "consolidation" with local therapeutic agents such as cryotherapy, infrared laser transpupillary thermotherapy, or radioactive plaques. Plaque brachyradiotherapy can be used safely because it does not predispose to secondary tumors; the radiation is delivered solely to the eye, sparing the adnexal tissues that are the substrate for secondary neoplasms. Called chemoreduction, this form of chemotherapy is used most commonly in the treatment of bilateral retinoblastoma. About 75% of eyes with unilateral retinoblastoma are still enucleated. Chemotherapy is not a totally innocuous therapy. There are risks associated with immunosuppression, and some have expressed concern that this systemic therapy in infants might have long term effects on development. Hence, it would seem prudent to enucleate a large unilateral sporadic tumor that has irrevocably destroyed the function of an eye rather than administer potentially deleterious systemic therapy. Although chemoreduction should prevent the development of secondary malignant neoplasms in the field of radiation by avoiding EBRT, it's possible that secondary tumors still might develop in some genetically predisposed patients as a response to chemotherapy. Particularly, there is concern that the chemotherapeutic agent etoposide might cause secondary acute myelogenous leukemia. Systemic chemotherapy does appear to prevent distant metastases, and preliminary results indicate that it may lead to a lower incidence of trilateral retinoblastoma, which is almost invariably fatal. Unfortunately, there are treatment failures with chemotherapy. The latter are caused by new clones of chemoresistant tumor cells.

The International Classification of Retinoblastoma

A new international classification of retinoblastoma (ICRB) was drafted at a meeting in Paris, France in 2003.[5,6] The ICRB is rapidly supplanting the older, ubiquitous Reese-Ellsworth classification in clinical practice. The Reese-Ellsworth classification for intraocular tumors does have prognostic significance for retention of an eye, maintenance of sight, and the control of local disease, but it recently has become less useful because it is based on the response to external beam radiotherapy, which, as noted above, is a treatment modality that is now used infrequently. The ICRB was designed to be a relatively simple, practical, more user-friendly classification based on clinical findings that was designed primarily to evaluate the potential response to modern therapy including chemoreduction. It is also called the ABC classification because it comprises five Groups A through E. Group A includes small tumors less than 3 mm in diameter that are located outside the macula. Group B tumors are larger than 3 mm in diameter without seeding. Group B also includes small tumors located in the macula, as well as tumors which have minor amounts of associated subretinal fluid. A tumor with localized subretinal or vitreous seeds is placed in Group C. Tumors with diffuse seeding are placed in Group D. Group E eyes contain extensive tumors occupying more than 50% of the eye, neovascular glaucoma, opaque media from hemorrhage in the anterior chamber, vitreous or subretinal space, and factors associated with poor prognosis including invasion of the postlaminar optic nerve, choroidal invasion greater than 2 mm in diameter, sclera, orbit or anterior chamber.

Initial studies from the Oncology Service at the Wills Eye Institute show that chemoreduction is successful in treating most patients with ICRB group A, B and C retinoblastoma, with success defined as avoidance of enucleation and/or external beam radiotherapy.[6] The success rate was 100% in group A, 93% in group B and 90% in group C with a mean 6.2 year follow-up. The effectiveness drops to 50% in group D tumors with diffuse seeding. Group E tumors generally require enucleation or EBRT. Patients tolerated chemoreduction well with no evidence of chemotherapy-related toxicities of renal or auditory function.

The Children's Oncology Group Study of High-Risk Histopathological Risk Factors

A variety of factors that can be evaluated on pathologic examination are used to assess the prognosis of retinoblastoma and the risk of developing distant metastases. These include invasion of the optic nerve and posterior uvea and, of course, the presence of extrascleral extension.

Optic nerve invasion is an extremely important prognostic factor in retinoblastoma. Retinoblastoma has a marked proclivity to invade the optic nerve, and optic nerve is the most common avenue for extraocular extension by retinoblastoma. Mortality rates correlate directly with the depth of optic nerve invasion. In an older series, the mortality rate was 10% if there was superficial invasion of the nerve head only (grade I) and 29% for involvement up to and including the lamina cribrosa (stage II). It rose to 42% when there was retrolaminar invasion (grade III) and 78% when the tumor extended to the surgical margin (grade IV).[7] Hence, surgeons should try to obtain as long a segment of optic nerve as possible when enucleating an eye that is known or suspected to contain a retinoblastoma. Furthermore, it is prudent that enucleation should not be performed by an inexperienced surgeon, if at all possible. Incomplete removal of tumor in the nerve or, even worse, soiling of orbital tissue with tumor caused by inadvertent "button-holing" of the sclera can have disastrous, fatal consequences.

The prognostic effect of posterior uveal invasion is less clear. The risk of hematogenous metastasis is thought to increase when tumor cells gain access to blood vessels in the uvea. In one series, the mortality rate was about 25% if choroidal invasion was minimal; this rose to 65% if the invasion was massive. However, another large retrospective multivariant analysis suggested that extrascleral extension is a much better indicator of poor prognosis than uveal invasion.[7,8] A factor that confounds the assessment of the effect of individual prognostic factors is the coexistence of multiple factors (eg, optic nerve and choroidal invasion, or choroidal invasion and extraocular extension) in a single eye. Many pathologists and ocular oncologists consider massive uveal invasion to be a risk factor, but there is some controversy about what actually constitutes massive invasion. The significance of other factors (ie, invasion of the iris stroma, anterior chamber and trabecular meshwork) is even less clear. The latter are thought to place patients at greater risk for metastasis, but these factors have never been evaluated prospectively in a systematic fashion.

A prospective multicenter clinical trial sponsored by the Children's Oncology Group currently is evaluating the effect of histopathologic prognostic factors such as uveal, anterior segment and optic nerve invasion on prognosis. The study, designated ARET 0332, is evaluating a series of patients undergoing enucleation for previously untreated unilateral retinoblastoma. Representative sections of the enucleated eyes are systematically evaluated by a committee of ocular pathologists, and the presence or absence of histopathologic features thought to be of prognostic significance are recorded in standard format. As part of this study, patients whose tumors have high risk features will be treated with chemotherapy. Indications for the latter include post-laminar optic nerve invasion and uveal invasion. In the study, massive choroidal invasion is defined as greater than 2 mm in diameter.

New Developments in Retinoma/Retinocytoma

Retinoblastomas occasionally undergo spontaneous regression. However, it was suggested that many lesions once classified as spontaneously regressed retinoblastomas actually are benign, generally nonprogressive retinal tumors also caused by mutation of at least one *RB1* allele, and an alternate name, retinoma, was proposed.[10,11] The term retinocytoma has also been used to describe these lesions in the ophthalmic pathology literature. Unfortunately, the latter term had also been used previously to describe retinoblastoma tumors with numerous Flexner-Wintersteiner rosettes.[12] Retinomas initially were thought to represent spontaneously regressed retinoblastomas on clinical grounds because they resemble retinoblastomas that have regressed after radiation therapy. The tumors have a translucent "fish flesh" appearance, contain abundant calcification that has been likened to cottage cheese, and are surrounded by a ring of retinal pigment epithelial (RPE) depigmentation. Retinomas generally are small tumors found in eyes that retain useful vision. They may be found incidentally, or are discovered in a parent or sibling when the detection of retinoblastoma in a child prompts examination of other family members. Rare cases of retinoma have been observed to undergo malignant transformation into retinoblastoma. Histopathologic examination in one such case confirmed the presence of benign cytology and photoreceptor differentiation in the initially observed basal part of the tumor.[13]

Histopathologically, viable areas of retinomas appear less cellular and relatively more eosinophilic than adjacent undifferentiated retinoblastoma during low-magnification microscopy of sections stained with hematoxylin and eosin (H&E). Necrosis is not observed, the nuclei of the tumor cells appear bland, mitoses and apoptosis are absent, and calcification occurs in viable parts of the tumor. However, the most characteristic feature is the presence of advanced degrees of photoreceptor-like differentiation that typically occur in aggregates called fleurettes, a term coined by Tso and Zimmerman.[14] The term 'fleurette' denotes a bouquet-like arrangement of cytologically benign cells joined by a series of zonulae adherentes that may form a short segment of neoplastic external limiting membrane. Bulbous eosinophilic processes that represent abortive photoreceptor inner segments form the "flowers" of the bouquet. Electron microscopy occasionally discloses stacks of cellular membranes representing early outer segment differentiation.

Foci of photoreceptor differentiation are found more frequently (40% of cases) in eyes that are enucleated after radiotherapy or chemoreduction. Presumably, the chemo- or radiotherapy preferentially kills the malignant part of the tumor and discloses the benign foci, which are relatively radio- or chemo-resistant. Retinal tumors composed entirely of fleurettes are thought to be a benign variant of retinoblastoma that is incapable of metastasis.

Recent molecular genetic studies of retinoma suggest the initial concepts concerning the RB1 tumor suppressor gene and its role in the pathogenesis of retinoblastoma are an oversimplification.[15] The *RB1* gene is the paradigmatic human recessive oncogene or tumor suppressor gene. The *RB1* gene is located in the 14 band of the q or long arm of chromosome 13 (13q14). Although retinoblastoma appears to be inherited in an autosomal dominant fashion, the gene actually is recessive at the molecular level. The protein product of the *RB1* gene, called pRB, is involved in control of the cell cycle. Absence of pRB causes continual cell division and lack of terminal differentiation. Classically, the *RB1* gene is thought to cause cancer when its protein product is absent or dysfunctional. Healthy persons have two normal or wild-type *RB1* genes, however, both alleles of the *RB1* gene are absent or inactivated in the retinoblastoma tumor cells. Carriers of familial retinoblastoma are heterozygous for the *RB1* gene. Although the pRB produced by a heterozygote's single functional gene is sufficient to inhibit tumorigenesis, heterozygotes are at substantial risk to develop retinoblastoma when the remaining functional copy of the gene is lost or inactivated in a cell in the developing retina.

Dimaras and colleagues, working in Brenda Gallie's laboratory in Toronto, have recently shown that both copies of the *RB1* gene are inactivated and pRB is absent in retinoma. It now appears that loss of function of both *RB1* alleles alone is insufficient for development of malignant retinoblastoma; additional mutations are necessary for malignant transformation of retinoma into retinoblastoma to occur. Although the cells of retinomas lack pRb retinoblastoma protein, proliferation markers Ki67 and PCNA are not expressed. In addition, retinomas show prominent cytoplasmic staining for the senescence marker p16^{INK4a}, which is absent in unaffected retina and retinoblastoma, and the cells appear to be arrested in the G1 phase of the cell cycle. In contrast, certain retinoblastoma candidate oncogenes such as *KIF14*, *E2F3* and *DEK*, are over-expressed in retinoblastoma, but not in retinoma, and another potential tumor suppressor gene *CDH11* is not expressed in retinoblastoma, but present in retinoma. Hence, it appears that additional progressive genetic changes occur when retinoblastoma develops from retinoma.

These new observations help to explain some interesting features of retinoblastoma. For instance, the *RB1* gene plays an important role in the regulation of cellular division in all cells in the body, yet only retinoblastoma, a relatively rare neoplasm that affects minute population of highly differentiated cells, results from the inactivation of both copies of the *RB1* gene. The highly retinal-specific predisposition imposed by mutations in the *RB1* gene is hypothesized to result from the specific pattern of expression of other genes in the unidentified cell of origin in the developing human retina rather than *RB1* alone.

The results from Dimaras et al strongly suggests that retinoma is the benign precursor lesion of retinoblastoma. Foci of photoreceptor differentiation consistent with retinoma were observed in 15% of a series of enucleated retinoblastoma, and Dimaras and colleagues. speculated that the incidence would be even higher if the tumors had been thoroughly sampled by serial sectioning. These foci were postulated to represent residual precursor retinomas that had undergone malignant transformation during a stepwise progression to cancer and subsequently had been overgrown by the resultant retinoblastoma. Based on the results of their molecular genetic studies, Dimaras and colleagues have redefined retinoma as a precancerous lesion characterized by the loss of function of both copies of the *RB1* gene, but lacking the additional genomic changes characteristic of retinoblastoma.

References

1. Wong FL, Boice JD, Abramson DH, et al: Cancer incidence after retinoblastoma: radiation dose and sarcoma risk. *JAMA* 278:1262-1267, 1997.
2. Moll AC, Imhof SM, Bouter LM, et al: Second primary tumors in patients with retinoblastoma. A review of the literature. *Ophthalm Genet* 18:27, 1997.
3. Shields CL, Mashayekhi A, Cater J, et al: Chemoreduction for retinoblastoma: analysis of tumor control and risks for recurrence in 457 tumors. *Trans Am Ophthalmol Soc* 102:35-44, 2004.
4. Shields CL, Meadows AT, Leahey AM, et al: Continuing challenges in the management of retinoblastoma with chemotherapy. *Retina* 24:849-862, 2004.
5. Shields CL, Shields JA: Basic understanding of current classification and management of retinoblastoma. *Curr Opin Ophthalmol* 17: 228-234, 2006.
6. Shields CL, Mashayekhi A, Au AK, et al: The International Classification of Retinoblastoma Predicts Chemoreduction Success. *Ophthalmology* 113:2276-2280, 2006.
7. Magramm I, Abramson DH, Ellsworth RM: Optic nerve involvement in retinoblastoma. *Ophthalmology* 96:217-222, 1989.
8. Kopelman JE, McLean IW, Rosenberg SH: Multivariate analysis of risk factors for metastasis in retinoblastoma treated by enucleation. *Ophthalmology* 94:371-377, 1987.
9. Messmer EP, Heinrich T, Hopping W, et al: Risk factors for metastases in patients with retinoblastoma. *Ophthalmology* 98:136-141, 1991.
10. Gallie BL, Ellsworth RM, Abramson DH, et al: Retinoma: spontaneous regression of retinoblastoma or benign manifestation of the mutation? *Br J Cancer* 45:513-521, 1982.
11. Gallie BL, Phillips RA, Ellsworth RM, et al: Significance of retinoma and phthisis bulbi for retinoblastoma. *Ophthalmology* 89:1393-1399, 1982.
12. Margo C, Hidayat A, Kopelman J, et al: Retinocytoma: A benign variant of retinoblastoma. *Arch Ophthalmol* 101:1519-1531, 1983.
13. Eagle RC Jr, Shields JA, Donoso L, et al: Malignant transformation of spontaneously regressed retinoblastoma, retinoma/retinocytoma variant. *Ophthalmology* 96:1389-1395, 1989.
14. Ts'o MO, Zimmerman LE, Fine BS: The nature of retinoblastoma. I. Photoreceptor differentiation: a clinical and histopathologic study. *Am J Ophthalmol* 69:339-349, 1970.
15. Dimaras H, Halliday W, Orlic M, et al: The Molecular Characterization of Retinoma. Presented at the International Society of Genetic Eye Disease and International Retinoblastoma Symposium, Whistler BC, September 2005.

The COMS Randomized Trial of Iodine 125 Brachytherapy for Choroidal Melanoma: V. Twelve-Year Mortality Rates and Prognostic Factors: COMS Report No. 28

Hawkins BS, for the Collaborative Ocular Melanoma Study (COMS) Group (COMS Coordinatoring Ctr, Baltimore, Md; et al)

Arch Ophthalmol 124:1684-1693, 2006   10–1

Objectives.—To report refined rates of death and related outcomes by treatment arm through 12 years after primary treatment of choroidal melanoma and to evaluate characteristics of patients and tumors as predictors of relative treatment effectiveness and time to death.

Design.—Randomized multicenter clinical trial of iodine 125 (^{125}I) brachytherapy vs enucleation conducted as part of the Collaborative Ocular Melanoma Study. Eligible patients were free of metastasis and other cancers at enrollment. All patients were followed up for 5 to 15 years at scheduled examinations for metastasis or another cancer or until death. Decedents were classified by the independent Mortality Coding Committee as having histopathologically confirmed melanoma metastasis, suspected melanoma metastasis without histopathologic confirmation, another cancer but not melanoma metastasis, or no malignancy.

Main Outcome Measures.—Deaths from all causes and deaths with histopathologically confirmed melanoma metastasis.

Results.—Within 12 years after enrollment, 471 of 1317 patients died. Of 515 patients eligible for 12 years of follow-up, 231 (45%) were alive and clinically cancer free 12 years after treatment. For patients in both treatment arms, 5- and 10-year all-cause mortality rates were 19% and 35%, respectively; by 12 years, cumulative all-cause mortality was 43% among patients in the ^{125}I brachytherapy arm and 41% among those in the enucleation arm. Five-, 10-, and 12-year rates of death with histopathologically confirmed melanoma metastasis were 10%, 18%, and 21%, respectively, in the ^{125}I brachytherapy arm and 11%, 17%, and 17%, respectively, in the enucleation arm. Older age and larger maximum basal tumor diameter were the primary predictors of time to death from all causes and death with melanoma metastasis.

Conclusion.—Longer follow-up of patients confirmed the earlier report of no survival differences between patients whose tumors were treated with ^{125}I brachytherapy and those treated with enucleation.

Application to Clinical Practice.—Estimated mortality rates by baseline characteristics should facilitate counseling of patients who have choroidal melanoma of a size and in a location suitable for enucleation or ^{125}I brachytherapy and no evidence of metastasis or another malignancy.

Trial Registration: clinicaltrials.gov Identifier: NCT00000124

▶ The latest long-term follow-up data from the COMS Group confirms, yet again, that survival of patients with medium-sized choroidal malignant melanomas treated with enucleation or ^{125}I plaque brachytherapy appears to be equivalent. Overall survival was somewhat better than predicted but still was significant. The results of this multicenter, multimillion dollar prospective study essentially confirmed what had been suggested by several prior retrospective studies. The study did not lead to any major changes in the therapy of uveal malignant melanoma; it merely validated prior therapy. In retrospect, the results of the COMS are not unexpected considering recent concepts of the biology of uveal melanoma. It is now thought that the melanoma will metastasize by the time that the patient becomes symptomatic and seeks ophthalmologic evaluation and treatment. Essentially, everything that the ophthalmologist or ocular oncologist does is local tumor control. Whatever treatment modality is employed—plaque brachytherapy, enucleation, local resection, or transpupillary thermotherapy—it really has no effect on patient survival. Whether or not a tumor metastasizes depends on the biology of its cells.

It now appears that certain nonrandom genetic abnormalities in melanoma cells, most notably monosomy of chromosome 3, put patients at extremely high risk for metastatic death. In one series from Germany, patients whose tumors had monosomy 3 had a 50% chance of dying in 3 years.[1] None of the patients whose tumors had 2 copies (disomy) of chromosome 3 died in the same time period. Currently, it is not known whether these genetic abnormalities, which have such a profound effect on survival, are present from the onset or accumulate as a small tumor grows. If the latter were true, early treatment of small tumors would seem to be justified to destroy them before this significant genetic event occurs. In that situation, treatment indeed might have systemic consequences.

Was the COMS worthwhile? It was quite costly and certainly led to no significant change in management. Unfortunately, it essentially was designed to test a hypothesis that later was shown to be false. I personally feel that our society would have been better served if only a small fraction of the money that was expended on the COMS had gone to train individuals who could bolster the steadily depleting ranks of ophthalmic pathologists.

R. C. Eagle, Jr, MD

Reference

1. Prescher G, Bornfeld N, Hirche H, et al: Prognostic implications of monosomy 3 in uveal melanoma. *Lancet* 347:1222-1225, 1996.

Immunohistochemical Evaluation of Conjunctival Fibrillin-1 in Marfan Syndrome

Ganesh A, Smith C, Chan W, et al (Univ of Toronto; Nebraska Med Ctr, Omaha)
Arch Ophthalmol 124:205-209, 2006   10–2

Objective.—To evaluate status of conjunctival fibrillin-1 in patients with Marfan syndrome with ectopia lentis.

Methods.—Frozen sections of conjunctiva from 6 patients with Marfan syndrome with ectopia lentis and from 15 age-matched control subjects were stained with mouse antihuman fibrillin-1 antibody, using an avidin biotin immunoperoxidase technique. The fibrillin-1 staining characteristics of conjunctiva were analyzed with the light microscope.

Results.—All the fresh frozen sections of conjunctival samples from control subjects demonstrated a characteristic pattern of fibrillin-1 staining. We observed a woven network of thin fibrils of uniform thickness surrounding collagen bundles. The fresh frozen samples from patients with Marfan syndrome showed consistent qualitative differences in fibrillin-1 staining when compared with samples from control subjects. The fibrils were longer and straighter than normal, varied in caliber, and showed fewer tendencies to form a woven pattern.

Conclusions.—Consistent, qualitative abnormalities in fibrillin-1 staining pattern can be seen in the conjunctiva of patients with Marfan syndrome with ectopia lentis. Conjunctival biopsy deserves further investigation as a diagnostic modality for Marfan syndrome in patients with ectopia lentis.

▶ Fibrillin-1 is a glycoprotein whose gene resides on chromosome 15. Fibrillin-1 is a major constituent of the elastic microfibrils that form the suspensory ligament of the lens and also serve as a nidus for the formation of elastic tissue. Ectopia lentis or heritable dislocation of the lens generally develops in patients who have heritable mutations in the fibrillin gene, most notably Marfan syndrome, or who have disorders of sulfur-containing amino acid metabolism such as homocystinuria or sulfite oxidase deficiency that affect the structure of fibrillin secondarily by interfering with disulfide bond formation. By far, the great majority of patients with ectopia lentis have Marfan syndrome, which is associated with more than 85 novel mutations in the fibrillin gene.

The authors of this article from The Hospital for Sick Children in Toronto sought to develop a relatively simple diagnostic test for Marfan syndrome based on conjunctival biopsy, a relatively simple office procedure. Molecular genetic testing for Marfan syndrome can be difficult because the fibrillin gene is complex and very large. The conjunctiva is rich in fibrillin and, of course, is readily accessible. Using antibodies against fibrillin, the authors were able to show characteristic qualitative abnormalities in the arrangement of fibrillin fibers in conjunctival biopsies from patients with Marfan syndrome as compared with normal controls. Unfortunately, quantitative assessment proved to be impossible, and the antifibrillin antibodies only worked on frozen-sectioned tissue, not conjunctival biopsies fixed in formalin and processed routinely by embedding in paraffin. The need for fresh tissue and frozen sections markedly decreases the ease and utility of this new test. Having to rely totally on qualitative assessment is also problematic, particularly if the findings are relatively subtle. Here again, experience of the observer would be a major factor.

R. C. Eagle, Jr, MD

Ocular and Systemic Pseudoexfoliation Syndrome

Schlötzer-Schrehardt U, Naumann GOH (Univ of Erlangen-Nürnberg, Erlangen, Germany)

Am J Ophthalmol 141:921-937, 2006   10–3

Purpose.—To provide an update on most recent developments regarding ocular and systemic manifestations and complications, clinical diagnosis and management, and molecular pathophysiology of pseudoexfoliation (PEX) syndrome, and to discuss future tasks and challenges in this field.

Design.—Perspective.

Methods.—Review of recent literature and authors' own clinical and laboratory studies.

Results.—PEX syndrome is a common age-related generalized fibrotic matrix process of worldwide significance, which may not only cause severe chronic open-angle glaucoma and cataract, but also a spectrum of other serious spontaneous and surgical intraocular complications (Table 1). Recent progress and advances have led to (1) improvements in clinical management by understanding the effects of the PEX process on ocular tissues, by refining diagnostic criteria, by applying new treatment regimes, and by developing preventive strategies to reduce surgical complications; (2) increasing evidence for systemic associations of PEX with cardiovascular and cerebrovascular morbidity; and (3) new insights into the molecular pathophysiology by analyzing the composition of PEX material, the differential gene expression of affected tissues, and key factors involved in pathogenesis. The current pathogenetic concept describes PEX syndrome as an elastic microfibrillopathy involving transforming growth factor-β1, oxidative stress, and impaired cellular protection mechanisms as key pathogenetic factors.

Conclusions.—Future tasks and challenges comprise epidemiologic prevalence and genetic studies of PEX syndrome, prospective randomized clinical and histopathological screening studies on its systemic manifestations and associations, and intensified basic research on differential protein and gene expression, animal and in vitro models, as well as potential biomarkers for PEX syndrome and its associated glaucoma.

▶ Drs Schlötzer-Schrehardt and Naumann have written a number of excellent articles on PEX syndrome that have increased our understanding of the pathology and clinical manifestations of this highly prevalent, yet poorly understood condition. This monumental review is highly recommended; I learned quite a few new facts about PEX. PEX appears to be the ocular manifestation of a systemic disorder of elastic tissue. PEX material may represent an elastotic material formed by the abnormal aggregation of elastic microfibrils that interact with a variety of ligands. Whether PEX predisposes to nonocular systemic abnormalities is not entirely clear. The article outlines some evidence that suggests that patients with PEX are at greater risk for cardiovascular and cerebrovascular disease.

Naturally, the ophthalmologist should be most familiar with the ophthalmic manifestations of the syndrome. The most important of these is the associa-

TABLE 1.—Diagnosis of Early Stages, and Clinical and Surgical Complications of Pseudoexfoliation (PEX) Syndrome

Tissue Involvement	Early Clinical Signs	Clinical Complications	Surgical Complications
Lens, ciliary body, and zonules	• Diffuse precapsular layer • Phacodonesis • PEX deposits on zonules (UBM)	• Cataract (nuclear) • Phacodonesis • Lens subluxation • Angle-closure glaucoma due to pupillary and ciliary block	• Zonular rupture/dialysis • Vitreous loss • Posterior capsule rupture • Decentration of the lens implant • Anterior capsule fibrosis • Secondary cataract
Iris	• Peripupillary atrophy and iris sphincter region transillumination • Melanin dispersion associated with pupillary dilation • Poor mydriasis, asymmetric pupil sizes	• Melanin dispersion • Poor mydriasis • Iris rigidity • Capillary hemorrhage • Blood-aqueous barrier defects, pseudouveitis • Anterior chamber hypoxia • Posterior synechiae	• Miosis/poor surgical access • Intra- and postoperative hyphema • Postoperative inflammation • Prolonged blood-aqueous barrier breakdown • Posterior synechiae and pupillary block
Trabecular meshwork	• Pigment deposition • Marked asymmetry of IOP • Marked IOP rise after pupillary dilation	• Intraocular hypertension • Open-angle glaucoma	• Postoperative IOP rise
Cornea	• Atypical cornea guttata	• Endothelial decompensation • Endothelial migration/proliferation	• Endothelial decompensation
Posterior segment		• Retinal vein occlusion	

IOP = Intraocular pressure; UBM = ultrasound biomicroscopy.
(Courtesy of Schlötzer-Schrehardt U, Naumann GOH: Ocular and systemic pseudoexfoliation syndrome. *Am J Ophthalmol* 141:921-937, Copyright 2006 by Elsevier Science Inc. Reprinted by permission of the publisher.)

tion of PEX and the relatively common form of secondary open-angle glaucoma, which initially was termed glaucoma capsulare by Vogt in 1926. In some regions of the world (eg, the eastern part of the Arabian peninsula), PEX glaucoma is the most common form of open-angle glaucoma, comprising 77% of cases. Glaucoma in patients with PEX is said to be more difficult to manage than primary open-angle glaucoma, with a higher incidence of treatment failures. Factors cited in this review that presumably are responsible for poorer prognosis include higher mean intraocular pressure levels, greater diurnal variations in intraocular pressure, and marked pressure spikes. Anterior displacement of the lens/iris diaphragm caused by zonular instability also can lead to secondary closed-angle glaucoma due to papillary or ciliary block mechanisms.

A higher incidence of surgical complications occurs in patients with PEX, most notably intra- or postoperative dislocation of the crystalline lens or lens capsular bag and intraocular lens after extracapsular surgery. Patients with PEX are prone to develop nuclear cataracts. Lens dislocation is related to zonular fragility and weakness, which is caused by the accumulation of PEX at the site of zonular attachment to the lens and ciliary body.

R. C. Eagle, Jr, MD

Fibrous Histiocytoma of the Conjunctiva
Kim HJ, Shields CL, Eagle RC Jr, et al (Thomas Jefferson Univ, Philadelphia)
Am J Ophthalmol 142:1036-1043, 2006   10–4

Purpose.—To review the clinical features and course of six patients with fibrous histiocytoma (FH) of the conjunctiva.

Design.—Retrospective, observational clinical case series.

Methods.—Chart review of six consecutive patients with unilateral cases of conjunctival FH was conducted. Clinical presentation, treatment, histopathologic condition, and follow-up information were recorded.

Results.—The mean patient age was 37 years (median, 38 years; range, 12 to 72 years). There were five white patients, one black patient, five male patients, and one female patient. The tumor was present for a mean of three months (median, five months; range, one to 12 months) and was unilateral (one right eye, five left eyes). In all cases, the tumor was a tan, dome-shaped limbal mass in the conjunctival stroma with visible intrinsic vessels. The mean tumor basal dimension was 7 mm (median, 5 mm; range, 4 to 11 mm). Surgical resection was performed in all cases, and histopathologic study demonstrated benign FH in four cases and malignant FH in two cases. Those cases with benign FH showed no recurrence over nine months (median, eight months; range, three to 18 months). One patient with malignant FH showed recurrence and required repeat excision. The other patient with malignant FH was treated with plaque radiotherapy to maintain control. There was no evidence of orbital invasion or remote metastasis in any case over the mean follow-up period of 21 months (median, 10 months; range, three to 80 months).

Conclusion.—FH is a rare conjunctival tumor that can show benign or malignant features. Complete resection is advised. Malignant FH can demonstrate recurrence that necessitates wide resection and radiotherapy.

▶ Spindle cell lesions of the conjunctiva are relatively rare and frequently are difficult to decisively diagnose histopathologically. In many instances, special procedures such as immunohistochemical stains are necessary for pathologic differential diagnosis. For example, positive immunoreactivity for cytokeratin can help to determine whether a spindle cell neoplasm is a poorly differentiated or sarcomatoid variant of conjunctival squamous cell carcinoma called spindle cell carcinoma. Spindle cell carcinoma behaves aggressively and may invade the eye or orbit. Many conjunctival melanomas have a prominent spindle cell component. The diagnosis of melanoma is readily established by positive staining for a variety of melanoma markers including S-100 protein, HMB-45, Melan A, tyrosinase, and MITF. Kaposi sarcoma usually is suspected clinically by its reddish appearance, which may be confused with subconjunctival hemorrhage, and its occurrence in individuals who are immunosuppressed by infection with HIV. Histopathologically, this malignant spindle cell tumor of lymphatic endothelial cell origin typically shows extravasation of erythrocytes in slit-like spaces.

The current series reports a fairly large clinicopathologic series of FH, one of the rarer conjunctival spindle cell tumors. The spindle cells in the substantia propria are arranged in a characteristic storiform or whorl-like pattern and stain positively for vimentin, smooth muscle actin, and factor XIIIa. The CD68 stain also demonstrates infiltration by histiocytes. Benign and malignant variants occur. Complete resection of this rare tumor is recommended therapy.

R. C. Eagle, Jr, MD

Adult xanthogranulomatous disease of the orbit and ocular adnexa: new immunohistochemical findings and clinical review
Sivak-Callcott JA, Rootman J, Rasmussen SL, et al (West Virginia Univ, Morgantown; Univ of British Columbia, Vancouver, Canada; Univ of Calgary, Alta, Canada; et al)
Br J Ophthalmol 90:602-608, 2006   10–5

Background/aims.—Adult xanthogranulomatous disease involving the ocular tissues is rare and poorly understood. Adult onset xanthogranuloma (AOX), adult onset asthma and periocular xanthogranuloma (AAPOX), necrobiotic xanthogranuloma (NBX), and Erdheim-Chester disease (ECD) are the four syndromes within this disorder, which is diagnosed by characteristic histopathology. Experience with eight cases prompted a multi-institutional effort to study the histopathology, immunohistochemistry, clinical findings, and systemic associations in this disorder.

Methods.—22 cases, including histopathological slides, were compiled. Published reports were identified by an English language Medline search (1966–2005) and review of reference citations. Each case in this series and the literature was classified as one of four syndromes and then analysed for age onset, sex, skin xanthoma, orbital location, immune dysfunction, internal organ and bone lesions, treatment, and outcome. The histopathology in each of these cases was reviewed by two pathologists. Immunhistochemical stains (CD3, CD4, CD8, L26) were performed in 14 cases where unstained slides were available.

Results.—137 cases were compiled. There was no sex or age difference between syndromes. AOX, AAPOX, NBX affect the anterior orbit, ECD tends to be diffuse and intraconal. Skin lesions are found in all the syndromes. Immune dysfunction was noted in all cases of AAPOX and NBX; 11% of NBX and all ECD patients had internal organ disease. Treatment included surgery, corticosteroids, other chemotherapeutic agents, radiotherapy, and combinations of these. No AOX or AAPOX deaths occurred; 66% of ECD patients died. All 22 cases had xanthoma cells; most had Touton giant cells. Lymphocytes were present in all cases and occurred as aggregates (mostly in AAPOX) or diffuse populations mixed with fibroblasts (mostly in ECD). Immunohistochemistry revealed the majority of these to be CD8 +. Necrosis was most marked in NBX.

Conclusion.—Adult xanthogranuloma of the orbit is rare, making prospective evaluation or meta-analysis impossible. The best treatment is unknown but seems to be with multiagent chemotherapy guided by histopathological, immunohistochemical, and systemic findings.

▶ The xanthogranulomatous disorders of the orbit described in this excellent review are rare, but they are encountered occasionally in clinical practice. Although most of the cases I have seen were treated by clinicians on the oculoplastic and oncology services at Wills Eye, the first case that I encountered was submitted by a comprehensive ophthalmologist from South Philadelphia. Clinically, these disorders typically present with atypical xanthelasma-like lesions. These are considered to be atypical because they tend to be much larger and more extensive than garden-variety xanthelasmas and are more indurated. Such lesions can be confused with xanthelasma histopathologically in a superficial skin biopsy if the pathologist lacks an adequate history, is unfamiliar with these conditions, or overlooks subtle variations in the histopathology.

Most of the cases that I have seen at Wills fall into the category of orbital xanthogranuloma with adult-onset asthma. We have seen several cases of ECD, however. In agreement with the current study, we found that patients with orbital xanthogranuloma and adult-onset asthma typically have reactive follicular lymphoid hyperplasia. Whether the 4 disorders discussed here represent distinct disease entities or are part of a disease spectrum remains uncertain. There definitely appears to be some overlap. For example, abnormal serum proteins evident as monoclonal spikes typically are associated with NBX, a potential eyelid marker for multiple myeloma, but they have also been reported in patients with orbital xanthogranuloma with adult-onset asthma. One of our adult-onset asthma cases at Wills has a small monoclonal spike.

The findings in ECD are somewhat dissimilar. The xanthogranulomatous infiltrate in that systemic disorder typically involves the muscle cone, and Touton giant cells are uncommon. Patients with this severe, relentlessly progressive disorder typically have bilateral orbital involvement and systemic involvement as well. The latter includes characteristic bone changes and retroperitoneal fibrosis, which can lead to death from obstructive uropathy. Although ECD is not thought to be a malignant neoplasm, it might as well be one from the aspect of patient survival. Sixty-one percent of the patients with ECD in this series died, a mortality rate far worse that that of most ocular tumors, including uveal melanoma. The ophthalmologist should carefully evaluate any patient who presents with atypical xanthelasma-like lesions, especially if they are large and indurated. They may be the ocular marker for a significant systemic disorder.

R. C. Eagle, Jr, MD

Langerhans Cell Histiocytosis of the Orbit: A Need for Interdisciplinary Dialogue
Harris GJ (Med College of Wisconsin, Milwaukee)
Am J Ophthalmol 141:374-378, 2006   10–6

Purpose.—To explore specialty-related perceptions and treatment strategies in Langerhans cell histiocytosis (LCH) of the orbit.

Design.—A perspective.

Methods.—We reviewed the reported ophthalmic experience with unifocal LCH of the orbit, analyzed current oncologic clinical trial protocols, and provided a brief summary of contemporary knowledge and theory of LCH pathogenesis.

Results.—Ophthalmic literature indicates that unifocal LCH of the orbit is usually responsive to local intervention. Current international oncologic protocols identify orbital LCH as a "central nervous system–risk" lesion (at risk for delayed-onset diabetes insipidus) and mandate a 6-month course of chemotherapy. Analysis suggests that the latter strategy is based on cases of orbital involvement in multifocal and multisystem disease. The pathologic Langerhans cell continues to define and unite the LCH variants, but cytokine activation of that cell may be an earlier pathogenetic determinant. Despite a common cellular mediator, LCH may be a heterogeneous process, with severity related to varied "upstream" trigger events.

Conclusion.—Treatment perspectives in LCH are influenced by dissimilar patient encounters and varied interpretations of the basic disease process. Pending documentation of linkage between unifocal orbital LCH and diabetes insipidus, we recommend local intervention, with systemic treatment reserved for incomplete response or local reactivation or the appearance of lesions elsewhere. LCH underscores the need for close interaction between specialists with intersecting clinical interests.

▶ This article shows that the standard of care for a disease may differ markedly depending on the specialty of the treating physician. The case in point is the localized form of LCH called eosinophilic granuloma, and the specialties in question are ophthalmology and pediatric oncology. I first became aware of this issue several years ago when I was the guest of the Canadian Ophthalmic Pathology Society at their meeting in Vancouver. A case of eosinophilic granuloma of bone was presented, and I was somewhat surprised to learn that the patient subsequently had received chemotherapy. I furthermore learned that chemotherapy appeared to be standard therapy in Canada. In the United States, a typical erosive lesion of the orbital bone that presents to the ophthalmologist generally responds successfully to curettage and/or intralesional steroid injection with rapid resolution, healing, and reossification and no evidence of systemic disease. Such patients generally do quite well and do not develop diabetes insipidis or other systemic abnormalities that characterize the more serious Hand-Schüller-Christian or Letterer-Siwe forms of the disease. This article notes that orbital involvement was considered to be a high-risk lesion in a major study conducted by pediatric oncologists because some patients who had orbital involvement developed diabetes insipidus. For this reason, orbital involvement was considered a risk factor for CNS involvement. However, all the patients with orbital involvement who were studied had systemic disease. None had the localized monostotic lesion of the orbital bone that typically presents to the ophthalmologist. In fact, no cases of eosinophilic granuloma with the typical ophthalmic presentation have been shown to develop diabetes insipidus. We agree that chemotherapy probably is not required in a patient who presents with a classic ocular lesion. Referral to a pediatric oncologist to exclude systemic disease would seem prudent, however.

R. C. Eagle, Jr, MD

Primary Synovial Sarcoma
Hartstein ME, Silver F-L, Ludwig OJ, et al (Saint Louis Univ)
Ophthalmology 113:2093-2096, 2006   10–7

Purpose.—To describe the clinicopathologic and immunohistochemical features and treatment of a rare case of primary synovial sarcoma of the orbit.

Design.—Retrospective interventional case report.

Participant.—A 14-year-old young man with histologically proven synovial sarcoma of the orbit. The diagnosis was confirmed by demonstration of a specific chromosomal translocation by polymerase chain reaction studies.

Methods.—The patient was treated with orbital exenteration and followed up for 18 months at regular intervals.

Results.—The tumor was excised completely, and the patient has done well during the initial 1-year follow-up with no sign of recurrence.

Conclusions.—We report the fourth case of synovial sarcoma of the orbit and, at 14 years of age, the youngest patient reported (Fig 5).

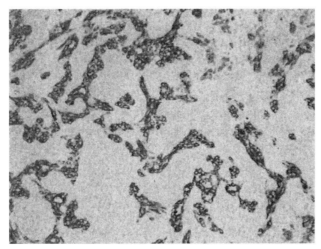

FIGURE 5.—Epithelial membrane antigen immunohistochemical staining highlights the epithelial component of this biphasic tumor. The cytokeratin stain showed similar findings. (Reprinted from *Ophthalmology*, 113, Hartstein ME, Silver F-L, Ludwig OJ, et al, Primary synovial sarcoma, pp 2093-2096, 2006. Copyright 2006, with permission from Elsevier Science.)

▶ This is the fourth reported case of orbital involvement by synovial sarcoma. This rare neoplasm occurs in relatively young individuals, and an orbital case could be confused with orbital rhabdomyosarcoma, the most common mesenchymal malignant tumor of the orbit in childhood. Although the biphasic form of synovial sarcoma reported here looks quite different histopathologically from rhabdomyosarcoma, some lesions are composed primarily of spindle cells. Synovial sarcomas and rhabdomyosarcomas can be readily differentiated by their pattern of immunoreactivity. The epithelioid cell component of a biphasic synovial sarcoma stains positively for epithelial membrane antigen and cytokeratin. In contrast, the cells of rhabdomyosarcoma are immunoreactive for muscle markers such as desmin, muscle-specific actin, or myogenin, a transcription factor involved in the regulation of myogenesis that stains the nuclei of muscle cells.

Another important test that led to the diagnosis of synovial sarcoma in this case was the use of polymerase chain reaction to detect a characteristic gene translocation that serves as a molecular genetic marker for the tumor. Consistent and specific, the t(X;18)(p11.2, q11.2) translocation is found in more than 90% of all synovial sarcomas. It involves the *SYT* gene on chromosome 18 and either the *SSX1* or *SSX2* genes on the X chromosome. The resultant fusion proteins are believed to function as aberrant transcriptional regulators, resulting in either activation of proto-oncogene or inhibition of tumor suppressor genes.

Polymerase chain reaction is also used to detect translocations that serve as specific markers for other malignancies. In the case of orbital rhabdomyosarcoma, it is important to submit tissue for analysis because 2 characteristic translocations are a marker for the alveolar variant of rhabdomyosarcoma, which is said to be more aggressive with a worse prognosis. These translocations result from fusion of the *PAX3* gene on chromosome 2 with the *FKHR* gene on chromosome 13 [t(2;13)], or from fusion of the *PAX7* gene on chromosome 1 with the *FKHR* gene. Other characteristic translocations occur in lymphoid lesions. Most cases of Burkitt lymphoma carry a translocation of the *c-myc* oncogene from chromosome 8 to either the immunoglobulin (Ig) heavy-chain region on chromosome 14 [t(8;14)] or one of the light-chain loci on chromosome 2 (kappa light chain) [t(8;2)] or chromosome 22 (lambda light chain) [t(8;22)]. These translocations result in the inappropriate expression of *c-myc*, an oncogene gene involved in cellular proliferation. The t(14;18)(q32;q21) translocation is the most common chromosomal abnormality associated with non-Hodgkin lymphoma. Found in 85% of follicular lymphomas and 28% of higher-grade non-Hodgkin lymphomas, this translocation results in the juxtaposition of the *bcl*-2 apoptotic inhibitor oncogene at chromosome band 18q21 to the heavy-chain region of the Ig locus within chromosome band 14q32.

R. C. Eagle, Jr, MD

Positron Emission Tomography in the Detection and Staging of Ocular Adnexal Lymphoproliferative Disease
Valenzuela AA, Allen C, Grimes D, et al (Univ of Queensland, Herston, Australia; Wesley Hosp, Auchenflower, Australia; Wesley Med Centre, Auchenflower, Australia)
Ophthalmology 113:2331-2337, 2006   10–8

Purpose.—To evaluate the role of fluorine 18 deoxyglucose positron emission tomography (FDG PET) in the initial staging of ocular adnexal lymphoma (OAL).

Design.—Retrospective nonrandomized case series.

Participants.—Eleven patients with OAL who underwent FDG PET at initial staging.

Methods.—Retrospective review of all the clinical and imaging records, including computed tomography (CT) and FDG PET.

Main Outcome Measures.—The ability of PET studies to detect OAL and distant disease was compared with CT.

Results.—Eleven patients with OAL who underwent FDG PET at initial staging were retrospectively reviewed having full access to their clinical and imaging data. Fluorine 18 deoxyglucose PET found distant disease in 5 of 6 lymphoma patients with systemic disease; 4 of these patients (66%) were upstaged, changing the clinical management. Orbital lesions were demonstrated in 3 of 11 patients, giving PET a sensitivity of 27% in the orbit and 83% systemically for detection of lymphoma.

Conclusion.—The ability of FDG PET to find systemic extranodal lymphomatous sites not detected with conventional imaging provides valuable information in OAL patients, which may result in important changes in staging and management. The technique does have limitations in detecting OAL compared with conventional imaging, possibly owing to background physiologic activity in the extraocular muscles in the orbit and the small volume of some orbital deposits.

Whole-Body Positron Emission Tomography/Computed Tomography Imaging and Staging of Orbital Lymphoma

Roe RH, Finger PT, Kurli M, et al (New York Eye Cancer Ctr; New York Univ; St Vincent's Comprehensive Cancer Ctr, New York; et al)
Ophthalmology 113:1854-1858, 2006   10–9

Objectives.—To report the use of whole-body positron emission tomography fused with computed tomography (PET/CT) for the diagnosis and staging of orbital lymphoma.

Design.—Retrospective observational case series.

Participants.—Four patients with biopsy-proven orbital lymphoma were evaluated by 18-fluoro-2-deoxyglucose whole-body PET/CT imaging.

Methods.—Positron emission tomography/CT images were studied for the presence of glucose uptake. Foci were considered suspicious based on their standardized uptake values (SUVs). Physiologic images (PET) and their anatomic counterparts (CT) were fused to allow form and function to be evaluated on the same diagnostic page.

Main Outcome Measures.—Positron emission tomography/CT images were assessed for foci with abnormally high SUVs that correlated with biopsy-proven lymphoma.

Results.—Positron emission tomography/CT detected orbital lymphoma in 3 patients (75%). It also revealed systemic lymphoma in 2 of the 4 patients. The 2 patients found to have systemic lymphoma were diagnosed to have extranodal marginal zone B-cell orbital lymphoma of the mucosa-associated lymphoid tissue (MALT) type. Similarly, the 2 with negative PET/CT results also had orbital MALT-type lymphoma. We found that PET/CT imaging helped guide further management in all 4 patients.

Conclusions.—Positron emission tomography/CT should be considered as a new method of diagnosing, staging, and restaging patients with orbital lymphomas.

▶ Many years ago, Knowles et al[1] concluded that the most important prognostic factor in the assessment of ocular adnexal lymphoma was the extent of the disease at the time of initial presentation disclosed by a thorough clinical staging. They reported that the vast majority of patients presenting with a clinical stage 1E ocular adnexal lymphoid proliferation have a benign, indolent clinical course regardless of histopathology or immunophenotypic analysis. The 2 articles highlighted here (Abstracts 10–8 and 10–9) discuss relatively new diagnostic tools that can demonstrate the presence of systemic disease, which typically remained hidden when clinical evaluation relied on older methods.

The new modalities include PET scanning and PET scanning combined with CT (PET/CT). In several instances, PET scanning disclosed foci of metabolically active cells consistent with lymphoma that had not been disclosed by the standard workup. This new information led to a change in the patient's systemic therapy.

Every patient with a lymphoid lesion of the eye or orbit needs a thorough systemic evaluation by a hematologist-oncologist. He or she has the expertise and experience to order these new, relatively expensive tests, interpret the results, and institute appropriate therapy.

R. C. Eagle, Jr, MD

Reference

1. Knowles DM, Jakobiec FA, McNally L, et al: Lymphoid hyperplasia and malignant lymphoma occurring in the ocular adnexa (orbit, conjunctiva, and eyelids): A prospective multiparametric analysis of 108 cases during 1977 to 1987. *Hum Pathol* 21:959-973, 1990.

Periocular and Orbital Amyloidosis: Clinical Characteristics, Management, and Outcome

Leibovitch I, Selva D, Goldberg RA, et al (Univ of Adelaide, Australia; UCLA, Los Angeles; Royal Brisbane Hosp, Australia)
Ophthalmology 113:1657-1664, 2006   10–10

Objective.—To present the clinical features and management outcome in a large series of patients with periocular and orbital amyloidosis.

Design.—Retrospective, noncomparative, interventional case series.

Patients.—All patients diagnosed with periocular and orbital amyloidosis in 6 oculoplastic and orbital units.

Methods.—Clinical records of all patients were reviewed.

Main Outcome Measures.—Clinical presentation, radiological and histological findings, treatment modalities, and outcome.

Results.—The study included 24 patients (15 female, 9 male) with a mean age of 57±17 years. Nineteen cases were unilateral, and 5 were bilateral. Clinical signs and symptoms included a visible or palpable periocular mass or tissue infiltration (95.8%), ptosis (54.2%), periocular discomfort or pain (25%), proptosis or globe displacement (21%), limitations in ocular motility (16.7%), recurrent periocular subcutaneous hemorrhages (12.5%), and diplopia (8.3%). Seven cases had orbital involvement, and 17 were periocular. Immunohistochemistry in 7 patients showed B cells or plasma cells producing monoclonal immunoglobulin chains that were deposited as amyloid light chains. Only 1 patient was diagnosed with systemic amyloid light chain amyloidosis. Treatment modalities were mainly observation and surgical debulking. During a mean follow-up period of 39 months, 21% showed significant progression after treatment, whereas 79% were stable or showed no recurrence after treatment.

Conclusion.—Periocular and orbital amyloidosis may present with a wide spectrum of clinical findings and result in significant ocular morbidity. Complete surgical excision is not feasible in many cases, and the goal of treatment is to preserve function and to prevent sight-threatening complications.

▶ The great majority of the patients in this large retrospective, multicenter study of periocular and orbital amyloidosis had the localized amyloid light-chain form of amyloidosis, which is unassociated with systemic disease. The amyloid deposits in this disorder are composed of monoclonal immunoglobulin light chains (kappa or lambda) that are produced locally by a clone of benign B cells or plasma cells. This form of amyloidosis is termed localized amyloid light-chain amyloidosis. The amyloid deposits in the more serious systemic disorder that previously were called primary systemic amyloidosis are also composed of immunoglobulin light chains. These usually are produced by a benign, low-grade, light chain–producing monoclonal gammopathy that causes widespread organ deposition and dysfunction. The latter disorder is now called primary amyloid light-chain amyloidosis. Only one patient in this series was confirmed to have systemic amyloidosis, although not all patients were extensively evaluated. I believe that one man who presented with bilateral periocular subcutaneous hemorrhages and died of cardiac arrest could have had systemic disease.

Several types of amyloid that affect other parts of the eye are composed of totally different amyloidogenic proteins. Vitreous amyloid always is associated with familial amyloidosis and is composed of mutant transthyretin, a transport protein for vitamin A and thyroid hormone. This type of amyloidosis is now called ATTR amyloidosis. Several corneal dystrophies are characterized by amyloid deposition. These include gelatinous drop-like dystrophy (or familial subepithelial amyloidosis), classic lattice corneal dystrophy type I, and lattice corneal dystrophy type II or Meretoja syndrome. The amyloid deposits in lattice dystrophy type I are composed of keratoepithelin, the protein product of the *TGFBI* gene on chromosome 5q31. Other mutant forms of the protein are found in granular corneal dystrophy. The amyloid deposits in Meretoja syndrome are composed of a protein involved in actin metabolism called gelsolin. Affected patients have systemic involvement including progressive cranial and peripheral neuropathies and skin changes, as well as mild lattice-like corneal deposits.

R. C. Eagle, Jr, MD

11 Socio-Economics

Ophthalmic Training

by Elisabeth J. Cohen, MD

Training in ophthalmology includes professionalism, as well as clinical and surgical competence. The shift in evaluation of training from experience and time spent to competence achieved is reasonable and appropriate, but much more difficult to document and enforce. Advances in technology have made surgical training much more challenging. Spreading out surgical training would be a first step in identifying challenged residents and providing more time for learning and career counseling if necessary. Professionalism can be taught, but it certainly helps if doctors are motivated first by a desire to help others. Cost-effective medicine and necessary business skills for survival in the current atmosphere of reduced reimbursement and increased malpractice costs should be learned after professional values are well established. Practicing physicians must be good professional role models consistently, not just when they are involved in formal teaching. The enthusiasm and good intentions of most doctors in training should be strengthened by their education.

The Developing Physician—Becoming a Professional
Stern DT, Papadakis M (Univ of Michigan, Ann Arbor; Univ of California, San Francisco)
N Engl J Med 355:1794-1799, 2006   11–1

Background.—The transition from student to a seasoned clinician caring for patients is the subject of this report. It is important for clinicians to reflect on that transitional period and to ask whether medical educators are cultivating in today's students and residents the professional behaviors they would seek should they require medical care.

Overview.—Included in the broad concept of "teaching" are 3 basic actions: setting expectations, providing experiences, and evaluating outcomes. The literature on professionalism is generally focused on one or another of these 3 tasks, but all 3 aspects of teaching must be addressed if an educational program is to be comprehensive. In most cases, the rules and expectations for medical students on the first day on the wards were unwritten and were discovered only after a mistake was made. It would make more sense to set explicit goals and expectations for students. A "white coat" ceremony is now performed for first-year students at most schools. At this ceremony, the meaning of the responsibility that accompanies the wearing of a white coat is taught, and expectations for humanism and professionalism are communicated. Continuing a public profession of principles into the years of residency and practice is unusual but important to ensure that physicians are committed to a common set of expectations for the profession. Until the late 1970s, the formal teaching of ethics, professionalism, and humanism was not part of the medical school curriculum. However, in the ensuing years, educators have developed curricular experiences to expose students to issues of professionalism and to promote knowledge of ethical principles, skills of moral reasoning, and the development of humanistic attitudes. The development of teamwork and leadership skills, which are critical aspects of professionalism, is one of the primary goals of problem-based learning. However, the informal experiences of medical students and residents may be more important than the formal elements of the curriculum. This sort of experience has been termed part of the "hidden curriculum"—rules, regulations, and routines transmitted mostly by residents rather than faculty. Role modeling is the most important factor in teaching the hidden curriculum. It is necessary for medical educators to set expectations, create appropriate learning experiences, and evaluate outcomes. The goal of evaluation should be to reward the best professional behavior, enhance professionalism in all students, identify those students who show deficiencies in professionalism, and dismiss the rare student who cannot practice professionalism.

Conclusions.—In the process of teaching students the core values of medicine, educators must consider the real world in which students will work and relax. The concept of teaching must include not only the formal but also the informal curriculum and include 3 basic actions: setting expectations, providing experiences, and evaluating outcomes.

▶ To be a professional requires putting the interest of the patient first. Many of the necessary attributes should be there before a person begins medical school. Altruism should be important in the desire to be a doctor. Caring for patients is still necessary. Unprofessional behavior is often hard to prove. Recently, we had a resident who we think wrote notes on patients without examining them. The resident denied it, and it was the resident's word against the patients, who were challenged by drug dependency, frailty, or both. When I failed as an intern to order a test (uric acid) that would have determined the cause of a patient's acute renal failure, the renal consultant told me in front of his team that my patient would have been better off in a hotel. This comment was somewhat unfair because the patient also had a resident, oncology fellow, and attending physician involved in his care. Being a role model for professionalism at all times is the highest responsibility of attending physicians, even if residents seem to learn more from their peers.

E. J. Cohen, MD

Ophthalmology Resident Surgical Competency: *A National Survey*
Binenbaum G, Volpe NJ (Univ of Pennsylvania, Philadelphia)
Ophthalmology 113:1237-1244, 2006   11–2

Purpose.—To describe the prevalence, management, and career outcomes of ophthalmology residents who struggle with surgical competency and to explore related educational issues.

Design.—Fourteen-question written survey.

Participants.—Fifty-eight program directors at Accreditation Council on Graduate Medical Education-accredited, United States ophthalmology residency programs, representing a total of 2179 resident graduates, between 1991 and 2000.

Methods.—Study participants completed a mailed, anonymous survey whose format combined multiple choice and free comment questions.

Main Outcome Measures.—Number of surgically challenged residents, types of problems identified, types of remediation, final departmental decision at the end of residency, known career outcomes, and residency program use of microsurgical skills laboratories and applicant screening tests.

Results.—One hundred ninety-nine residents (9% overall; 10% mean per program) were labeled as having trouble mastering surgical skills. All of the programs except 2 had encountered such residents. The most frequently cited problems were poor hand-eye coordination (24%) and poor intraoperative judgment (22%) (Table 1). Most programs were supportive and used educational rather than punitive measures, the most common being extra practice-laboratory time (32%), scheduling cases with the best teaching surgeon (23%), and counseling (21%). Nearly one third (31%) of residents were believed to have overcome their difficulties before graduation. Other residents were encouraged to pursue medical ophthalmology (22%) or to obtain further surgical training through a fellowship (21%) or a supervised practice setting (12%); these residents were granted a departmental statement of satisfactory completion of residency for Board eligibility. Twelve percent were asked to leave residency. Of reported career outcomes, 92% of residents were practicing ophthalmology, 65% as surgical and 27% as medical ophthalmologists. Ninety-eight percent of residency programs had mi-

TABLE 1.—Types of Problems Learning Surgical Skills

	n	%
Poor hand–eye coordination	78	24
Poor intraoperative judgement	71	22
Inability to listen to supervising surgeon	51	16
Tremor	45	14
Questionable behavior (e.g., poor case selection)	34	11
Inappropriate reaction to stress of the operating room	32	10
Visual problems	10	3
Total	321	100

crosurgical practice facilities, 64% had a formal teaching course, and 36% had mandatory practice time. Most programs (76%) did not perform applicant vision or dexterity screening tests; questions existed about the legality and validity of such tests.

Conclusions.—The issue of ophthalmology residents who struggle to develop surgical competency appears common. Although many problems appear to be remediable with time, practice, and dedicated, patient teachers, more specific guidelines for a statement of surgical competency are likely necessary to standardize the Board certification process.

▶ This article reports that "9 to 10% of ophthalmology residents in this study are surgically challenged." It is interesting that one of the approaches used for this problem is to obtain additional surgical training through a fellowship. As a corneal specialist with a large fellowship program, I think this is a suboptimal solution. It is very sad to have a cornea fellow who struggles in surgery because of a lack of depth perception when this issue should have been dealt with earlier. Ideally, the problems should be worked out during residency, and, if they do not resolve, ophthalmic surgical subspecialty training is not in the best interest of the resident or the patients. I think the idea of starting surgical training early in the residency so it is not primarily done in the third year is a good one to promote early detection of problems, time for resolution, and career counseling, if indicated. It is interesting that surgically challenged residents may or may not be problem residents in general. I suspect that surgically challenged residents who are otherwise good or great residents are more likely to successfully work through these issues than those who are problem residents in general. It is also noteworthy that legal ramifications are less likely for surgical/academic dismissals than disciplinary/problem resident dismissals. Screening for problems at the time of application is probably illegal, according to the Americans with Disabilities Act.

E. J. Cohen, MD

Teaching Surgical Skills—Changes in the Wind
Reznick RK, MacRae H (Univ of Toronto; Mount Sinai Hosp, Toronto)
N Engl J Med 355:2664-2669, 2006   11–3

Background.—A German-style residency training system with an emphasis on graded responsibility was introduced at Johns Hopkins Hospital in 1889 by Sir William Halsted. This system has remained the cornerstone of surgical training in North America to the present. However, advances in educational theory and increasing pressures in the clinical environment have led to questions about the reliance on this approach for teaching technical skills. The potential changes to the teaching of surgical skills were reviewed.

Overview.—Among the pressures on the current resident training model are a move toward a shorter workweek for residents and an emphasis on operating room efficiency, both of which reduce teaching time. However, the patients in this country's teaching hospitals are generally much sicker than in the past and have more complex problems. A high volume of exposure, rather than specifically designed curricula, is the hallmark of current surgical training. However, as opportunities for learning through work with "real" patients have diminished, interest in laboratories with formal curricula has increased dramatically. In this new model, basic surgical skills are learned and practiced on models and simulators to better prepare trainees for the operating room experience. These new training techniques are based on established theories of the acquisition of motor skills and development of expertise, including Fitts and Posner's 3-stage theory of motor skill acquisition. The 3 stages are the cognitive, integrative, and autonomous stages. In the cognitive stage, the task is intellectualized. In the integrative stage, knowledge is translated into appropriate motor behavior. In the autonomous stage, practice gradually results in smooth performance. The implications of this model for surgical training are that the earlier stages of teaching technical skills should occur outside the operating room; practice is the rule until automaticity in basic skills is achieved. Valid and reliable assessments of technical skills are needed to facilitate better planning of instruction and assessment of the efficacy of curricular interventions. There is also a need to address important motor-learning issues, such as whether it is preferable to practice whole operations or segments of operations, building to the whole from the segments.

Conclusions.—In light of the advances in technology and the increasing evidence of their effectiveness, it is appropriate to critically evaluate the changes that must be made to improve the assessment and training of surgeons in the future.

▶ It is comforting that the increased challenges of teaching ophthalmic surgery are also present in teaching general surgery. In corneal training, the shift to sutureless cataract surgery has produced fellows with limited experience in tying knots. Practice eyes are necessary, but often the best surgeons like to practice the most, so it is hard to know which comes first. The shift is now toward model eyes and next it will be virtual training. The new paradigm of competency in place of time spent in training is a challenge to document and enforce. It is difficult to rule that doctors who spent the required year(s) in training are not competent, but it can be true. Currently, there are no readily available avenues for additional training if needed to achieve competence. Career counseling at this stage is rather late in a profession with already very long training and delayed gratification.

E. J. Cohen, MD

Resident Physician Mentoring Program in Ophthalmology: The Tennessee Experience

Tsai JC, Lee PP, Chasteen S, et al (Columbia Univ, New York; Vanderbilt Univ, Nashville, Tenn; Duke Univ, Durham, NC; et al)
Arch Ophthalmol 124:264-267, 2006   11–4

Objective.—To establish a mentoring program to provide resident physicians in ophthalmology with career guidance in practice management and to identify new and creative ways to involve future eye physicians in the legislative and political process.

Methods.—A multicenter prospective study was conducted of the mentorship experiences of 24 (88.9%) of 27 resident physicians in Tennessee during the 2000-2001 academic year. Participants were assigned into 1 of 3 groups: an active mentorship group, a passive mentorship group, and a no mentorship group. The active mentorship group participated in preceptorship activities with "mentor" community-based eye physicians and scheduled meetings with state legislators and regulators. The active mentorship and passive mentorship groups attended a 1-day practice management seminar, but the no mentorship group received no formal mentorship during the 4-month study period. A survey instrument was given to all participants before and after the 4-month study period.

Results.—Following completion of the mentorship program, the active mentorship group had favorable changes in perceptions and attitudes toward medical organizations (*P*<.03) when compared with baseline prementorship responses. Compared with the no mentorship group, the active mentorship group also reported an increased willingness to make political campaign donations (*P*<.05) and expressed an increased desire for the Tennessee Academy of Ophthalmology to offer practice management programs (*P*<.02).

Conclusion.—A short 4-month mentorship program can elicit favorable changes in residents' perceptions and attitudes toward medical professional organizations. Additional opportunities may lie with a lengthier and more intensive mentoring program.

▶ It is not surprising that mentoring has a positive impact on resident attitudes. In this study, mentoring was used to encourage interest in organized medicine. Different mentoring programs have different purposes. One can use them to promote interest in academic medicine and research as well. I think personal contact with residents and fellows can have a huge, positive impact. Each resident should have a mentor appropriate for his or her interests, and frequent contact throughout training should be encouraged. We all can remember doctors who shaped our careers, and we should hope to do the same for others.

E. J. Cohen, MD

Can Massachusetts Lead the Way in Health Care Reform?

Altman SH, Doonan M (Brandeis Univ, Waltham, Mass)
N Engl J Med 354:2093-2095, 2006   11–5

Background.—The number of uninsured persons in the United States is rapidly approaching 50 million. Numerous polls have reported that a majority of Americans, whether Democrats, Republicans, or independents, support universal health care coverage. The problem is that there is no consensus on any specific solution to the problem of inadequate health care coverage. The state of Massachusetts may be emerging as a leader in meaningful health care reform in the United States. The Massachusetts legislature has recently passed health care reform that is designed to cover 90% to 95% of the state's uninsured citizens over the next 3 years. The components of

---

TABLE 1.—Key Components of the Massachusetts Plan

Individual health insurance mandate. All state residents 18 years of age or older will be required to carry a minimum level of health insurance, which will be confirmed and enforced through the state tax return. Parents will be responsible for meeting the obligation for children. A database of insurance coverage for all persons will be established. The financial penalty for noncompliance will eventually be 50 percent of what a person would have paid toward an "affordable" insurance premium.

Employer responsibilities. There will be a $295 annual charge per employee to businesses with 11 or more full-time employees that do not provide health insurance for workers or contribute to it. Such employers must offer "cafeteria plans," which allow the purchase of insurance on a pretax basis. These employers will also be subject to a "free-rider surcharge" when their employees use more than a specified amount of care from a state "health safety-net fund."

Creation of the Commonwealth Health Insurance Connector. This state authority will administer many of the insurance aspects of the reforms, including the new subsidized and affordable policies and the annual setting of a sliding scale for "affordable" coverage. The exchange will connect persons and businesses with 50 or fewer employees with insurance products. Policies cannot be sold through the connector unless they receive its seal of approval. Those who are elibible to purchase coverage will include people who are self-employed, not working, not eligible for coverage through work, or working at companies that do not offer insurance. Insurance can be purchased with pretax dollars. People can keep their policies even if they change jobs.

Premium assistance for individuals and families with low incomes. Persons who earn less than 300 percent of the federal poverty guidelines and who are ineligible for other public insurance will be eligible for subsidized policies through the Commonwealth Care Health Insurance Program. Premiums will be on a sliding scale based on household income, with no premiums for those who earn less than 100 percent of the federal proverty guidelines. No plans will have deductibles.

New insurance products. In July 2007, the individual and small-group insurance markets will be merged, reducing the cost of nongroup premiums. There will be new insurance products for people whose incomes make them ineligible for the subsidized plans. These plans may have deductibles, limited networks of physicians and hospitals, and substantial out-of-pocket costs. Young adults will be able to stay on their parents' insurance plans until two years after the loss of their dependent status or until they turn 25 (whichever occurs first). Specially designed products with lower costs and limited coverage will be available for people between the ages of 19 and 26 years.

Medicaid expansion. Eligibility for MassHealth, as Medicaid is known in Massachusetts, will be expanded to include children of families who earn up to 300 percent of the federal poverty guidelines. Medicaid providers will receive rate increases.

Cost and quality measures. Cost and quality data for physicians, hospitals, and specific procedures will be collected and made public. Hospitals will be required to collect and report data on racial and ethnic health disparities. Medicaid rate increases will be tied to achievement of performance goals.

Massachusetts' health care reform plan were reviewed, and its potential role as a model for other states and the federal government was discussed.

Overview.—The legislation approved in Massachusetts included several measures designed to make insurance more affordable. Beginning in July 2007, all residents of the state are required to carry a minimum level of health insurance. This mandate will be enforced through the state's tax returns. Assistance in the payment of premiums will be provided for low-income persons and families who are not eligible for other public assistance. The state's Medicaid program will cover all children in families with incomes of up to 300% of the poverty level, or about $60,000 for a family of 4. A new state marketplace will allow residents to purchase approved health insurance with pretax dollars. Businesses with more than 10 employees will be required to pay an assessment of $295 per employee per year if they do not provide insurance for their workers (Table 1). There are several concerns about the Massachusetts plan. First, it is unclear whether the current financing package will generate enough funds to sustain the program. The requirement is for a minimal level, not an optimal level, of health insurance. Improving access to medical care for previously uninsured persons may increase the demand for needed services, which would improve health but would also increase costs. However, it is often the case that holding out for the best plan will kill efforts to make real reforms.

Conclusions.—The health care reform legislation passed in Massachusetts is not perfect, but there is agreement that it represents significant progress toward meaningful health care reform in this country.

▶ It is encouraging that Massachusetts has passed health care reform legislation so that more than 90% of their uninsured population will have coverage within 3 years. It has been a huge failure of both Democratic and Republican administrations to deal effectively with the intolerable problem of uninsured Americans, presently approaching 50 million. Perhaps reforms at the state level are a good way to start to solve this serious problem. Ultimately, nationwide insurance makes more sense than statewide insurance, which is more complicated, bureaucratic, and therefore, expensive because patients often live in one state and get medical care in another. Involvement of, and compromise among health care providers, business payers, and patient advocates were necessary to get the ball rolling in the right direction. Providing insurance for the uninsured will indeed increase demand for health care services and should be expected to increase health care costs, at least in the short run.

E. J. Cohen, MD

Medical Professional Liability Insurance and its Relation to Medical Error and Healthcare Risk Management for the Practicing Physician

Abbott RL, Weber P, Kelley B (Univ of California, San Francisco; Ophthalmic Mutual Insurance Co, San Francisco)
Am J Ophthalmol 140:1106-1111, 2005   11–6

Purpose.—To review the history and current issues surrounding medical professional liability insurance and its relationship to medical error and healthcare risk management.

Design.—Focused literature review and authors' experience.

Methods.—Medical professional liability insurance issues are reviewed in association with the occurrence of medical error and the role of healthcare risk management.

Results.—The rising frequency and severity of claims and lawsuits incurred by physicians, as well as escalating defense costs, have dramatically increased over the past several years and have resulted in accelerated efforts to reduce medical errors and control practice risk for physicians. Medical error reduction and improved patient outcomes are closely linked to the goals of the medical risk manager by reducing exposure to adverse medical events. Management of professional liability risk by the physician-led malpractice insurance company not only protects the economic viability of physicians, but also addresses patient safety concerns.

Conclusions.—Physician-owned malpractice liability insurance companies will continue to be the dominant providers of insurance for practicing physicians and will serve as the primary source for loss prevention and risk management services. To succeed in the marketplace, the emergence and importance of the risk manager and incorporation of risk management principles throughout the professional liability company has become crucial to the financial stability and success of the insurance company. The risk manager provides the necessary advice and support requested by physicians to minimize medical liability risk in their daily practice.

▶ This article was published late in 2005, after this section was completed last year, but it is interesting and important enough to include in the 2006 selections. It explains the evolution toward physician-owned malpractice insurance companies and the importance of the risk manager in these companies. Medical errors contribute to malpractice claims. When errors occur, their cause should be determined and discussed so action can be taken to prevent their recurrence and enhance patient safety. Fear of malpractice suits discourages discussion of errors and adverse outcomes. The goals of risk management are to prevent and reduce the severity of losses from claims. The risk manager and the insurance company work with the physicians and not against them.

Risk management can be a win-win proposition insofar as it can be used to identify causes of errors and implement changes to prevent them to the benefit of the insurance company, the physicians and patients. For example, in anesthesia, a review of claims showed that more meticulous monitoring of patients during anesthesia would help prevent occurrences resulting in claims. Changes were made, and anesthesia is no longer a high-risk medical specialty, such as neurosurgery, obstetrics, or orthopedics. In ophthalmology, it has been shown that high surgical volume and prior claims or law suits are associated with increased risk of having malpractice claims or law suits related to refractive surgery.

Risk management principles are also used to develop underwriting guidelines to determine who gets insurance coverage. These guidelines related to patient selection, informed consent, postoperative care, and advertising have been used successfully to avoid catastrophic losses by insurers, such as OMIC (Ophthalmic Mutual Insurance Company), from refractive surgery claims. It is comforting to know that the risk managers provide support to physicians facing malpractice suits who are under a great deal of stress.

E. J. Cohen, MD

Claims, Errors, and Compensation Payments in Medical Malpractice Litigation

Studdert DM, Mello MM, Gawande AA, et al (Harvard School of Public Health, Boston; Brigham and Women's Hosp, Boston; Harvard Risk Management Found, Boston)
N Engl J Med 354:2024-2033, 2006   11–7

Background.—In the current debate over tort reform, critics of the medical malpractice system charge that frivolous litigation—claims that lack evidence of injury, substandard care, or both—is common and costly.

Methods.—Trained physicians reviewed a random sample of 1452 closed malpractice claims from five liability insurers to determine whether a medical injury had occurred and, if so, whether it was due to medical error. We analyzed the prevalence, characteristics, litigation outcomes, and costs of claims that lacked evidence of error.

Results.—For 3 percent of the claims, there were no verifiable medical injuries, and 37 percent did not involve errors. Most of the claims that were not associated with errors (370 of 515 [72 percent]) or injuries (31 of 37 [84 percent]) did not result in compensation; most that involved injuries due to error did (653 of 889 [73 percent]). Payment of claims not involving errors occurred less frequently than did the converse form of inaccuracy—nonpayment of claims associated with errors. When claims not involving errors were compensated, payments were significantly lower on average than were payments for claims involving errors (313,205 dollars vs. 521,560 dollars, P=0.004). Overall, claims not involving errors accounted for 13 to 16 percent of the system's total monetary costs. For every dollar spent on compensation, 54 cents went to administrative expenses (including those involving lawyers, experts, and courts). Claims involving errors accounted for 78 percent of total administrative costs.

Conclusions.—Claims that lack evidence of error are not uncommon, but most are denied compensation. The vast majority of expenditures go toward litigation over errors and payment of them. The overhead costs of malpractice litigation are exorbitant.

▶ One can look at the glass as half full or half empty. The authors conclude that claims without errors are uncommon, but they account for 37% of all claims! Only 3% of claims had no medical injuries, but that number should be zero. Most claims without errors did not get compensation, but 28% of these claims did! Frivolous lawsuits may not be driving the cost of malpractice, but given that claims take an average of 5 years to be resolved, defendants in the claims suffer a lot of unnecessary "uncertainty, acrimony, and time away from patient care." The high overhead of malpractice litigation includes legal fees. Non-error claims accounted for 21% of this overhead. It is reassuring that the majority of malpractice costs involve medical errors, but it would be absurd if this were not the case. Streamlining the process for claims involving errors is a reasonable goal so that overhead is reduced and delays until resolution are decreased for both patients and doctors.

E. J. Cohen, MD

Reform of Drug Regulation—Beyond an Independent Drug-Safety Board
Ray WA, Stein CM (Ctr for Education and Research on Therapeutics, Nashville, Tenn; Veterans Affairs Med Ctr, Nashville, Tenn; Vanderbilt Univ, Nashville, Tenn)
N Engl J Med 354:194-201, 2006   11–8

Background.—The recent withdrawal of several high-profile drugs has stimulated a reassessment of the process of drug regulation in the United States and provoked concerns that the current process is inadequate for protection of the public health. There is a perception by some that the Food and Drug Administration and the pharmaceutical industry are unable to impartially evaluate drugs and to respond adequately to signals indicating potential drug-safety problems. This perception has fostered growing support for the establishment of an independent drug-safety board. More extensive reforms to the current drug regulation system are proposed to provide better protection for the American public.

Overview.—At present, there are no systematic provisions for postmarketing studies of drugs. Thus, there often is insufficient information on the safety of widely used drugs, the effects of long-term exposure, and the frequency of rare adverse effects. In addition, the present system of drug regulation is susceptible to the influence of conflicts of interest. The Prescription Drug User Fee Act (PDUFA) has led to significantly decreased review times for new drug applications, but its strict timetables and detailed requirements for communication with manufacturers are controversial because they may promote hasty approvals and divert resources from postmarketing surveillance. There is also a perception that the pharmaceutical industry is the customer of the Food and Drug Administration. A consensus is emerging in favor of an independent drug-safety board. This proposed reformed regulatory authority would have 3 distinct functions: approval of new drugs; postmarketing studies; and drug information. Three independent but cooperative centers would be established within a unified agency and would be funded by a tax on pharmaceutical sales. The Center for New Drug Approval would regulate the initial licensing of new drugs; the Center for Postmarketing Studies would specify and oversee mandatory postapproval studies; and the Center for Drug Information would coordinate the communication of accurate, unbiased information to patients and practitioners promoting the use of drugs in accordance with the best available data.

Conclusions.—There are serious flaws in the current system of drug regulation in the United States. Implementation of the proposed reforms will not be easy or inexpensive, but the costs of inaction will be much greater.

▶ This article proposes major reform of the drug regulatory process into 3 parts: one for new drugs similar to the Food and Drug Administration, with some modifications, one for postmarketing studies, and one for drug information. Postmarketing relative efficacy studies would compare new drugs with alternative drugs instead of placebos. The performance of postmarketing studies independent of the manufacturer is a good idea that may get approved. However, it may be harder to find acceptance for phasing in the release of new drugs, which could be seen as bureaucratic delay. Communication of drug information beyond the current use of the drug label is very important, since the drug label is not read very often. One would think that there could be weekly communication to physicians somewhat analogous to the *Morbidity and Mortality Weekly Report* from the Centers for Disease Control and Prevention. The cyclooxygenase-2 (COX-2) disaster should be used as an opportunity for acceptance of fundamental change and improvement in drug safety monitoring in the United States. As Dr David Worthen instructed incoming members, including me, of the Ophthalmic Device Panel of the Food and Drug Administration in the 1980s, the critical issue is safety, since efficacy can be determined by the marketplace.

E. J. Cohen, MD

System Failure versus Personal Accountability—The Case for Clean Hands
Goldman D (Harvard Med School)
N Engl J Med 355:121-123, 2006   11–9

Background.—Hand hygiene is an important component in preventing the spread of antibiotic-resistant bacteria. The focus on patient safety programs is often on improving systems, yet there is a need to emphasize the lower-profile steps that can be taken, such as thorough hand washing by health care practitioners.

Overview.—Infections with methicillin-resistant *Staphylococcus aureus,* which are difficult to treat, are transmitted primarily by the contaminated hands of health care providers who have touched a colonized patient or something in the patient's environment. Caregivers who leave the bedsides of colonized patients without washing their hands may carry thousands or even hundreds of thousands of colony-forming units of antibiotic-resistant bacteria on their hands. Even if these caregivers wear gloves, they frequently contaminate their hands when they remove the gloves. Fortunately, the remedy is simple and straightforward: proper hand hygiene. If every caregiver would reliably practice simple hand hygiene when leaving the bedside of every patient and before touching the next patient, there would be an immediate and significant reduction in the spread of resistant bacteria. This task has been made even easier in recent years by the introduction of waterless, alcohol-based hand antiseptics. Performing hand hygiene with these products will kill bacteria (with the exception of *Clostridium difficile*) in less time than is required with traditional hand washing and is gentler on the skin than repeated use of soap and water. However, compliance with hand hygiene is poor in most institutions, often in the range of 40% to 50%. It is important that staff members are not so seriously overworked that they do not have time to perform important standard procedures, and that caregivers be adequately educated on effective hand hygiene. Once educated, caregivers should have their hand hygiene competency evaluated and certified. They then must be provided with reliable access to alcohol-based antiseptics at the point of care, which requires a foolproof system for refilling containers before they are empty. Finally, there must be accountability in the system to ensure that violations of an institution's hand hygiene policy result in consequences to offending caregivers.

Conclusions.—Each caregiver has a duty to perform hand hygiene perfectly every time to prevent the spread of antibiotic-resistant organisms.

Selling Soap: How do you get doctors to wash their hands?
Dubner SJ, Levitt SD (New York)
Freakonomics in The New York Times September 26:22-23, 2006   11–10

Background.—The recent experience of a Los Angeles urologist on a vacation cruise in the South Seas is illustrative of a significant problem in health care. The crew of the ship wouldn't allow passengers who had gone ashore to reboard until they had squirted some waterless antibiotic cleanser on their hands. In fact, the crew even dispensed the cleanser to passengers lined up at the buffet table. Why, he wondered, was a cruise ship more diligent about killing germs than his own hospital? The Institute of Medicine has estimated that 44,000 to 98,000 Americans die each year because of hospital errors, and that one of the leading errors was the spread of bacterial infections. Numerous studies have shown that hospital personnel wash or disinfect their hands in fewer than half the instances they should. And doctors are the worst offenders, according to these reports. There is a need for some kind of incentive to increase compliance with hand hygiene policies without alienating physicians. The experience at one institution was presented.

Overview.—Even excellent hospitals, such as Cedars-Sinai Medical Center in Los Angeles, pass along bacterial infections. It may seem a mystery as to why doctors, of all people, would practice poor hand hygiene, but a meeting of the hospital leadership identified several reasons. The doctors are busy, and sinks are often inconveniently located. The introduction of an alcohol-based disinfectant, however, did not appreciably increase compliance with hand hygiene protocols. Psychological factors were also cited as reasons for noncompliance with hand washing. An Australian study found that doctors self-reported their rate of hand washing at 73%, while observation of these same doctors found their actual rate was just 9%. Cedars-Sinai devised an incentive schedule that would increase compliance, beginning with gentle exhortations via faxes and posters. When that failed, hospital administrators began handing out bottles of an alcohol-based disinfectant at the physician parking lot entrance. A Hand Hygiene Safety Posse began to roam the wards, handing out $10 Starbucks cards to physicians who were caught washing up. Compliance rose from 65% to 80%, but still fell short of the 90% required by the Joint Commission. The final step was culture and photograph of agar plates into which doctors had pressed their palms. The images, showing numerous colonies of bacteria, were loaded as screen savers into every computer in the medical center. Hand hygiene compliance rose to nearly 100%.

Conclusions.—This case is an example of the efforts often required to solve a seemingly simple problem—how to get physicians to wash their hands. It must be remembered, however, that microbes can thrive on just about any surface in a hospital room, including stuffed animals.

▶ It still amazes me that doctors do not wash their hands before and after every patient. I usually emphasize hand washing before examining each patient, in front of the patient, but this article emphasizes hand washing afterward. Both are necessary. Methicillin-resistant *Staphylococcus aureus* infections are on the rise, and hospital personnel are known to be carriers and at risk of infecting themselves or patients. The alcohol-based hand antiseptics are more user friendly than sinks and much easier on the skin. They work except when soil is present, in which case hand washing remains necessary. According to *The New York Times* article, at Cedars-Sinai Hospital, $10 Starbucks cards raised hand washing to 80%, but a photo of a culture plate of a hand as a screen saver on every computer in the hospital raised the rate to 100%! Physicians should have as their New Year's resolution to hand wash before and after every patient—as I am sure we all want our doctors to do when they take care of us.

E. J. Cohen, MD

After the Storm—Health Care Infrastructure in Post-Katrina New Orleans
Berggren RE, Curiel TJ (Tulane Univ Health Sciences Ctr, New Orleans, La)
N Engl J Med 354:1549-1552, 2006   11–11

Background.—Our television sets showed the desperate times immediately after Hurricane Katrina hit New Orleans. However, of the months of health care since the hurricane, the first week was the easiest seen at Charity Hospital by medical personnel from Louisiana State University (LSU) School of Medicine. The chronic phase of the crisis is worse; even today there is unacceptably primitive health care in the city.

The Problems.—How extensively the health care infrastructure was damaged was not apparent when patients and staff were evacuated September 2, 2005. Survival depended on initiating self-rescue and professional teamwork. These same principles guide recovery, but local needs are unmet. New Orleans is 24% smaller than before the storm, but only 15 of its 22 hospitals are open. Diminished total hospital capacity is the primary problem, with 2000 available beds rather than the prestorm 4400.

A second problem is uncompensated health care. Because of job loss, many persons in the city are transient workers with no health insurance. Since the storm, the level of uncompensated care has tripled and reimbursement for uncompensated care is lacking. In addition, the Centers for Medicare and Medicaid Services (CMS) has held up funds to pay the medical residents who remain in the city.

A third concern stems from complications related to untreated chronic diseases, especially hypertension, diabetes, and AIDS. Complications develop when health care regimens are abandoned. Caring for such patients in acute care facilities costs more than in chronic care sites, but these facilities are closed. Death notices increased 25% over a year's time. Suicide and post-traumatic stress disorder are prevalent, but mental health facilities and providers are not sufficient.

Medical education is a fourth problem, with faculty layoffs at both Tulane and LSU. Medical residents provide care for most underinsured patients in all major US cities, and New Orleans obviously needs them now. Historically, physicians trained at LSU and Tulane remain in the area. However, financial issues, including government aid and bureaucratic CMS holdups, are only slowly addressed, hurting training programs.

Solutions.—Creative approaches to provide services and increase available beds include collaborations between Touro Infirmary, LSU, Tulane, Ochsner Clinic, and the Veterans Affairs (VA) hospital. Tulane and LSU maintain their graduate medical education (GME) programs. Medical students have transferred to Baylor Medical School, other hospitals have picked up house staff, and LSU moved temporarily to Baton Rouge. Only 6 of 90 internal medicine residents left Tulane's program, although 11 of 24 pediatric trainees at Charity Hospital were lost with a declining pediatric population. Protecting GME programs seems to be a low priority for government help, but the Hospital Corporation of America is funding residents' salaries. CMS dollars for GME salaries must be tied to residents rather than institutions and health care reimbursements should follow patients rather than hospitals to improve the situation.

Conclusions.—Without speedy and coordinated help from government sources that effectively addresses the problems, New Orleans will continue to have insufficient health care for its residents. However, through this experience, residents have learned personal and character lessons that should strengthen them as physicians.

► This is a grim picture of the current state of medical care, hospitals, and resident training in New Orleans, 7 months after Katrina. It is sad to hear from the Vice-Chairman for Education at LSU School of Medicine that "The desperate week we spent inside Charity after Katrina . . . was the easiest week of the last 6 months." It sounds like a perfect storm now with too few hospital beds, too many uninsured very sick patients, and no government help. It should not be so difficult to get graduate medical education salaries to residents instead of hospitals. "The pace of bureaucratic change could be lethal to training programs," and much more in New Orleans.

E. J. Cohen, MD

Fighting HIV—Lessons from Brazil
Okie S (Waltham, Mass)
N Engl J Med 354:1977-1981, 2006   11–12

Background.—The government of Brazil has launched a nationwide public health campaign to encourage the use of condoms. In 2006, in the week leading up to Carnaval, Brazilians venturing out in public to catch a bus, buy a beer, or mail a letter were reminded of the importance of condoms. Coca-Cola distributors delivered condom posters to bars along with the soft drink, and a television commercial on the country's most popular soap opera promoted condom usage. A prostitute's organization in an urban business district began working with the local health department on preventing HIV infection by passing out free condom samples to spectators during a Carnaval parade. The efforts to fight HIV in Brazil were highlighted, and the lessons that can be learned from that country's fight to slow and ultimately prevent the spread of HIV infection and contain the country's epidemic were discussed.

Overview.—Brazil is best known for its pioneering decision to offer free combination antiretroviral therapy to all citizens with AIDS. This program has saved the country an estimated $2.2 billion in hospital costs. However, the country's aggressive efforts to prevent the spread of new HIV infections have likely played an equal or greater role in slowing the spread of HIV and containing the country's epidemic. At the beginning of the 1990s, the epidemics in Brazil and South Africa were at a similar stage, with a prevalence of infection of about 1.5%. However, by 1995, the prevalence of infection in South Africa was greater than 10%, while the infection rate in Brazil had declined by half. Brazil's emphasis on prevention has included steps that in the United States have sometimes ignited political controversy. Brazil is also pursuing HIV prevention in prisons, an environment that has been neglected in the United States and in most other countries. Doctors and patients have stated that access to free treatment transformed public attitudes about HIV. Between 1996 and 2002, mortality from AIDS was reduced by 50% in Brazil, and AIDS-related hospitalizations fell by 80%. However, there has not been enough research into which aspects of the country's program have been most responsible for its success thus far.

Conclusions.—The success of HIV prevention programs in Brazil can provide valuable lessons in the effective prevention and treatment of this disease.

▶ The success of Brazil's programs to prevent and treat HIV is impressive. The United States can certainly learn from Brazil. It is striking that this Catholic country has been so successful at educating high-risk populations to use condoms. It is very sad that our government still emphasizes abstinence as the main way to prevent HIV. Needle exchange programs have decreased the number of AIDS cases acquired through drug injection, with IV drug users accounting for only 10% of new cases in Brazil in 2003, compared with 22% in the United States during the same year. The prevention programs have successfully customized their message for the specific target populations, rather than doing mass campaigns that some might find inappropriate.

E. J. Cohen, MD

For Sale: Physicians' Prescribing Data
Steinbrook R (Waltham, Mass)
N Engl J Med 354:2745-2747, 2006   11–13

Background.—For nearly 2 decades, health care information companies have purchased electronic records of prescriptions from pharmacies and other sources and linked them with information about physicians that is licensed from the Physician Masterfile of the American Medical Association (AMA). These health care information companies have then sold individual physician's prescribing data to pharmaceutical manufacturers. This is a lucrative business, but a growing number of physicians have rebelled against the sale of their prescribing data after becoming aware that drug companies have access to their data. The practice of selling physicians' prescribing data was reviewed, and the changes proposed or enacted by the AMA and state legislatures regarding these sales were discussed.

Overview.—In some cases, overzealous sales agents for some health care information companies have confronted physicians with their prescribing histories. Such incidents have occurred despite "best practice guidelines" from the AMA that include admonitions that industry and its representatives should keep prescribing data confidential, that companies should not allow disclosure by sales representatives to any other party, and that the use of prescribing data to pressure or coerce physicians to prescribe a particular drug is absolutely inappropriate. One of several consequences of the turmoil over this issue is the creation of a Prescribing Data Restriction Program. Physicians are now able to deny all sales representatives access to their individual prescribing data. The California State Medical Association, in conjunction with the largest information company, is developing a program that will allow physicians who do not restrict access to their information to see their own data, comparative data, and educational material that will focus on prescribing for common diseases as well as categories of medications that are heavily prescribed.

Conclusions.—Broad notification efforts are planned, yet many physicians are unaware that they can restrict access to their own data, so it is unknown how many will do so or whether the proposed monitoring system will be effective in preventing abuses. If the AMA were to stop licensing the Masterfile to aid the compilation of prescribing data, it would separate itself from the practice, but its revenue would decline, and information companies would turn to other medical societies and commercial entities to obtain similar data. The sale of physicians' prescription data and efforts to restrict access to these data will be a controversial issue for the foreseeable future.

▶ I was rather surprised when a senior employee of a major drug company visited me from the central office and expressed concern about the number of prescriptions I had written for a certain allergy drop. It is worth knowing that one can register through the AMA to restrict access to individual prescribing data at www.ama-assn.org/ama/pub/category/12054.html.

E. J. Cohen, MD

Subject Index

275

Author Index